AF789645

Mild Traumatic Brain Injury

Mild Traumatic Brain Injury

A Clinician's Guide

. . . .

Edited by
Michael J. Raymond,
Thomas L. Bennett,
Lawrence C. Hartlage,
and
C. Munro Cullum

pro-ed
An International Publisher
8700 Shoal Creek Boulevard
Austin, Texas 78757-6897
800/897-3202 Fax 800/397-7633
Order online at http://www.proedinc.com

pro·ed
An International Publisher
© 1999 by PRO-ED, Inc.
8700 Shoal Creek Boulevard
Austin, Texas 78757-6897
800/897-3202 Fax 800/397-7633
Order online at http://www.proedinc.com

All rights reserved. No part of the material protected by this copyright notice may be reproduced or used in any form or by any means, electronic or mechanical, including photocopying, recording, or by any information storage and retrieval system, without prior written permission of the copyright owner.

Library of Congress Cataloging-in-Publication Data

Mild traumatic brain injury : a clinician's guide / edited by Michael J. Raymond
. . . [et al.].
p. cm.
Includes bibliographical references and indexes.
ISBN 0-89079-809-5 (alk. paper)
1. Brain damage—Diagnosis. 2. Brain damage—Patients—Rehabilitation. 3. Brain damage—Law and legislation.
I. Raymond, Michael J., 1952–
[DNLM: 1. Brain Injuries—diagnosis. 2. Brain Injuries—therapy. 3. Brain Injuries—rehabilitation. 4. Jurisprudence. WL 354 M6408 1999]
RC387.5.M527 1999
617.4'81044—dc21
DNLM/DLC
for Library of Congress 98-46594
CIP

This book is designed in Italia and New Century Schoolbook.

Production Director: Alan Grimes
Production Coordinator: Dolly Fisk Jackson
Managing Editor: Chris Olson
Art Director: Thomas Barkley
Designer: Jason Crosier
Print Buyer: Alicia Woods
Preproduction Coordinator: Chris Anne Worsham
Staff Copyeditor: Martin Wilson
Project Editor: Jennifer Knoblock
Publishing Assistant: John Means Cooper

Printed in the United States of America

1 2 3 4 5 6 7 8 9 10 03 02 01 00 99

Contents

Contributors *xi*

Preface *xiii*

1 Introduction and Overview *1*
Michael J. Raymond and Thomas L. Bennett

Introduction to Mild Traumatic Brain Injury *1*

Societal Impact *2*

Research Findings *2*

Pathophysiology of TBI *3*

Definition of Mild Brain Injury *4*

Preview and Organization of Text *5*

Part I: Diagnostic and Assessment Issues *9*

2 Neuroimaging in Mild Traumatic Brain Injury *11*
Erin D. Bigler

Fundamentals of Image Analysis *12*

Typical Imaging Abnormalities Associated with Trauma *12*

Quantitative Neuroimaging in Cerebral Trauma *19*

SPECT Imaging *19*

Permanent Versus Transient Neuroimaging Findings *23*

Conclusions *26*

3 Evaluation of Neuropsychological Status Following Mild Traumatic Brain Injury *31*
C. Munro Cullum and Laetitia L. Thompson

Biomechanical Forces and Brain Injury *32*

Acute Symptomatology *33*

Accuracy of Event Recall *36*

Neuropsychological Findings *37*

Recovery from Mild TBI *40*

Consequences of Inaccurate Diagnosis *41*

False-Positive and False-Negative Diagnostic Issues in Mild TBI *42*

Conclusions *43*

4 The Influence of Age and Education on Neuropsychological Performances of Persons with Mild Traumatic Brain Injuries *49*
Ralph M. Reitan and Deborah Wolfson

Brief Literature Review *51*

Recent Studies *53*

Conclusions *73*

5 Assessment of Mild Traumatic Brain Injury in Children for Neuropsychological Rehabilitation *77*
Cynthia A. Riccio and Cecil R. Reynolds

Neuropsychological Assessment Process *80*

Test Selection and Behavioral Domains in TBI Assessment *87*

Psychometric Issues *88*

Translating Assessment Information to Rehabilitation *103*

Conclusions *105*

6 Mild Traumatic Brain Injury in Sports *117*
Robert A. Ruchinskas, Joseph P. Francis, and Jeffrey T. Barth

Introduction *117*

What Is Mild Head Injury? *119*

Severe Brain Injury in Boxing *121*

Mild Concussion in Boxing *122*

Mild Concussion in Football *123*

Concussion in Soccer *125*

Head Injuries in Other Sports *125*

Conclusions *126*

Part II: Medicolegal Issues *133*

7 Forensic Aspects of Mild Traumatic Brain Injury *135*
Lawrence C. Hartlage

Recognition *135*

Documentation *137*

Neuropsychologist's Role in Documentation *139*

8 Litigation Perspectives for the Health Professional *147*
Rex D. Smith and Ian R. Rapaport

The Claims Process *147*

The Complaint and Answer *149*

Discovery—Subpoenas and Request To Produce *150*

Independent Medical Exam *151*

Testimony *154*

Conclusions *156*

9 Forensic Misconceptions in Mild Traumatic Brain Injury *159*
Anjali Palav, Kevin Duff, and Robert J. McCaffrey

Introduction *159*

Role of the Clinical Neuropsychologist as an Expert *159*

Selection and Interpretation of Neuropsychological Tests *167*

Forming Opinions Within a Reasonable Degree of Neuropsychological Certainty *171*

Conclusions *179*

10 Social and Legal Impact of Malingered Mild Traumatic Brain Injury *187*
Kay B. Stevens and J. Randall Price

Introduction *187*

Roles of the Neuropsychologist *188*

Role of the Plaintiff *193*

Implications for the Legal System *195*

Implications for the Trier of Fact *197*

Conclusions *199*

Part III: Treatment and Rehabilitation Issues *201*

11 Effective Treatment of Mild Traumatic Brain Injury and Understanding its Neurological Consequences *203*
Michelle Kibby and Charles J. Long

Defining Mild TBI *203*

Determination of Brain Injury Severity *204*

Posttraumatic, Noncognitive Factors *210*

Conclusions *214*

12 Psychotherapeutic Interventions for Individuals with Mild Traumatic Brain Injury *219*
Thomas L. Bennett and Michael J. Raymond

Nature and Basis for Emotional Changes Following Brain Injury *220*

Psychotherapy for Individuals with Mild TBI *224*

Conclusions *228*

13 Efficacy of Cognitive Rehabilitation in the Treatment of Mild Traumatic Brain Injury *231*
Keith D. Cicerone

The Nature of Cognitive Impairments After Mild TBI *234*

Postconcussive Symptoms and Cognitive Deficits *238*

Remediation of Cognitive Disability After Mild TBI *241*

Conclusions *249*

14 The Medical Management of Noncognitive Sequelae of Mild Traumatic Brain Injury *255*
Gerald C. McIntosh

Posttraumatic Headache *256*
Posttraumatic Seizures *258*
Posttraumatic Dizziness *259*
Posttraumatic Tinnitus and Hearing Impairment *260*
Posttraumatic Anosmia *260*
Posttraumatic Tremor *261*
Posttraumatic Neck Pain and Back Pain *261*
Posttraumatic Visual Symptoms *262*
Posttraumatic Depression and Emotional Lability *262*
Management of Sports-Related Injuries *263*
Conclusions *264*

15 Outpatient Rehabilitation Program for Individuals with Persisting Mild to Moderate Symptoms Following Mild Traumatic Brain Injury *267*
Christy Dittmar

Critical Features of Rehabilitation *268*
Program Design *270*
Efficacy of Treatment *274*
Conclusions *275*

About the Editors *277*

Author Index *279*

Subject Index *289*

Contributors

Jeffrey T. Barth, PhD
University of Virginia Medical School
Psychiatric Medicine
PO Box 203
Charlottesville, VA 23452

Thomas L. Bennett, PhD
Brain Injury Recovery Program
1049 Robertson
Ft. Collins, CO 80524

Erin D. Bigler, PhD
Brigham Young University
1086 SWKT
Provo, UT 84602

Keith D. Cicerone, PhD
JFK Medical Center
2048 Oak Tree Road
Edison, NJ 08820

C. Munro Cullum, PhD
University of Texas Southwestern
Medical Center at Dallas
Department of Psychiatry
5323 Harry Hines Boulevard
Dallas, TX 75235

Christy Dittmar, MS, OTR
Brain Injury Recovery Program
1049 Roberston
Fort Collins, CO 80524

Kevin Duff, MA
SUNY Albany
Psychology Department
Albany, NY 12222

Joseph P. Francis, PsyD
704 Queen Elizabeth Drive
Virginia Beach, VA 23452

Lawrence C. Hartlage, PhD
4227 Evans-Lock Road
Evans, GA 30809

Michelle Kibby, PhD
2215 Ridgecrest Dr.
Augusta, GA 30907

Charles J. Long, PhD
University of Memphis
Psychology Department
Memphis, TN 38152

Robert J. McCaffrey, PhD
SUNY Albany
Psychology Department
Albany, NY 12222

Gerald C. McIntosh, MD
1247 Riverside, Suite 4
Fort Collins, CO 80524

Anjali Palav, MA
SUNY Albany
Psychology Department
Albany, NY 12222

J. Randall Price, PhD
1221 Abrams Road, Suite 109
Richardson, TX 75081

Ian R. Rapaport, Esq.
Chambers Mabry, 10th Floor
220 Century Parkway NE
Atlanta, GA 30345

Michael J. Raymond, PhD
Allied Services, John Heinz Institute of Rehabilitation Medicine
150 Mundy Street, PO Box 2096
Wilkes-Barre Township, PA 18702

Ralph M. Reitan, PhD
Reitan Neuropsychology Laboratory
2920 S 4th Avenue
Tucson, AZ 85713

Cecil R. Reynolds, PhD
Texas A & M University
Educational Psychology
704 Harrington Education Center
College Station, TX 77843

Cynthia A. Riccio, PhD
Texas A & M University
Educational Psychology
704 Harrington Education Center
College Station, TX 77843

Robert A. Ruchinskas, PsyD
Temple University Hospital
Department of Physical Medicine & Rehabilitation
Philadelphia, PA 19140

Rex D. Smith, Esq.
Chambers Mabry, 10th Floor
220 Century Parkway NE
Atlanta, GA 30345

Kay B. Stevens, EdD
University of Kentucky
Department of Special Education
229 Taylor Education Building
Lexington, KY 40506

Laetitia L. Thompson, PhD
UCHSC Neuropsychology Lab
North Pavillion, #A-011-08
4455 E 12th Avenue, #129
Denver, CO 80220

Deborah Wolfson, PhD
Reitan Neuropsychology Laboratory
2920 S 4th Avenue
Tucson, AZ 85713

Preface

In 1997 a special issue on mild brain injury was published in *Applied Neuropsychology* (Bennet & Raymond, 1997). This issue included 10 articles which provided an overview of mild brain injury including epidemiology, etiology, diagnostic criteria, and clinical symptoms. The contributing authors discussed various issues related to this topic and presented divergent views on causes, symptoms, assessment, and recovery from mild traumatic brain injury. Rehabilitation and forensic aspects of mild brain injury were also discussed.

This text is an extension of those original 10 articles and is divided into three main parts: diagnostic and assessment issues; medicolegal issues; and treatment and rehabilitation issues. This text will provide the clinician with information to enhance his or her understanding of the consequences of mild traumatic brain injury. Moreover, this text should help stimulate additional interest and research into this phenomenon.

Michael J. Raymond
Thomas L. Bennett
Lawrence C. Hartlage
C. Munro Cullum

Reference

Bennett, T. L., & Raymond, M. J. (1997). Mild brain injury [Special issue]. *Applied Neuropsychology, 4*(1), 1–88.

Introduction and Overview

1

Michael J. Raymond
and Thomas L. Bennett

Introduction to Mild Traumatic Brain Injury

This text on mild brain injury covers a number of issues related to the topic and presents divergent views. This underscores the fact that there is far from universal agreement regarding what a mild brain injury is and what the outcome from such an injury will be. A number of terms are used interchangeably with mild traumatic brain injury: mild brain injury; mild head injury, minor head injury, minor traumatic brain injury, concussion, and postconcussive syndrome.

Traumatic brain injury (TBI) is a major health problem in the United States. Variations with regard to the incidence of TBI are noted throughout research literature. It has been estimated that 7 million brain injuries occur annually in the United States, with about 500,000 individuals requiring hospitalization and follow-up medical treatment (Caveness, 1977; Frankowski, 1986). The numbers are staggering; the consequences often tragic.

Approximately 300,000 people lose their lives due to brain injury each year (Rimel, Giordani, Barth, Boll, & Jane, 1981). Probably more than 70% of individuals who sustain TBIs have what would be classified as a mild brain injury, according to a well conceptualized epidemiological investigation by Kraus and Nourjah (1989), who studied TBI victims in San Diego County, California. According to the National Center of Health Statistics, approximately 85% of all brain injuries are classified as mild. Unfortunately, the majority of these "mild" injuries are not identified, and consequently, not treated effectively.

Reprinted, with changes, from "Mild Brain Injury: An Overview," by Thomas L. Bennett and Michael J. Raymond, 1997, *Applied Neuropsychology, 4*(1), pp. 1–5. Copyright 1997 by Lawrence Erlbaum Associates, Inc.

Most individuals with mild brain injury have uneventful recoveries, but it has been estimated that as many as 25% to 35% of individuals who sustain mild brain injury will continue to have cognitive and emotional difficulties when reevaluated 3 to 6 months later. As Kibby and Long point out in Chapter 11 of this text, many of these individuals with persisting problems who were classified as mild TBI victims may have actually sustained a moderate degree of brain injury; they may have been misclassified because duration of loss of consciousness was the only criterion used to evaluate severity of injury.

Societal Impact

The impact of TBI on our society is underscored by the fact that 70% of injured individuals are 30 years old or less at the time of their TBI. The peak incidence is among 15- to 24-year-olds (Rimel, Jane, & Bond, 1990). Many of these individuals will need lifelong care, and even among TBI victims with supposedly "mild" brain injuries, significant disability (although usually temporary) can result. Younger people are undoubtedly more likely to sustain brain injury because of their risk-taking behavior, their experimentation with alcohol and drugs, their participation in contact sports, and the typical adolescent's and young adult's belief that he or she is invincible. The rate of brain injuries in males is 2 to 3 times higher than in females, and alcohol has been implicated in at least one third of all TBIs (Rimel, Jane, & Bond). For individuals with persisting problems after even mild brain injury, the effects of the injury can result in a permanent, if mild, reduction of an individual's preinjury potential. As Symonds (1962) suggested, "it is questionable whether the effects of concussions, however slight, are ever completely reversible" (p. 4).

Research Findings

Research regarding mild brain injuries began in Europe, with additional studies conducted in the United States in the early 1980s. The general consensus is that mild brain injury typically occurs following a mild to moderate blow to the head. The majority of these injuries are related to motor vehicle accidents, whereas others may result from falls, sports, physical fights, or various other forms of trauma. However, in some cases, a mild brain injury occurs without a direct blow or contact to the head. Whiplash amnesia and electroencephalographic alterations may occur following a sudden stop or change in direction of a relatively stationary head position (Torres & Shapiro, 1961). Individuals sustaining such injuries may shortly thereafter complain of headache, blurred vision, dizziness, confusion, disorientation, and forgetfulness. According to Fisher (1985), these symptoms are consistent from patient to patient; however, the degree and duration of symptoms, as well as the extent to which they prove disabling, may vary greatly.

Kraus and Nourjah (1989) concluded that 42% of all mild brain injuries were the result of a motor vehicle accident. With that in mind, it is helpful to understand what happens to the brain when a TBI results from a motor vehicle accident.

Pathophysiology of TBI

When a person is in an automobile that collides with another vehicle or other object (e.g., parked vehicle, utility pole, tree), forces are applied to the brain, producing injury. Two things are important to know when trying to understand the mechanics of TBI. First, the brain is soft tissue. It has a consistency something like gelatin, cooked oatmeal, or soft cheese. Second, the inside of the skull is very rough, particularly above the eyes and in the temporal regions. The skull is certainly a magnificent device to protect the brain if one is merely struck on the head, but because of these rough areas (bony contours), the skull is less than optimal for protecting the brain from sudden forces applied to the head. Neither air bags nor any other protective device will prohibit a brain from being injured when an automobile suddenly comes to a stop, and the head and brain are still traveling at a rate of about 50 miles per hour.

Gennarelli (1986), Reitan and Wolfson (1986), and others suggested the pathophysiology of these injuries is such that the brain moves within the skull through linear and rotational forces, resulting in shear–strain damage to brain tissue along with possible changes at the cellular and neuronal level. Damage is produced when the brain is set into motion within the skull, rubbing over and colliding with the rough surfaces. Damage is also produced when this 3½ pound mass rotates unevenly, stretching and disconnecting axons which normally conduct information within the brain. Although loss of consciousness is certainly an indication of a concussion or TBI, it is very clear that an individual can experience a serious brain injury without losing consciousness. As previously noted, an individual can experience persisting cognitive problems after a brain injury without ever striking the head (Yarnell & Rossie, 1988). This is because damage is produced by deceleration and rotational forces as the brain strikes the inside of the skull and rotates unevenly in the course of a motor vehicle accident.

This shear–strain phenomenon, as originally observed by Holbourn (1943) and later by Strich (1961), was the result of rapid brain movement within the cranial vault, causing stretching of white matter fibers and eventual degeneration. These "microscopic" injuries were attributed to even mild brain trauma and eventually verified by Nevin (1967) and Oppenheimer (1968) through their histological (cell) staining techniques. Damage at the cellular level was often diffuse, involving both cortical and subcortical regions. Loss of consciousness often occurs following alterations of the brain stem and subsequent interference of the ascending reticular activating pathways. In addition to the upper and lower brain stem, the frontotemporal regions are especially prone to damage due to bony contours of the skull. Multifocal involvement is evidenced at the site of impact (coup), an opposite site (contre coup), or surrounding brain regions.

Because mild brain injuries may result in microscopic (cellular) alterations, controversy continues to exist regarding their sequelae. Rarely are focal neurologic deficits found on physical examinations, or structural changes reported on sophisticated neurodiagnostics (e.g., computerized tomography or CT scan, magnetic resonance imaging or MRI, electroencephalogram or EEG). This paucity of objective abnormal findings leaves only the clinical symptomatology on which to base diagnostic impressions. Nevertheless, brain injury researchers and clinicians have recently compiled data that support the existence of a constellation of physical, cognitive, and emotional symptoms associated with postconcussive syndrome. Undoubtedly, the symptom complex observed in many individuals reflects a blend of microscopic brain damage, reactive emotional stress secondary to the traumatic event, pre-injury personality characteristics, and developmental variables.

More significant TBIs (moderate, severe) obviously produce different and more prolonged symptoms in conjunction with a poorer prognosis. The degree of severity is generally associated with the level of altered consciousness: the greater length of unconsciousness, the more severe the injury (Jennett, 1990).

Severity of brain injury has traditionally been rated using a variety of medical classifications (Bennett, 1992). Medical classifications of TBI include skull and brain trauma descriptors, duration of loss of consciousness, and duration of posttraumatic amnesia. Teasdale and Jennett (1974) developed a scale to measure alterations of consciousness, the *Glasgow Coma Scale* (GCS).

Definition of Mild Brain Injury

Although the exact definition of mild brain injury will vary somewhat among specialists in TBI, we have found it helpful to use a definition of mild brain injury that was developed by The Mild Traumatic Brain Injury Committee of The Head Injury Interdisciplinary Special Interest Group of The American Congress of Rehabilitation Medicine (1993). According to these criteria, a person with mild brain injury is a person who has traumatically induced physiological disruption of brain function as manifested by *at least one* (not necessarily all) of the following:

1. any loss of consciousness up to approximately 30 minutes in duration; within 30 minutes after the injury, the person must have progressed to a Glasgow Coma Scale score of 13 to 15 (of a possible 15)
2. any loss of memory for events immediately before or after the accident (retrograde or anterograde amnesia)
3. any alteration of mental state at the time of the accident (e.g., feeling dazed, disoriented, or confused)
4. focal neurological deficit which may or may not be transient (in the past, a mild head injury was ruled out if focal signs persisted)
5. posttraumatic amnesia not greater than 24 hours

This definition includes instances in which TBI is produced when the head is struck, or during a whiplash injury in which the head is not hit. Cerebral CT scans or MRIs may be read as normal. Although it is unusual, it is important to note that CT and MRI studies may at times detect intracranial lesions following mild brain injury (Jenkins, Teasdale, Hadley, McPhearson, & Rowan, 1986; Levin et al., 1987), even in individuals with no documented loss of consciousness (Levi, Guildburd, Lemberger, Soustiel, & Feinsod, 1990). Although we continue to use the term mild brain injury to describe TBIs that meet the criteria set forth by the Head Injury Interdisciplinary Special Interest Group, such findings of detectable neurological injury when there is no documented loss of consciousness certainly question the validity of calling such injuries "mild."

Preview and Organization of Text

As previously noted, this text is divided into three major parts. Part I addresses diagnostic and assessment issues, Part II addresses medicolegal issues, and Part III addresses treatment and rehabilitation issues. In Part I a number of issues related to symptoms, assessment, and recovery from mild brain injury are discussed. In Chapter 2, Bigler reviews current aspects of neuroimaging and how it relates to the assessment of mild brain injury. In Chapter 3, Cullum and Thompson discuss diagnostic issues for neuropsychology in cases of mild brain injury. They describe biomechanical forces that produce brain injury in impact and nonimpact accidents. They also discuss the importance of considering such factors as the normal base rate of symptom complaints in the general population, normal deficits in recall of details of events (such as an automobile accident), and preexisting difficulties of the injured person when evaluating the complaints of individuals presenting with apparent postconcussive syndrome. The consequences of incorrectly diagnosing the presence or absence of brain injury are also covered. In Chapter 4, Reitan and Wolfson report results of a study in which they examined the relationship between age and education and the *General Neuropsychological Deficit Scale* (GNDS) for individuals with mild brain injury. The results of their study raise serious questions about the validity of adjusting neuropsychological or intellectual test scores for participants with brain damage by using results for normal participants, when the rational bases for making such adjustments are limited or absent. Chapter 5, by Riccio and Reynolds, addresses assessment issues in the diagnosis and rehabilitation of children with TBI. The authors stress the need for serial neuropsychological assessments to monitor progress and evaluate intervention methods, with specific emphasis on school reintegration. In Chapter 6, Ruchinskas, Francis, and Barth discuss mild brain injury resulting from professional and amateur sports. They pay particular attention to mild brain injuries and their sequelae resulting from participation in football and boxing.

Because a majority of mild traumatic brain injuries result from motor vehicle accidents or work-related accidents, many cases involve litigation. Part II of this text covers medicolegal aspects of mild brain injury. In Chapter 7, Hartlage discusses the difficulty of documenting mild brain injury from a medicolegal perspective. He emphasizes the importance of a competent neuropsychological evaluation in helping to clarify the presence or absence of brain injury and how the injury will affect a person's activities of daily living. In Chapter 8, Smith and Rapaport provide an attorney's perspective in cases involving mild brain injury. They specifically discuss the claims process, the complaint and answer, the discovery phase, and the independent medical examination. They stress the importance of health care professionals being properly prepared during all aspects of litigation. In Chapter 9, Palav, Duff, and McCaffrey discuss additional guidelines for mild brain injury litigation. They outline specific guidelines for the expert witness (neuropsychologist) while dispelling myths about forensic neuropsychology. They include actual courtroom testimony to illustrate topics, including the role of the neuropsychologist in legal proceedings, the formation of opinions within a reasonable degree of neuropsychological certainty, and selection and interpretation of neuropsychological tests. In Chapter 10, Stevens and Price examine the implications of invalid brain injury claims in both the psychological health care and legal systems. Because neuropsychological test data depend on the person being assessed, if the person is not motivated to do his or her best or tries to exaggerate difficulties, then testing will indicate more dysfunction than is actually present. A conscious attempt to exaggerate or feign deficits is called malingering, and this can result in invalid brain injury claims.

This text concludes with Part III, which covers issues related to the treatment and rehabilitation of individuals with documented or suspected mild brain injury. In Chapter 11, Kibby and Long directly address the issue of the minimum criteria for a brain injury. They also discuss noncognitive and preinjury factors that can influence the rate of recovery. In Chapter 12, Bennett and Raymond discuss neuropsychological counseling for individuals with mild brain injury. This therapy focuses on two goals: (a) educating the person about the effects of brain injury and providing strategies to compensate for day-to-day difficulties, and (b) helping the person develop and maintain good strategies for coping with the cognitive and emotional consequences of his or her injuries. The authors make important distinctions between psychotherapy for individuals with brain injury and traditional psychotherapy. The importance of supportive counseling, education, and cognitive rehabilitation in the treatment of mild brain injury is addressed by Cicerone in Chapter 13. To illustrate effective treatment, the author discusses two case examples in detail, with specific emphasis on the design and implementation of individual treatment methods. In Chapter 14, McIntosh, a neurologist who specializes in neurorehabilitation, addresses medical management of a number of posttraumatic physical symptoms including headaches, seizures, dizziness, tinnitus and hearing impairment, anosmia, tremor, head and back pain, visual symptoms, depression, and emotional lability. In Chapter 15, Dittmar discusses a neuropsychologically based, interdisciplinary outpatient rehabilitation program for individuals who have suffered mild to moderate brain injuries and have significant persisting problems. Rehabilitation services include the patient's family members in the rehabilitation treatment team. The interdisciplinary program includes neuropsychological assessment, cognitive rehabilitation, occupational therapy, speech and language therapy, neuropsychological counseling, biofeedback, vocational rehabilitation, and neurological services.

We enjoyed editing this text on mild traumatic brain injury. It is our hope, and that of the contributing authors, that this text will help to clarify the nature of mild brain injury and also stimulate additional interest and research into this phenomenon. It is certainly clear that our present ways of classifying brain injury severity are inadequate; we would argue that severity is best evaluated through assessments that quantify postinjury deficits and relate them to specific activities of daily living (Bennett, 1992; Raymond, 1989).

References

Bennett, T. L. (1992). Conceptualizing traumatic brain injuries. *The Journal of Head Injury, 3*(1), 21–28.

Caveness, W. (1977). Incidence of craniocerebral trauma in the United States. *Transitions of the American Neurological Association, 102,* 136–138.

Fisher, J. (1985). Cognitive and behavioral consequences of closed head injury. *Seminars on Neurology, 5,* 197–204.

Frankowski, R. F. (1986). Descriptive and epidemiological studies of head injury in the United States: 1974–1984. *Advances in Psychosomatic Medicine, 16,* 153–172.

Gennarelli, T. (1986). Mechanisms and pathophysiology of cerebral concussion. *Journal of Head Trauma Rehabilitation, 1,* 23–30.

Holbourn, A. (1943). Mechanism of head injuries. *Lancet, 2,* 438–441.

Jenkins, A., Teasdale, G., Hadley, M., MacPhearson, P., & Rowan, J. (1986). Brain lesions detected by brain magnetic imaging in mild and severe head injuries. *Lancet, 2,* 445–446.

Jennett, B. (1990). Scale and scope of the problem. In M. Rosenthal, E. R. Griffith, M. R. Bond, & J. D. Miller (Eds.), *Rehabilitation of the adult and child with brain injury* (2nd ed., pp. 3–7). Philadelphia: F. A. Davis.

Kraus, J. F., & Nourjah, P. (1989). The epidemiology of mild head injury. In H. S. Levin, H. M. Eisenberg, & A. L. Benton (Eds.), *Mild head injury* (pp. 8–22). New York: Oxford University Press.

Levi, L., Guildburd, J. M., Lemberger, A., Soustiel, J. F., & Feinsod, M. (1990). Diffuse axonal injury: Analysis of 100 patients with radiological signs. *Neurosurgery, 27,* 429–432.

Levin, H. S., Amparo, E. G., Eisenberg, H. M., Williams, D. H., High, W. M., McArdle, C. B., & Weiner, R. L. (1987). Magnetic resonance imaging and computerized topography in relation to the neurobehavioral sequelae of mild and moderate head injuries. *Journal of Neurosurgery, 66,* 706–713.

Mild Traumatic Brain Injury Committee of the Head Injury Interdisciplinary Special Interest Group of the American Congress of Rehabilitation Medicine (1993). Definition of mild traumatic brain injury. *Journal of Head Trauma Rehabilitation, 8,* 86–87.

Nevin, N. (1967). Neuropathological changes in the white matter following head injury. *Journal of Neuropathology and Experimental Neurology, 26,* 77–84.

Oppenheimer, D. (1968). Microscopic lesions in the brain following head injury. *Journal of Neurology, Neurosurgery, & Psychiatry, 31,* 299–306.

Raymond, M. J. (1989). Major consequences of minor head injury. *JMA Bulletin, 2,* 4–7.

Reitan, R., & Wolfson, D. (1986). *Traumatic brain injury* (Vol. 1). Tuscon, AZ: Neuropsychology Press.

Rimel, R. W., Giordani, B., Barth, J. T., Boll, T. J., & Jane, J. A. (1981). Disability caused by minor head injury. *Neurosurgery, 9,* 221–228.

Rimel, R. W., Jane, J. A., & Bond, M. R. (1990). Characteristics of the head injured patient. In M. Rosenthal, E. R. Griffith, M. R. Bond, & J. D. Miller (Eds.), *Rehabilitation of the adult and child with brain injury* (2nd ed., pp. 8–16). Philadelphia: F. A. Davis.

Strich, S. (1961). Shearing of nerve fibers as a cause of brain damage due to head injury: A pathological study of twenty cases. *Lancet, 2,* 443–448.

Symonds, C. (1962). Concussion and its sequelae. *Lancet, 1,* 1–5.

Teasdale, G., & Jennett, B. (1974). Assessment of coma and impaired consciousness: A practical scale. *Lancet, 2,* 81–84.

Torres, F., & Shapiro, S. (1961). Electroencephalograms in whiplash injury. *Archives of Neurology, 5,* 40–47.

Yarnell, P. R., & Rossi, G. V. (1988). Minor whiplash head injury with major debilitation. *Brain Injury, 2,* 255–258.

Diagnostic and Assessment Issues

I

Neuroimaging in Mild Traumatic Brain Injury

2

Erin D. Bigler

Because of the clinical utility and ready availability of neuroimaging techniques in assessing both acute and chronic effects of head injury, the majority of individuals who receive a head injury have some type of neuroimaging study performed (Gean, 1994). The two most common studies performed are computerized tomography (CT) and magnetic resonance imaging (MRI). However, other imaging techniques that involve MRI methods such as functional MRI (fMRI), magnetic resonance spectroscopy (MRS), and diffusion-weighted MRI (Bigler, 1996a, 1996b; Prichard, 1998), along with single photon emission computed tomography (SPECT) and magneto-encephalography, are also being applied to the clinical and research evaluation of the head injured subject (Orrison, Lewine, Sanders, & Hartshorne, 1995; Thatcher, Hallett, Zeffiro, John, & Huerta, 1994).

There are several detailed texts and chapters that deal with neuroimaging in moderate to severe head injury (Bigler, 1996b; Gean, 1994). The reader who wishes greater detail on the entire subject of brain imaging in neuro-trauma can refer to these texts. This chapter provides an overview of the field of imaging in cases of mild head injury or mild TBI. Although there are various definitions of mild head injury, in this chapter, a mild TBI subject will be one who had a Glasgow Coma Scale (GCS) score of 13 or higher when first assessed by emergency personnel at the scene and when evaluated in the emergency room (ER). Some patients who sustain mild TBI may not even receive neuroimaging studies if their GCS score is 15 at the scene or has improved to 15 by the time evaluated in the ER, and they have no other neurologic signs or abnormalities (Osborn, 1994).

In the ER the imaging modality of choice is the CT scan because of its rapid imaging time and ability to detect most gross structural abnormalities associated with trauma. In addition, movement artifact distortion is minimal, and most life support equipment is compatible with the CT imaging environment. The problem with CT imaging in mild TBI is that the lesions associated with such injury are often below the threshold of detection, and/or the day-of-injury (DOI) scan occurs too early in the evolution of the lesion (Bigler, 1990, 1997). As such, the DOI CT scan in mild TBI may yield little if any clinically relevant information. As Alexander (1995) clearly stated, in the majority of mild TBI cases the CT will be clinically read as "normal," but this does not necessarily mean that abnormalities of structure or function are not present; they simply may be undetectable by the CT scan.

Fundamentals of Image Analysis

Although there are many major and subtle factors in neuroimaging interpretation, there are two key elements to any evaluation: (a) normal symmetry of the brain and (b) similarity (normal structural configuration of the brain compared to other brains). These two points are amply illustrated in Figure 2.1, wherein three normal subjects are presented in axial (horizontal) view at the level of the head of the caudate nucleus and anterior horn of the lateral ventricle. There is close symmetry between right and left cerebral structures in each individual. Thus, if an individual's two hemispheres are not mirror images, then there may be underlying pathology. Figure 2.1 also demonstrates the consistency of brain structure across different individuals when MRI is performed at a similar level and plane. Thus, when examining two brains at a similar level, the major forms of the brains should be similar. Any deviation from these two principles of symmetry and similarity may indicate underlying brain abnormalities associated with cerebral trauma.

Typical Imaging Abnormalities Associated with Trauma

Although the events of cerebral injury typically involve complex physical forces of acceleration and deceleration, mechanical deformation and force, certain brain regions are more commonly involved than others. These brain regions are frontal and temporal lobe areas at the brain–skull interface, white matter–gray matter junction, or long coursing white matter pathways. These pathological substrates of traumatic injury apply whether the injury is mild or severe.

Brain–Skull Interface

Figure 2.2 presents axial, coronal, and sagittal views from a subject who sustained a mild TBI. The arrows point to regions of prior cortical surface

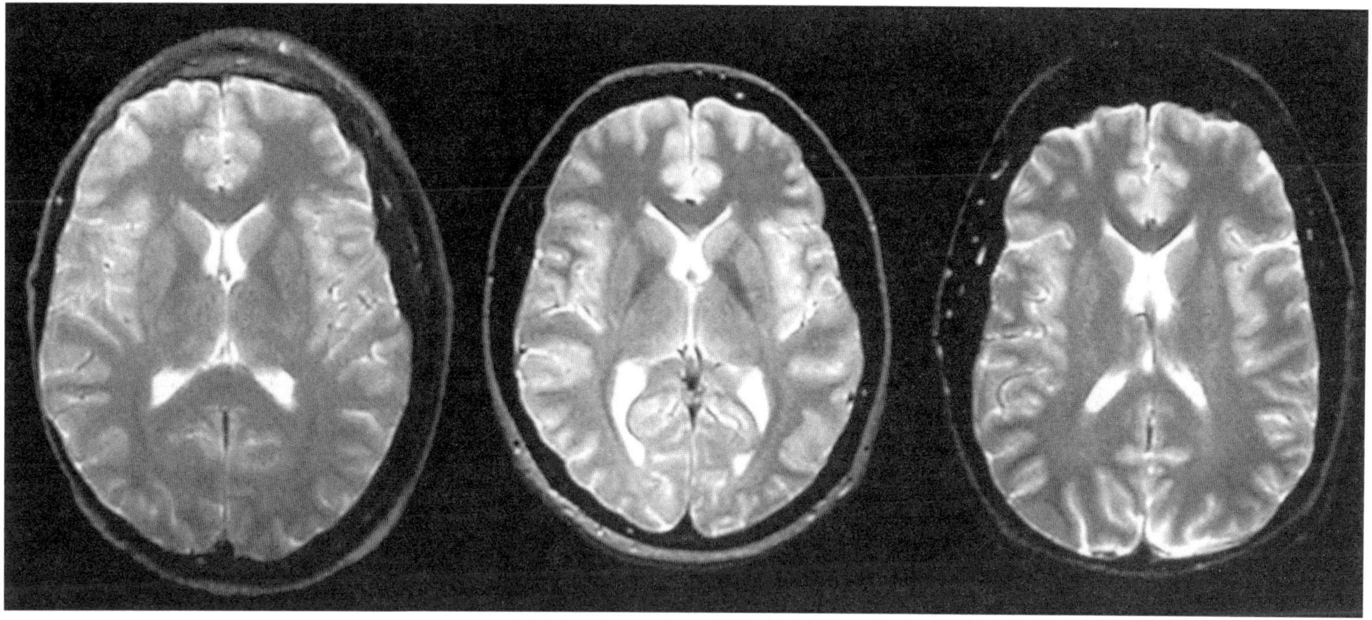

Figure 2.1. Three T2 weighted MRIs taken from three individuals without brain damage, obtained at the level of the head of the caudate nucleus and anterior (or frontal horns) and third ventricle of the lateral ventricle system. With this type of MRI weighting, white matter is represented by darker shades of gray, and gray matter is a lighter shade of gray. Cerebral spinal fluid (CSF) is represented by white. This figure illustrates the principles of symmetry and similarity. Even though these three individuals are unrelated and of different ages (left, 31; middle, 50; right, 25), images taken at this level appear similar.

contusions that occurred in the fall and are now visible on follow-up MRI performed months after the injury. The observable structural damage occurred in the inferior frontal region. Another case is presented in Figure 2.3. In this subject, the subtle abnormalities are in the frontotemporal regions. Because the inferior and anterior-mesial aspects of the frontotemporal region of the brain come into contact with rough, bony edges, these regions represent areas easily contused, particularly in more severe TBI (see Figure 2.4). Because of the probability of frontotemporal damage in any TBI, it is likely that injury in these regions causes some of the common problems observed in TBI patients such as disrupted memory, variable attention span, and impaired executive and emotional ability. These functions are thought to be mediated, in part, by frontotemporal systems.

White Matter–Gray Matter Junction

Tissue differences between gray matter (condensed cell bodies) and white matter (coursing myelinated axons projecting from cell bodies) provides a gradient wherein acceleration/deceleration movements may allow for a disruption in the integrity of the axon and/or provide a focal point of shearing. The damage depicted in Figure 2.2 occurred at the white–gray matter junction, in addition to the surface contusions. Just as with the cortical contusions, these white–gray matter junction injuries occur most often in the frontotemporal regions of the brain (see also Figures 2.8, 2.9, and 2.10).

White Matter Atrophy

Although the exact neuropathological mechanisms that underlie axonal injury from head trauma are not fully understood, axons are particularly vulnerable (Maxwell, Povlishock, & Graham, 1997). The largest white matter structure of the brain is the corpus callosum; corpus callosum atrophy following brain injury is commonplace (Johnson, Bigler, Burr, & Blatter, 1994). Atrophy of the corpus callosum probably occurs because of one or a combination of two factors:

1. Because the corpus callosum is centrally located in the brain, connecting the two cerebral hemispheres, traumatic rotational forces cause opposite movement of the hemispheres and put particular strain on the corpus callosum, potentially resulting in shearing action.
2. Transneuronal degeneration, in which cell bodies and/or axons damaged distally from the corpus callosum die, and axonal degeneration across the corpus callosum occurs.

In either case the midsagittal view of the corpus callosum is the best MRI view for examining callosal atrophy. The fornix is another white matter

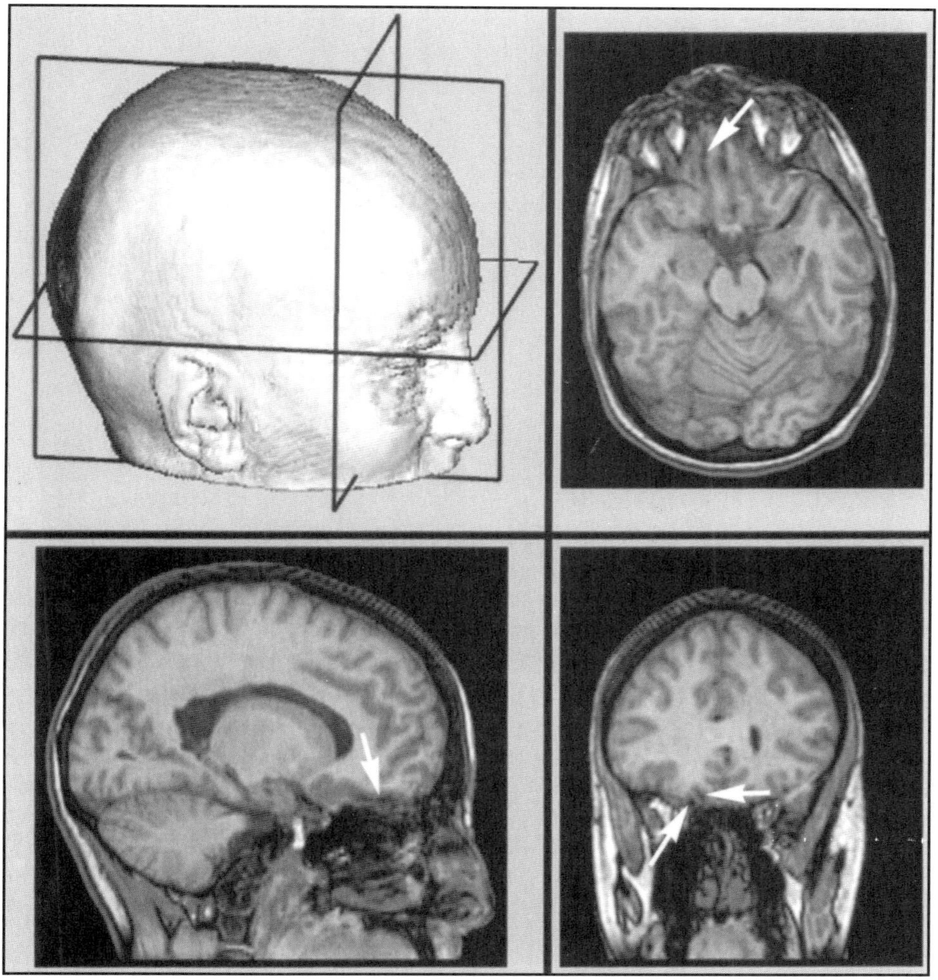

Figure 2.2. Three-dimensional MRI reconstruction of the head of a subject injured in a fall, demonstrating the position of the three planes of images (sagittal, lower left; axial, upper right; and coronal, lower right). In the sagittal view note that in the most inferior aspect of the frontal region (olfactory grove/gyrus rectus region; see arrow) there is a much darker appearance to the tissue than in surrounding gray matter structures. This dark signal on a T1 weighted image is an indication of necrosis or loss of tissue. Similarly, this can be viewed in the axial and coronal planes (arrows point to identical regions). Such inferior lesions typically disrupt smell, and this patient was anosmic. Likewise, important pathways involved in regulating emotion course through the inferior frontal region of the brain. After sustaining the TBI, this patient was plagued with problems in mood regulation. Often in such cases there are not major cognitive sequelae; this patient's assessed level of cognitive functioning was within the broad range of normal. The pathology associated with mild TBI in this patient was predominately affective, in addition to the loss of smell.

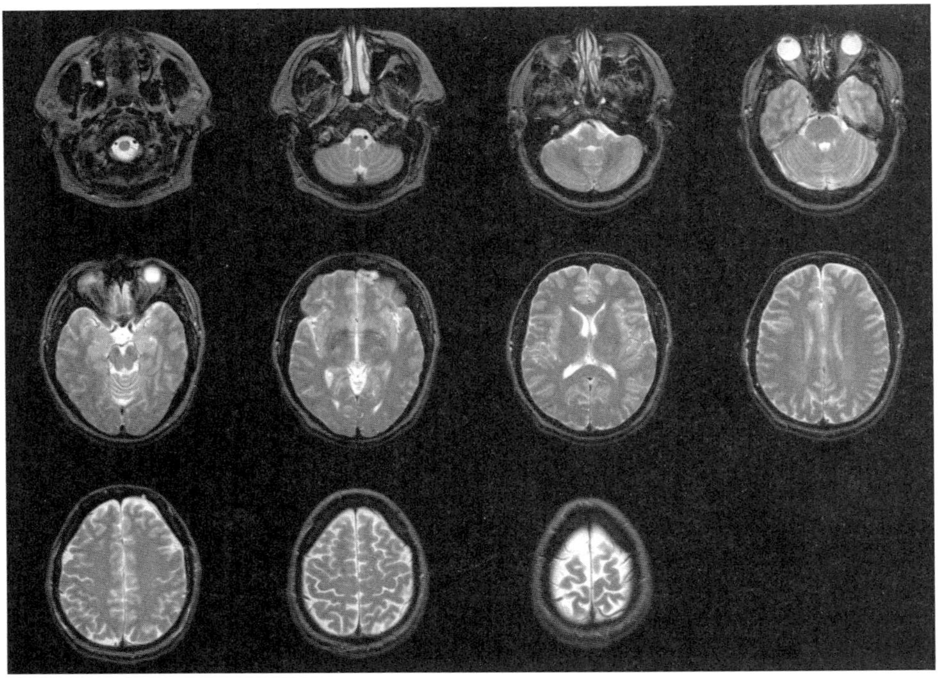

Figure 2.3. Serial axial MRIs from spinal cord (top left) to vertex (bottom right) in a patient with mild TBI from a fall. Some subtle abnormalities are evident. For example, in the middle row the left image shows an asymmetry of the temporal horn and a greater amount of regional CSF in the anterior pole of the left temporal lobe (left is on the viewer's right, as images are in radiological perspective). This type of asymmetry in head injury is thought to indicate subtle, but focal damage to the left temporal lobe. In the next image, there is a definite asymmetry in the frontal lobe. There is a focal area in the left frontal lobe that has an excessive amount of CSF and an apparent hemosiderin deposit (blood byproduct likely from a hemorrhegic contusion). This is a probable indication of underlying atrophy in the frontal pole region. Thus, although the abnormalities are subtle, this patient's MRIs demonstrate the presence of definite abnormalities in frontal and temporal regions of the brain. As discussed elsewhere in this chapter, when such abnormalities are detected, it is likely that there are other nonspecific abnormalities elsewhere in the brain. Damage observed on MRI studies is detected only when it reaches a certain threshold, typically that which would be visible to the eye on gross anatomic inspection.

structure vulnerable to atrophy due to head injury, and is visualized in the same midsagittal plane (Gale, Burr, Bigler, & Blatter, 1993; Gale, Johnson, Bigler, & Blatter, 1995). Figure 2.5 shows common findings of corpus callosum atrophy from brain injury and degeneration that can occur between the DOI scan and the follow-up MRI. This illustration demonstrates that an initially

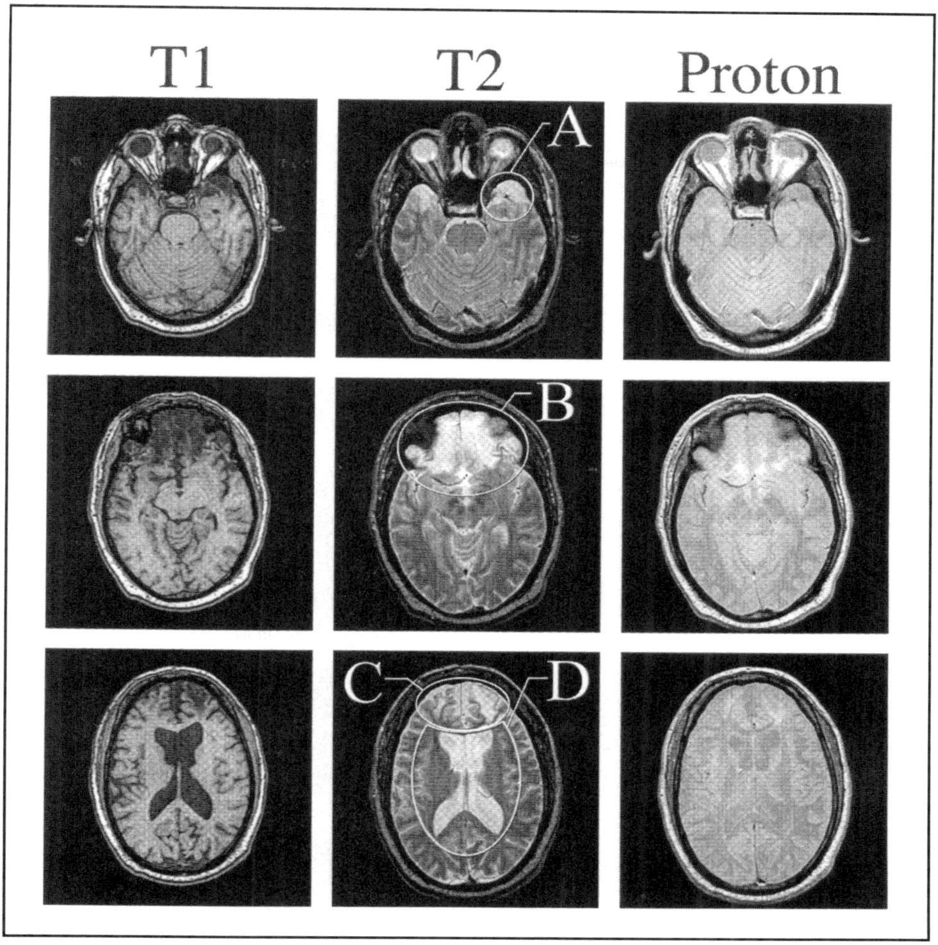

Figure 2.4. MRIs of a patient who sustained a moderate to severe TBI when thrown from a horse. This figure demonstrates the three most common weightings in MRI and how these different weightings depict the trauma-induced lesion. Note the differences in depiction of white, gray, and CSF spaces. Also, note the extensive involvement of the anterior and inferior frontal regions along with the anterior aspect of the temporal lobes. Lastly, note the generalized dilation of the ventricular system. As in Figure 2.2, this patient's clinical picture was dominated by affective and behavioral changes, rather than cognitive deficits, despite the extensive brain damage present. This illustration also depicts the three main types of clinical images: T1, T2, and proton density of mixed-weighted MRIs. (A) Temporal lobe encephalomalcia, (B) inferior frontal encephalomalcia, (C) anterior-frontal encephalomalcia, (D) ventriculomegaly.

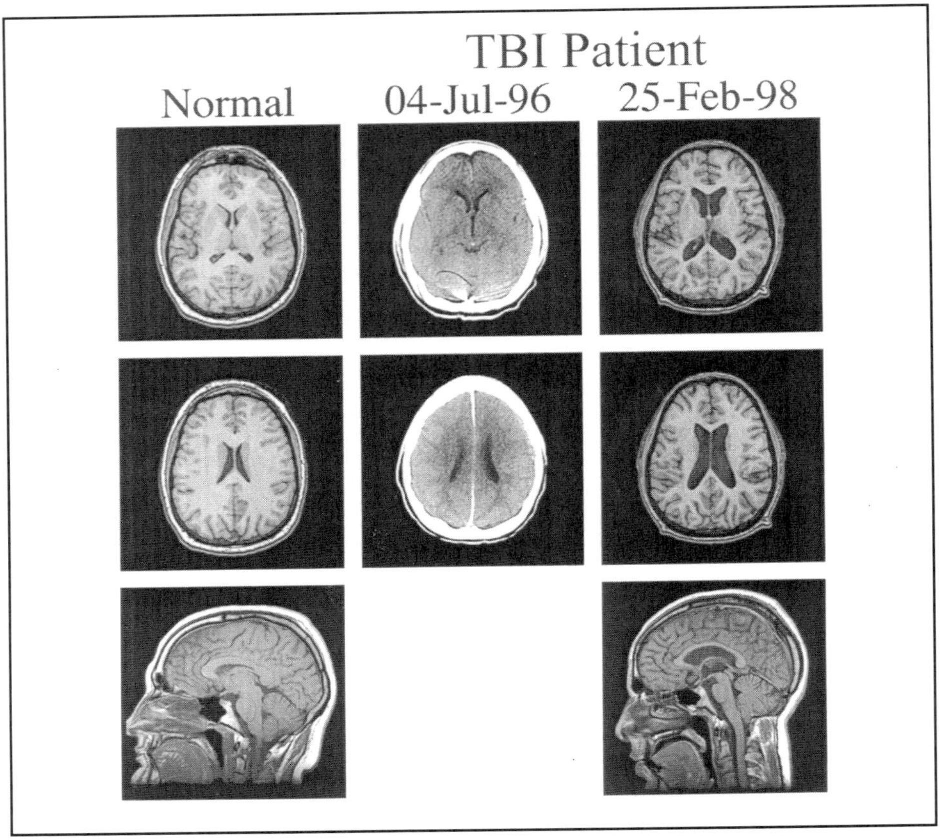

Figure 2.5. From left to right, normal axial T1 weighted MRI at the level of the anterior horn, third ventricle (top), body of the lateral ventricle (middle), and sagittal (bottom), from an individual with no history of brain injury; DOI CT scan taken within 2 hours of a moderate to severe head injury (GCS = 8); axial MRIs representing the chronic imaging findings approximately 1½ years later. The DOI scan indicates generally normal symmetry of the ventricular system without significant midline shift. Although not readily visible in this figure, when this scan was interpreted clinically by a radiologist, some areas appeared to represent localized regions of poor definition between white and gray matter, often an indication of some localized edema. Otherwise, the scan was normal. In the top axial CT scan, the radiologist had circled an area of artifact in the occipital skull region. This represents a defect from an operation for congenital skull deformity that took place in infancy and was unrelated to the head injury. The axial MRI on the right demonstrates the chronic damage observed in severe trauma, compared to the DOI scan as well as the normal MRI on the left. The DOI scan does not reveal the level and degree of damage that has taken place. In contrast, by approximately 18 months postinjury, there are marked structural changes in the form of ventricular dilation, more prominent sulcal width, and thinning of the corpus callosum. All of these findings are indicators of generalized atrophy that accompanies TBI.

"normal" CT does not mean that no significant pathology is present. The pathology is below the threshold for CT detection, and pathological changes may take significant time to evolve.

Quantitative Neuroimaging in Cerebral Trauma

Contemporary imaging methods can not only produce exquisitely refined images of the brain, but also quantify anatomy and pathology. For example, Blatter et al. (1995) analyzed a large number of normal subjects from age 16 to 65, then compared normal brain volumetrics from these control subjects to patients who sustained a TBI (Blatter et al., 1997; see also Bigler et al., 1997). Figures 2.6 and 2.7 provide examples of how MRI images can be quantified. Results of such quantitative analyses typically demonstrate that significant structural changes occur throughout the brain, and the severity of injury directly relates to the amount of structural change (see Figure 2.8). Particularly germane is that although gross structural changes assessed by quantitative analysis were clearly evident in TBI subjects with at least moderate head injury (GCS < 13), quantitative structural changes were not systematically observed in subjects with mild TBI (GCS 13–15). Furthermore, in a series of four cases wherein brain imaging was available both before and after mild head injury, quantitative analysis yielded no significant difference (Bigler & Snyder, 1995). However, this should not be misinterpreted as indicating that mild TBI patients do not have some underlying pathology. As Bigler and Snyder pointed out, one patient who had normal imaging before head injury had clear evidence of white matter shear injury, but no volume loss. Thus, gross brain pathology typically does not evolve from mild TBI, but focal lesions can nonetheless be observed in some mild TBI patients. Likewise, the pathology in mild TBI may be primarily at the ultrastructural level. Functional brain imaging that either directly or indirectly assesses metabolic activity and/or blood flow may be more sensitive in detecting certain cerebral pathologies in mild TBI than structural imaging using CT or MRI. SPECT imaging is the most common functional imaging method in assessing mild TBI.

SPECT Imaging

SPECT imaging is a radiological procedure based on cerebral blood flow. Because cerebral metabolism relates to regional cerebral blood flow (rCBF), metabolism/rCBF should be relatively uniform across the brain when the

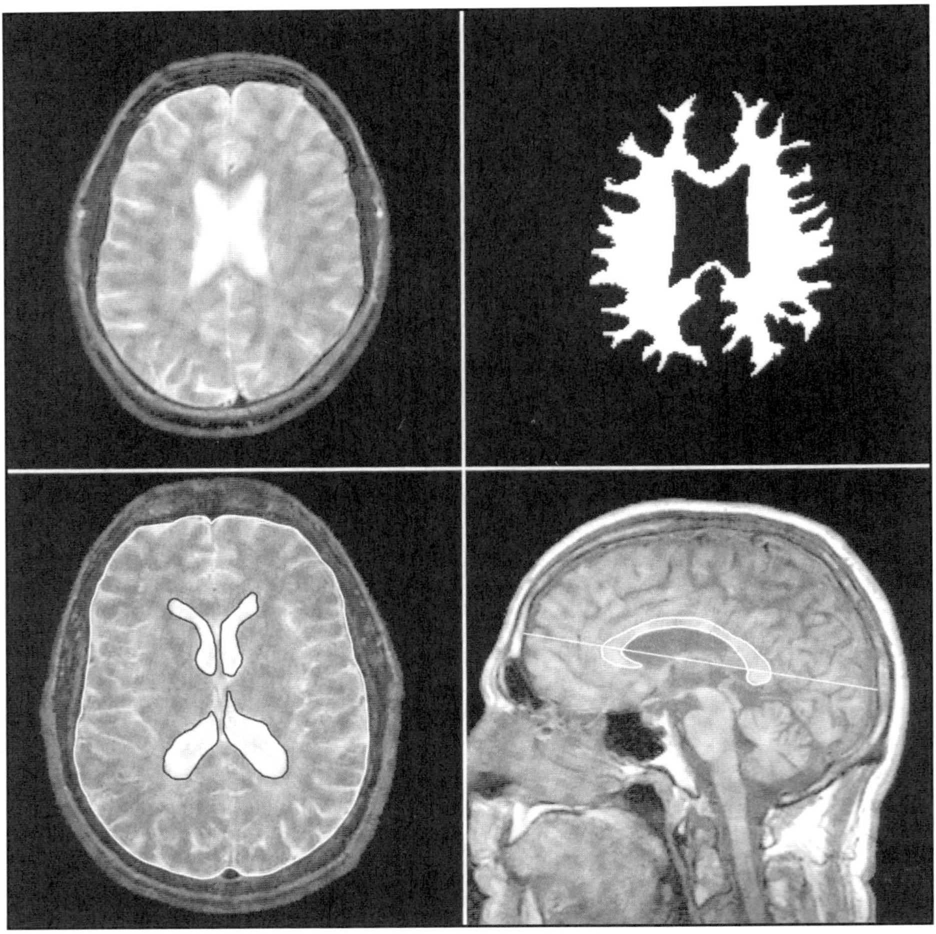

Figure 2.6. Typical axial view of a T2 weighted MRI. Note the delineation of CSF space compared to brain parenchyma. By using a technique that separates different tissues by the pixel value on a gray scale (which provides the basis for coloration of the MRI), CSF is separated from brain parenchyma, and gray matter is extracted, leaving just white matter (upper right). In the axial image on the lower left, the ventricular system is traced, as is the corpus callosum in the lower right image. Using such tracing techniques, any critical structure can be outlined and quantified. Also, in the lower right image, a linear anterior–posterior distance is measured to correct for head size differences across subjects. These methods can be used to quantify any brain structure.

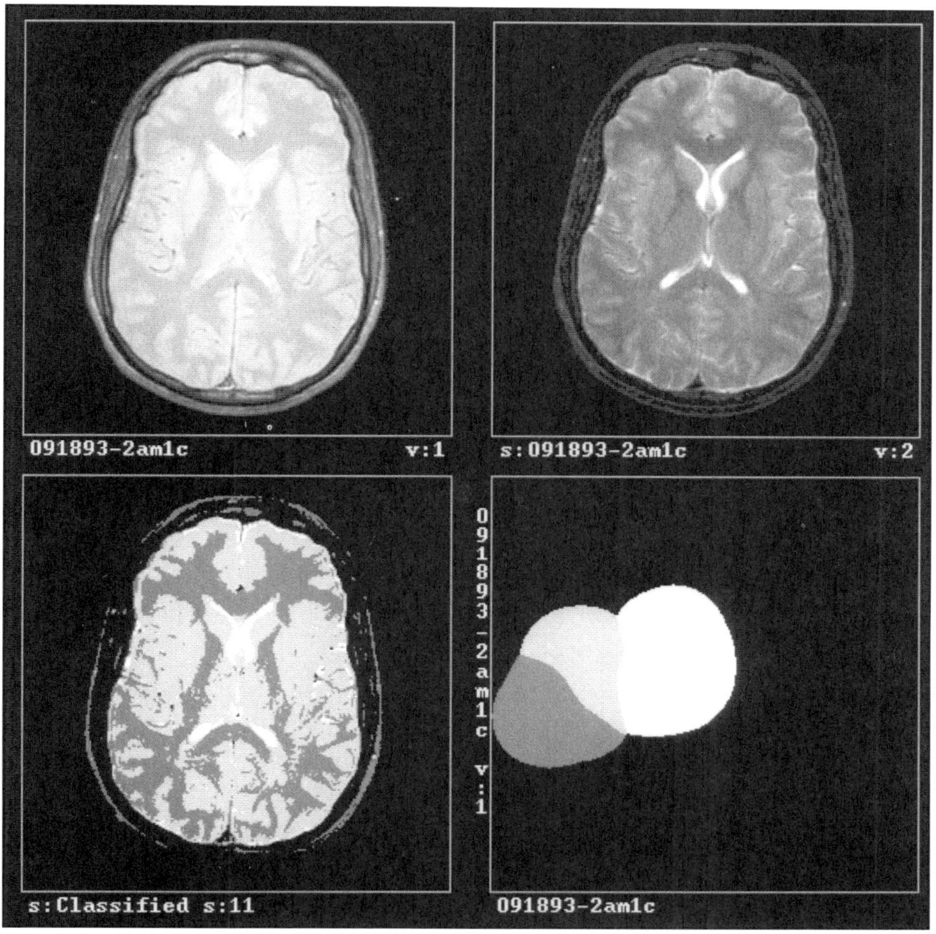

Figure 2.7. Two co-registered images: mixed weighted or proton density (upper left) and T2 weighted (upper right). This figure demonstrates the quantification method of image segmentation. A coordinate system is established (lower right), in which each individual pixel value from the mixed weighted image (*y* axis) is compared to the identical pixel value from the T2 weighted image (*x* axis). An algorithm is applied that aids in segmenting white from gray matter and brain parenchyma from CSF-filled spaces. The final product (lower left) demonstrates the separation of gray and white matter and CSF. Regions of interest or whole brain measures of any structure can then be calculated.

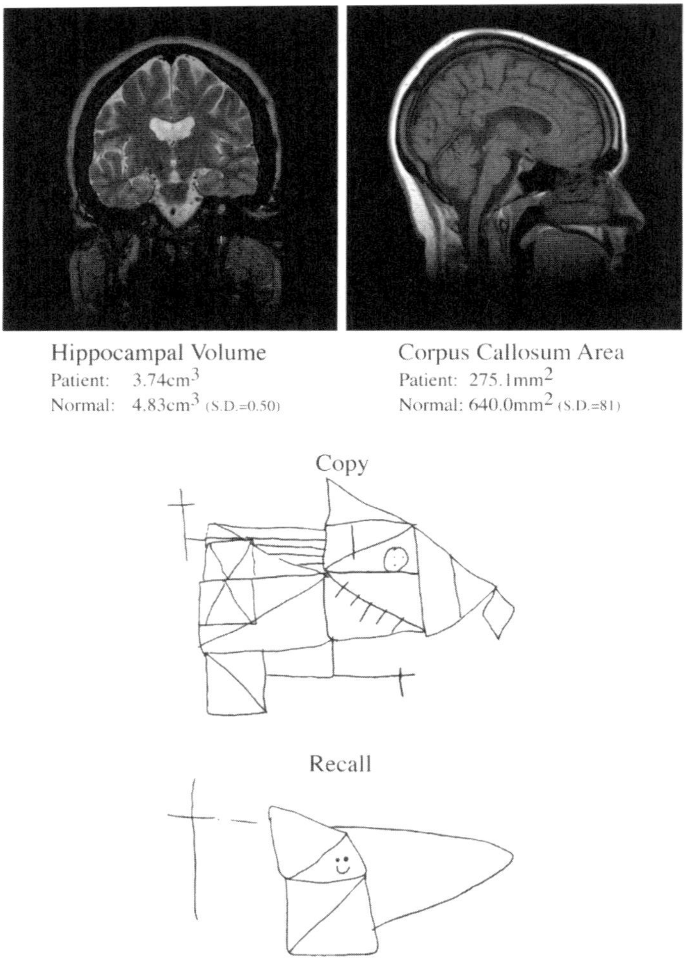

Figure 2.8. Significant atrophic effects of a head injury along with memory impairment in retention of the Rey-Osterrieth Complex figure in a TBI victim. The hippocampus and corpus callosum have been quantified where the patient's morphometric values are compared to normal controls. Note that the quantitative analyses demonstrated significant atrophy (for the corpus callosum, visually compare these images to the normal images shown in Figure 2.5). In addition to the obvious problems with retention of the complex figure, note the piecemeal drawing of the figure. Some of the graphomotor problems may be secondary to the generalized white matter atrophy that accompanies more severe injuries, which disrupts the integrative pathways of the brain (see Gale et al., 1995). Copying requires the integration of visual–perceptual and perceptual–motor functions, so a relationship might exist between white matter atrophy and the loss of perceptual–motor speed or integration.

brain is at rest. Any deviation in the expected pattern of resting perfusion of a radiotracer may be an indication of damage or dysfunction. Figure 2.9 shows obvious pathology in a case of severe brain injury, where corresponding MRI identified lesions are present. It is more challenging when a lesion is not present on MRI, but the patient is experiencing significant neurobehavioral sequelae. In such cases SPECT imaging may be the method of choice. For example, Kant, Smith-Seemiller, Isaac, and Duffy (1997) examined 43 mild TBI cases. Only 9% of these subjects had an MRI abnormality, and less than 5% had an abnormality identified on CT imaging. However, 53% had abnormal SPECT findings. Varney et al. (1995) found similar results. Jacobs, Put, Ingels, Put, and Bossuyt (1996) found that a positive SPECT scan in patients with mild head injury carried with it a poorer prognosis (see also Goldenberg, Oder, Spatt, & Podereka, 1992; Gray, Ichise, Chung, Kirsh, & Franks, 1992; Oder et al., 1992; Varney & Bushnell, in press). It should be noted that SPECT imaging does have its foibles, and careful clinical correlation is required to judge whether a particular SPECT finding relates to the patient's clinical condition and history of head injury (see "Assessment of Brain SPECT," 1996).

Permanent Versus Transient Neuroimaging Findings

Traumatically induced, acute hemorrhage in the brain may present as a transient lesion (Osborn, 1994). Although the ultrastructure perturbations associated with TBI hemorrhagic lesions may be below the threshold of detection, their presence on any postinjury imaging study likely indicates associated structural damage in the vicinity of the hemorrhagic lesion, even when such small lesions are not observed on subsequent imaging studies. Thus, if in acute imaging there is detection of punctate or petechial hemorrhaging, there is certainly the likelihood of surrounding axonal disruption (see Figure 2.10). Such hemorrhagic findings in imaging at any stage can be viewed as indicators that there are permanent structural abnormalities in the region of the hemorrhage, even when follow-up imaging does not show the abnormality (the new diffusion weighted and other techniques may ultimately lead to such detection) (Prichard, 1998).

Substantial lesions on acute imaging typically give rise to permanent changes on follow-up imaging. Blatter et al. (1997) has demonstrated that it may take several months for the full impact of such lesions to be detected. This is also true for the nonspecific degenerative findings associated with TBI (i.e., increased sulcal width, ventricular dilation).

Another issue concerning the permanence of the effects of head injury is raised by Schofield et al. (1997). In this study, subjects who met the criteria

(A)

(B)

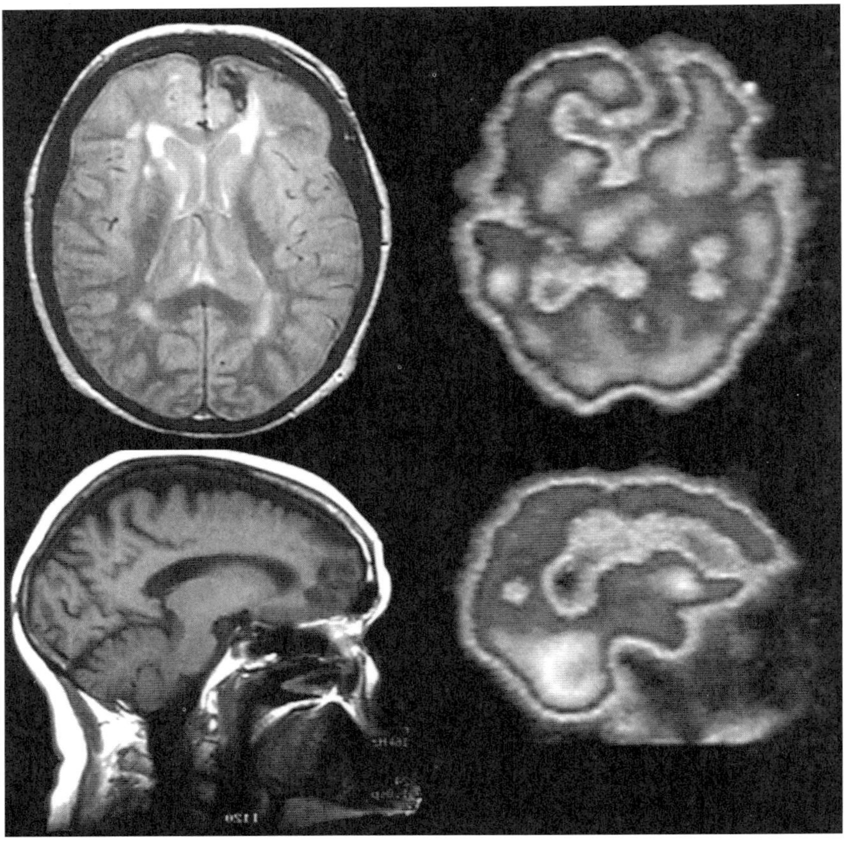

Figure 2.9. (A) SPECT imaging (right) in a patient with significant structural damage secondary to TBI, compared to the MRI (mixed weighted) (left); (B) Sagittal view of MRI (left) and SPECT imaging (right). The MRI demonstrates several classic abnormalities associated with TBI. The dark signal in the left frontal region (viewer's right) is hemosiderin, a blood product that is left as a residual deposit when intraparenchymal hemorrhage occurs. In both frontal regions there are multiple areas of signal hyperintensity (different areas of prominent white). Also note that these areas of white matter hyperintensity tend to be in border regions where white–gray matter interface. These are probably areas of traumatic shearing. In the SPECT imaging, a large defect in cortical perfusion in seen in the left frontal region, compared to the right. Thus, the MRI demonstrates the locus of structural damage, and the SPECT imaging demonstrates metabolic or functional changes associated with the damage. Note further in the SPECT imaging the differences in comparing the activation pattern of the right frontal region (on the reader's left) to the left frontal defect. The obvious major defect where there is no activation is readily apparent, but the entire left frontal region demonstrates defective perfusion. Thus, SPECT imaging demonstrates an even larger area of abnormality, involving much of the left frontal lobe, than that depicted by the MRI.

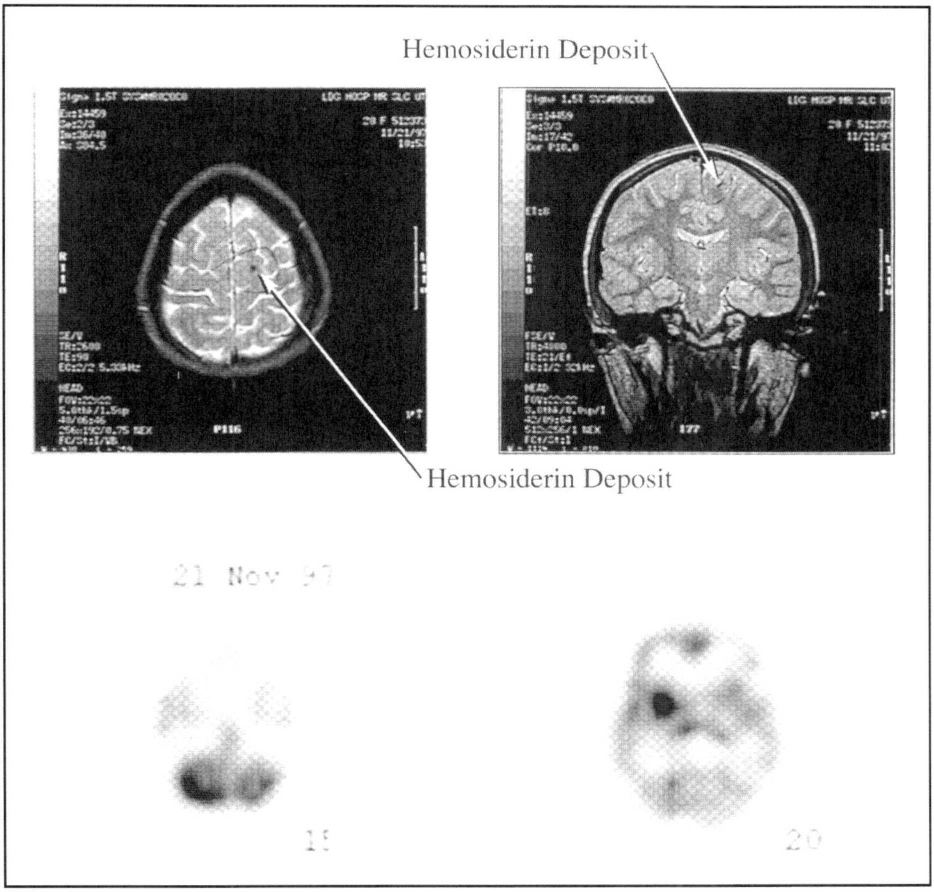

Figure 2.10. Single area of hemosiderin deposit observed on MRI performed more than 3 years postinjury. This 17-year-old patient was in a motor vehicle accident in which she was thrown from the vehicle. DOI CT imaging was negative. The patient met all criteria for a mild TBI. Because the only likely explanation for a hemosiderin deposit in such a young individual would be from the trauma, the presence of hemosiderin in this case is likely an indication of at least a single focus of shearing detected by brain imaging. Behaviorally, she had the typical affective lability and mild neurocognitive problems. A single punctate lesion such as this may reflect pathology that is below the structural imaging threshold of MRI. In this case, SPECT imaging did indicate areas of diminished perfusion in the frontal region and overactivation in the right basal ganglia.

of loss of consciousness (LOC) for a minimum of 5 minutes had an increased likelihood of developing Alzheimer's disease. As of this writing, we do not know if there are neuroimaging correlates to this relationship. However, given the vulnerability of the hippocampus to injury, even in mild TBI (Bigler et al., 1997; Bigler et al., 1996) it would seem that neurochemical and/or structural changes may ultimately lead to an adverse interaction with aging or a late-life disorder such as Alzheimer's disease. In any event, any permanent lesions that can be detected by contemporary neuroimaging methods will be superimposed on a brain that will exhibit dynamic changes with age, and will likely exaggerate any age-related effects.

Conclusions

Neuroimaging studies provide a means to evaluate gross structural abnormalities that may be associated with trauma. In mild TBI, clinically defined abnormalities may not be observed, even though injury is present at the ultrastructure level. When abnormalities are present in TBI, they tend to be located in the inferior frontal, anterior, and/or mesial temporal lobe and at junctions between gray and white matter (see Figure 2.11). The fact that these lesions occur in these particular areas likely represents, at least in part, the pathophysiological basis for some of the cognitive (particularly memory and attention) and behavioral (particularly affective) changes so often associated with mild TBI.

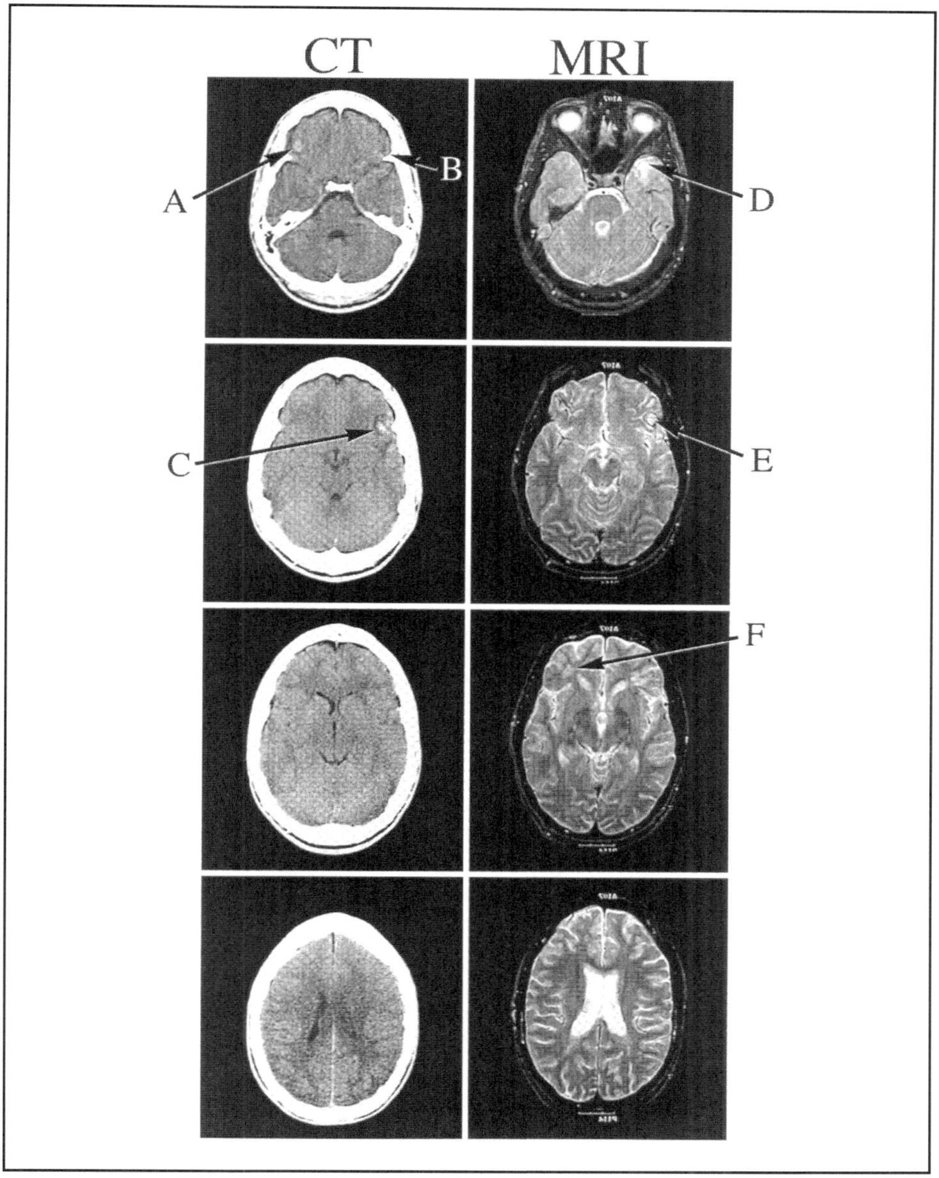

Figure 2.11. From left to right, CT imaging performed on the day of injury representing areas of acute contusion in the inferior frontal region (A and B), and an area of frontotemporal contusion (C); MRI over 2 years postinjury demonstrating the chronic lesions (D, E, and F) that accompany the acute pathology observed in CT imaging on the left. Note the expansion of the ventricular system in the lower right-hand MRI. The classic lesions in TBI occur in frontotemporal areas, along with diffuse, nonspecific white matter changes as reflected in ventricular dilation.

References

Alexander, M. P. (1995). Mild traumatic brain injury: Pathophysiology, natural history, and clinical management. *Neurology, 45,* 1253–1260.

Assessment of brain SPECT: Report of the therapeutics and technology assessment subcommittee. (1996). *Neurology, 46,* 278–285.

Bigler, E. D. (1990). Neuropathology of traumatic brain injury. In E. D. Bigler (Ed.), *Traumatic brain injury: Mechanisms of damage, assessment, intervention, and outcome* (pp. 13–49). Austin, TX: PRO-ED.

Bigler, E. D. (1996a). Introduction. In E. D. Bigler (Ed.), *Neuroimaging I: Basic science* (pp. 1–6). New York: Plenum Press.

Bigler, E. D. (1996b). Neuroimaging in traumatic brain injury. In E. D. Bigler (Ed.), *Neuroimaging II: Clinical applications* (pp. 261–278). New York: Plenum Press.

Bigler, E. D. (1997). Brain imaging and behavioral outcome in traumatic brain injury. In E. D. Bigler, E. Clark, & J. E. Farmer (Eds.), *Childhood traumatic brain injury: Diagnosis, assessment, and intervention* (pp. 7–29). Austin, TX: PRO-ED.

Bigler, E. D., Blatter, D. D., Anderson, C. V., Johnson, S. C., Gale, S. D., Hopkins, R. O., & Burnett, B. (1997). Hippocampal volume in normal aging and traumatic brain injury. *American Journal of Neuroradiology, 18,* 11–23.

Bigler, E. D., Johnson, S. C., Anderson, C. V., Blatter, D. D., Gale, S. D., Russo, A. A., Ryser, D. K., Macnamara, S. E., Bailey, B. J., Hopkins, R. O., & Abildskov, T. J. (1996). Traumatic brain injury and memory: The role of hippocampal atrophy. *Neuropsychology, 10,* 333–342.

Bigler, E. D., & Snyder, J. L. (1995). Neuropsychological outcome and quantitative neuroimaging in mild head injury. *Archives of Clinical Neuropsychology, 10,* 159–174.

Blatter, D. D., Bigler, E. D., Gale, S. D., Johnson, S. C., Anderson, C. V., Burnett, B. M., Parker, N., Kurth, S., & Horn, S. (1995). Quantitative volumetric analysis of brain MR: Normative database spanning five decades of life. *American Journal of Neuroradiology, 16,* 241–251.

Blatter, D. D., Bigler, E. D., Gale, S. D., Johnson, S. C., Anderson, C. V., Burnett, B. M., Ryser, D., Macnamara, S. E., & Bailey, B. J. (1997). MR-based brain and cerebrospinal fluid measurement after traumatic brain injury: Correlation with neuropsychological outcome. *American Journal of Neuroradiology, 18,* 1–10.

Gale, S. D., Burr, R. B., Bigler, E. D., & Blatter, D. (1993). Fornix degeneration and memory in traumatic brain injury. *Brain Research Bulletin, 32,* 345–349.

Gale, S. D., Johnson, S. C., Bigler, E. D., & Blatter, D. D. (1995). Nonspecific white matter degeneration following traumatic brain injury. *Journal of the International Neuropsychological Society, 1,* 17–28.

Gean, A. D. (1994). *Imaging of head trauma.* New York: Raven Press.

Goldenberg, G., Oder, W., Spatt, J., & Podereka, I. (1992). Cerebral correlates of disturbed executive function and memory in survivors of severe closed head injury: A SPECT study. *Journal of Neurology, Neurosurgery, & Psychiatry, 55,* 362–368.

Gray, B. G., Ichise, M., Chung, D. G., Kirsh, J. C., & Franks, W. (1992). Technetium-99m-HMPAO SPECT in the evaluation of patients with a remote history of traumatic brain injury: A comparison with x-ray computed tomography. *Journal of Nuclear Medicine, 33,* 52–58.

Jacobs, A., Put, E., Ingels, M., Put, T., & Bossuyt, A. (1996). One-year follow-up of Technetium-99m-HMPAO SPECT in mild head injury. *Journal of Nuclear Medicine, 37,* 1605–1609.

Johnson, S. C., Bigler, E. D., Burr, R. B., & Blatter, D. D. (1994). White matter atrophy, ventricular dilation, and intellectual functioning following traumatic brain injury. *Neuropsychology, 8,* 307–315.

Kant, L., Smith-Seemiller, L., Isaac, G., & Duffy, J. (1997). Tc-HMPAO SPECT in persistent postconcussion syndrome after mild head injury: Comparison with MRI/CT. *Brain Injury, 11,* 115–124.

Maxwell, W. L., Povlishock, J. T., & Graham, D. L. (1997). A mechanistic analysis of nondisruptive axonal injury: A review. *Journal of Neurotrauma, 14,* 419–440.

Oder, W., Goldenberg, G., Spatt, J., Podreka, I., Binder, H., & Deecke, L. (1992). Behavioural and psychosocial sequelae of severe closed head injury and regional cerebral blood flow: A SPECT study. *Journal of Neurology, Neurosurgery, and Psychiatry, 55,* 475–480.

Orrison, W. W., Lewine, J. D., Sanders, J. A., & Hartshorne, M. F. (1995). *Functional brain imaging.* St. Louis, MO: Mosby.

Osborn, A. G. (1994). *Diagnostic neuroradiology.* St. Louis, MO: Mosby.

Prichard, J. W. (1998). Neurorehabilitation: Three new NMR tools. *The Neuroscientist, 4,* 231–235.

Schofield, P. W., Tang, M., Marder, K., Bell, K., Dooneief, G., Chun, M., Sano, M., Stern, Y., & Mayeux, R. (1997). Alzheimer's disease after remote head injury: An incidence study. *Journal of Neurology, Neurosurgery, and Psychiatry, 62,* 119–124.

Thatcher, R. W., Hallett, M., Zeffiro, T., John, E. R., & Huerta, M. (1994). *Functional neuroimaging: Technical foundations.* San Diego: Academic Press.

Varney, N. R., & Bushnell, D. (in press). NeuroSPECT findings in patients with post-traumatic anosmia: A quantitative analysis. *Journal of Head Trauma Rehabilitation.*

Varney, N. R., Bushnell, D. L., Nathan, M., Kah, D., Roberts, R., Rezai, K., Walker, W., & Kirchner, P. (1995). NeuroSPECT correlates of disabling mild head injury: Preliminary findings. *Journal of Head Trauma Rehabilitation, 10,* 18–28.

Evaluation of Neuropsychological Status Following Mild Traumatic Brain Injury

3

C. Munro Cullum and
Laetitia L. Thompson

The concept of mild or "minor" TBI remains an area of controversy. Even though it has been demonstrated that brain damage and even serious medical complications can result from apparently minor injuries (Dacey, Alves, Rimel, Winn, & Jane, 1986), we have limited understanding of how much force is required to cause such an injury. Furthermore, there is often a question of whether it is likely an individual sustained **any** brain injury in a particular incident (i.e., "possible" TBI). This can pose a significant challenge from a clinical diagnostic standpoint, particularly in cases of apparently minor "bumps" to the head and/or whiplash types of injuries, where the neuropsychologist is asked to determine whether a TBI likely occurred. Obviously, the brain is relatively well protected by the skull, meninges, and cerebrospinal fluid; a significant injury to the brain requires an exceptional force. Considering the various sports-related falls, occasional blows to the head, and/or whiplash injuries we have all experienced, we can acknowledge that the vast majority of these relatively common insults to the cerebrum tend to be neurobehaviorally innocuous. In contrast, mild TBI should not be considered "trivial," and acute symptoms following mild TBI are well established (e.g., see Levin, Eisenberg, & Benton, 1989). Much of the controversy centers around longer term sequelae and chronic postconcussive symptomatology. Accordingly, a number of apparently discrepant findings with respect to residual mild TBI sequelae have been reported in the literature. Such discrepancies probably relate to a variety of definitional and methodological issues (e.g., see Bohnen & Jolles, 1992; Jacobson, 1995; Kay, Newman, Cavallo, Ezrachi, & Resnick, 1992), but nevertheless underscore the complexities of the problem at hand.

Reprinted, with changes, from "Neuropsychological Diagnosis and Outcome in Mild Traumatic Brain Injury," by C. Munro Cullum and Laetitia L. Thompson, 1997, *Applied Neuropsychology, 4*(1), pp. 6–15. Copyright 1997 by Lawrence Erlbaum Associates, Inc.

Biomechanical Forces and Brain Injury

As noted, the forces required to cause concussion or residual cerebral dysfunction are still poorly understood (Melvin, Lighthall, & Ueno, 1993). Whereas the brain is relatively well protected, it has been clearly demonstrated that brain injury can occur in the absence of physical trauma to the skull (Gennarelli et al., 1982; Ommaya & Gennarelli, 1974). Furthermore, relatively mild percussional forces have been associated with demonstrable cerebral damage and neurobehavioral deficits in cats, with a significant correlation between the severity of injury and the degree of subsequent memory impairment (Hilton et al., 1993). Nevertheless, knowledge about what constitutes sufficient force to cause brain damage remains largely speculative and often open to debate. This is further complicated by the fact that neuroimaging results are usually, but not always (Levin, Williams, Eisenberg, High, & Guinto, 1992), normal in cases of mild TBI (Bigler & Snyder, 1995).

Nonimpact Brain Injury

Recent definitions of mild TBI include whiplash as a potential etiological factor (Mild Traumatic Brain Injury Committee, American Congress of Rehabilitation Medicine, 1993). However, there is still controversy over the neurocognitive effects of nonimpact brain injury. This is at least partly due to the general paucity of studies on nonimpact brain injury and the fact that no adequately controlled neuropsychological investigations in this area exist (Sweeney, 1992).

One of the most thorough investigations to date found that acutely injured whiplash victims performed more poorly than demographically matched control subjects on measures of attention and concentration, in addition to showing otoneurological and/or EEG abnormalities. In contrast, MRI and auditory-evoked response findings were uniformly normal. Although most patients returned to normal functioning by 1 year, several remained symptomatic (Ettlin et al., 1992).

Di Stefano and Radanov (1995) examined a series of whiplash patients and found no demonstrable deficits in memory at 1 year, although there was some variability in aspects of attention that could not be easily explained by pain or medication effects. Other cases of cognitive abnormalities in post-whiplash patients have been reported (Bohnen, Jolles, & Verhey, 1993; Yarnell & Rossie, 1988), although there is significant debate over these infrequent case reports. Nevertheless, as with most of the mild TBI literature, there is an emerging sense that when cognitive complaints are present after whiplash, a majority of patients recover completely, and mitigating factors must be carefully considered in interpreting cognitive test results (e.g., see Radanov, Di Stefano, Schnidrig, Sturzenegger, & Augustiny, 1993).

Another complicating issue is that the evidence for nonimpact brain injury in humans is largely theoretical and based on animal models. Several animal studies have documented microscopic shear–strain effects with repeated rapid acceleration–deceleration of the cerebrum in the absence of physical trauma (Gennarelli, 1986). It has been suggested that compared to a direct impact to the head, a nonimpact concussion requires approximately twice the velocity (Hirsch, Ommaya, & Mahone, 1970). It has also been demonstrated that high g-force acceleration can induce loss of consciousness probably related to a transient reduction in blood flow (Whinnery & Whinnery, 1990). The challenge lies in how to translate such information to an enhanced clinicopathological understanding of how specific whiplash injuries or mild TBI affect individual patients.

Acute Symptomatology

Reconstructed information about the likely biomechanical forces of an accident can be helpful, but because of limited knowledge about biomechanical variables in a particular accident, such data may be of limited utility. For the neuropsychologist, therefore, consideration of acute and subsequent symptomatology is crucial (Stuss, 1995).

Duration of loss of consciousness (LOC) is often used as an index of TBI severity, but LOC is not a sufficient indicator of residual brain injury. "Concussion," defined as the temporary interruption in normal consciousness, is also nonspecific and tells little about the likelihood of residual, underlying cerebral dysfunction. The staging of concussion severity has been addressed by several groups, and most recently outlined by the Quality Standards Committee of the American Academy of Neurology (Report of the Quality Standards Committee of the American Academy of Neurology, 1997). LOC can be an important neurobehavioral factor in assessing the likely severity of TBI, although some data suggest that the presence or absence of brief LOC in mild TBI may be of limited clinical utility (Leininger, Gramling, Farrell, Kreutzer, & Peck, 1990). The "second impact syndrome" is the occurrence of a second concussion prior to recovery from an initial concussion, resulting in neurobehavioral sequelae. As with the potential cumulative effects of multiple TBIs, it appears that the second impact syndrome can have serious consequences in some cases. To take an extreme example, serial concussions without loss of consciousness have been associated with diffuse brain swelling and death in at least one case (Kelly et al., 1991). Although cases are rare, the syndrome is only beginning to be recognized, and there is little specific information regarding its frequency or likelihood of occurrence.

Whereas the duration of LOC can be difficult to reconstruct and quantify, it is most commonly assessed by the Glasgow Coma Scale (GCS). The

GCS enjoys widespread use and is frequently implemented by paramedics and emergency room personnel. Thus, GCS scores in the acute stages of TBI are often available in patients' medical records. However, the GCS was developed to assess LOC across a wide range of severity and provides limited information about subtle alterations in consciousness. In the case of mild TBI, scores generally range from 13 to 15 (15 is the highest score on the GCS).

The presence or extent of posttraumatic amnesia (PTA) is another commonly examined indicator of brain injury severity. PTA refers to the period following a brain injury or concussion wherein new memories are not consistently formed. Definitions of mild TBI include a maximum period of PTA ranging from minutes to hours. Whereas the length of PTA has shown a significant relationship with cognitive dysfunction (Dikmen, Machamer, Winn, & Temkin, 1995; Levin et al., 1992), the relationship is far from perfect because a small proportion of mild TBI patients show evidence of residual cognitive difficulties, yet a few individuals with more severe injuries show complete recovery. PTA is typically assessed by asking patients to indicate their first memories following TBI. It is important to note that both anterograde and retrograde amnesia should be assessed as carefully as possible. In the acute setting, more quantifiable data regarding PTA can be gathered by using instruments such as the *Galveston Orientation and Amnesia Test* (GOAT; Levin, O'Donnell, & Grossman, 1979), which consists of some simple questions about current orientation and short-term memory.

Despite its clinical utility, one should use caution in assessing PTA. For example, it is not uncommon in accident situations for people to have difficulty recalling events. This often occurs in the absence of any potential brain injury, and reflects situational emotional distress rather than PTA symptoms per se. Along these lines, it is also important to assess posttraumatic stress-related symptoms, using formal diagnostic criteria for posttraumatic stress disorder (PTSD).

Postconcussive Syndrome

Following mild TBI, a number of neurobehavioral symptoms are reported with enough frequency to be referred to as the postconcussive syndrome (PCS) (Alves, Macciocchi, & Barth, 1993). Some of the classic symptoms include headaches, photosensitivity, dizziness, fatigue, irritability, problems with attention and concentration, and depression, although other complaints are reported with some frequency. Most of these cognitive, emotional, and physical symptoms typically improve over time, and the majority of mild TBI patients recover within a few months after injury (Barth, Macciocchi, & Giordani, 1983; Binder, 1986; Levin et al., 1987). However, a small proportion of patients continue to complain of symptoms over a longer period (Dikmen, Temkin, & Armsden, 1989; Gronwall & Wrightson, 1980; Rimel, Giordani, &

Barth, 1981; Rutherford, Merrett, & McDonald, 1979), and sometimes these complaints alone result in a late, retrospective diagnosis of mild TBI.

Recovery from PCS appears to be a complex process, and may be further mitigated by a host of psychological variables and/or secondary gain issues, particularly in cases involving litigation (Youngjohn, Burrows, & Erdal, 1995). Persistent PCS is less common in sports-related than in accident-related TBI (Barth et al., 1989), which suggests an additional level of complexity in the maintenance of PCS. Although recovery from PCS is clearly the norm following mild TBI, some individuals seem to experience more persistent symptoms (e.g., see Bohnen, Twijnstra, & Jolles, 1993). It remains to be seen whether any type of early intervention may decrease the severity or duration of PCS, although some promising data on early, brief psychological/educational interventions have recently been reported (Mittenberg, Tremont, Zielinski, Fichera, & Rayls, 1996).

It is important to note that PCS and PTSD share some symptoms, although PTSD is relatively uncommon in mild TBI (Ruff, Wylie, & Tennant, 1993). Because of the symptom overlap, it can be difficult to sort out complaints that are neurologically or psychologically based. PTSD involves the reexperiencing of a traumatic event; thus, it may not be an appropriate diagnosis when there is significant amnesia for the event in question. A diagnosis of PTSD in cases of mild TBI should be made conservatively, as there may be a tendency of overdiagnosis in complex cases. Other obvious issues in the assessment of PCS are symptom exaggeration and malingering (e.g., see Ruff et al., 1993).

Symptom Base Rates

There has recently been interest in the examination of base rates of common TBI symptoms in non-TBI conditions. For example, it is important to know whether an individual's complaints of headaches or poor concentration are new or predated the TBI. If the symptoms developed after the accident, it is important to consider their nature and etiology: Is the headache due to a brain injury or to a neck or back injury? Is the complaint of poor concentration due to cognitive impairment related to a brain injury, or to depression or chronic pain or fatigue? If symptoms arise months after a possible TBI, is there a causal relationship, or might other factors account for the symptoms? Few PCS symptoms are exclusive to concussion, and therefore may have other causes. Many such symptoms may occur in individuals who have not sustained a brain injury, or may have another cause even in individuals with a brain injury.

The potential role of expectancy or symptom attribution should also be carefully considered; benign or "normal" lapses in mental efficiency may be automatically attributed to TBI. This can be a particularly important issue for patients who suffer persistent PCS, because they can become attuned to or overly focused on these benign lapses. This can in turn lead to further emotional distress, in addition to providing ongoing "evidence" of their brain impairment. Accordingly, feelings of stress following TBI may lead to hyperarousal, which may subsequently contribute to decreased attention (Gronwall, 1987). Such attributions or expectations can be key factors in the development and maintenance of PCS (Mittenberg, DiGiulio, Perrin, & Bass, 1992). The discussion of such psychological factors is not meant to infer malingering or conscious attempts to exaggerate symptoms, although all of these factors certainly may coexist and merit careful consideration.

Knowing how common specific symptoms are in the general population can be quite useful in the assessment of TBI sequelae. Gouvier, Uddo-Crane, and Brown (1988) used questionnaires to assess base rates of neuropsychological, psychological, and physical symptoms among head injured and non–head injured groups. They found no significant differences between the groups, establishing that a number of symptoms commonly associated with TBI occur with some frequency in the general population. Dikmen, McLean, & Temkin (1986) obtained essentially the same results in their study of mild TBI. More recently, Fox, Lees-Haley, Earnest, and Dolezal-Wood (1995) found high rates of postconcussive types of symptoms in a survey of individuals referred for outpatient psychological treatment. Although those who reported a history of TBI with loss of consciousness showed the highest reporting of certain symptoms, results of this survey suggest that some classic postconcussive symptoms (e.g., headaches, fatigue, irritability) may be more strongly associated with nonneurological factors in many cases. Thus, the presence or absence of some symptoms in mild TBI may be of limited diagnostic utility.

Accuracy of Event Recall

When mild TBI is not initially diagnosed, and one needs to determine whether or not a brain injury occurred, one can obviously ask the patient about the event and his or her acute and subsequent symptomatology. However, it can be difficult to know how much to rely on this information, particularly when the patient's report is somewhat inconsistent over time and/or is inconsistent with reports of witnesses, investigating officers, emergency room personnel, etc. Clearly, asking the patient to provide much information regarding loss of consciousness is difficult. First of all, the patient cannot differentiate between actual loss of consciousness and PTA. Second, if there is a lapse of memory, the patient cannot know how long it lasted. Information from a variety of sources must be pieced together to estimate how long the patient may have been unconscious and/or in PTA.

Research regarding healthy, non–brain injured subjects' recall of events also provides useful information about patients' ability to recall details about an accident and how specific recollections can change over time. Loftus and her colleagues (Hall & Loftus, 1984; Loftus, 1979; Wells & Loftus, 1984), for example, have conducted numerous studies on memory and memory distortion. In the classic paradigm, subjects witness a staged event such as an accident or crime and then are asked to recall aspects of what they saw. Such scenarios are obviously different from accidents involving a TBI, because these subjects are not hurt, dazed, and/or confused. Nevertheless, this research has shown that significant errors in recall can occur, particularly when subjects are asked direct questions about specific details (Loftus). Further, it has been shown that incorrect details can be introduced through others' questions or comments and incorporated into subjects' recall of events without their awareness (Hall & Loftus). Loftus, Miller, and Burns (1978) also found that recall for remote events was more susceptible to alteration than recall for more recent events.

This research calls into question how much a patient's report of details should be relied upon in determining the likelihood of a TBI. It also suggests that self-reports may be more accurate shortly after an accident than later. However, some inconsistencies in reporting over time should not necessarily be viewed as intentional distortions of events.

Neuropsychological Findings

Most of the carefully controlled group studies of single, uncomplicated, mild TBI show that when acute impairment is found, differences between patients and control subjects are no longer discernible after a few months (Barth et al., 1983; Dikmen et al., 1995; Levin et al., 1987). This does not mean that prolonged neuropsychological impairment cannot result from mild TBI, because this clearly does occur (e.g., Bigler & Snyder, 1995). However, improvement usually occurs following mild TBI, typically to a baseline or normal level (Alexander, 1995).

With much attention being given to the prolonged difficulties experienced by some individuals with mild TBI, it is worth noting that preliminary data from an ongoing study at the University of Colorado Health Sciences Center revealed no differences in performance among mild TBI patients with or without previous mild TBI and control subjects who had also been involved in an accident but without any injury to the head, neck, or back (L. Thompson, A. Naplin, & J. Kelly, personal communication, November, 1993). Subjects were tested within 1 week of the accident and then again 2 months later, with a brief battery of standard measures including the Digit Vigilance Test, Category Test, Trail Making Test, Story Memory Test, Figure Memory Test, and Grooved Pegboard (Heaton, Grant, & Matthews, 1991). The criteria for mild TBI used in this study are presented in Table 3.1.

Table 3.1

Mild TBI Study Inclusion Criteria

1.	Trauma resulting in a blow to the head
2.	LOC for up to 20 minutes **or** evidence of some period of PTA up to 24 hours
3.	Acute symptoms of concussion, including persisting headache and feeling dazed or confused
4.	No significant history of alcohol or other substance abuse, severe TBI, or disease affecting the central nervous system

Figure 3.1 depicts group means for the verbal learning and memory results as an illustration of preliminary findings. The relative performances of groups and the lack of change over time were quite similar on the other measures as well. Also, although prior TBI has been reported as a risk factor for increased impairment following mild TBI, this was not supported by the preliminary data in this study.

Base Rates of Neuropsychological Impairments

Clearly neuropsychological test results must not be interpreted in isolation. Furthermore, it is critical to examine the pattern of findings in addition to levels of performance. With these caveats in mind, normative reference bases must be carefully used as interpretive guidelines. In addition to considering basic demographic factors (e.g., age, education, gender, ethnicity, socioeconomic status, dominant language), one must remember that everyone has relative cognitive strengths and weaknesses, and no two individuals are alike. Even within the normal range of neuropsychological performance, there is tremendous heterogeneity. Furthermore, cognitive skills lie on a distribution, with some abilities falling above and below individual and group means. Some individuals will fall at the lower and the upper ranges of any given ability distribution, and an individual may show variability across cognitive domains.

One example of base rates of neuropsychological impairment can be found in Heaton, Grant, and Matthews (1991). Normative scores from many common neuropsychological measures can be found in this reference. Whereas this work represents a significant clinical advancement in test score interpretation, it also provides information regarding neuropsychological base rates. Specifically, based on a comprehensive battery of popular neuropsychological measures, comprised of 40 primary test scores, the median number of scores falling in the "impaired" range (i.e., one standard deviation or

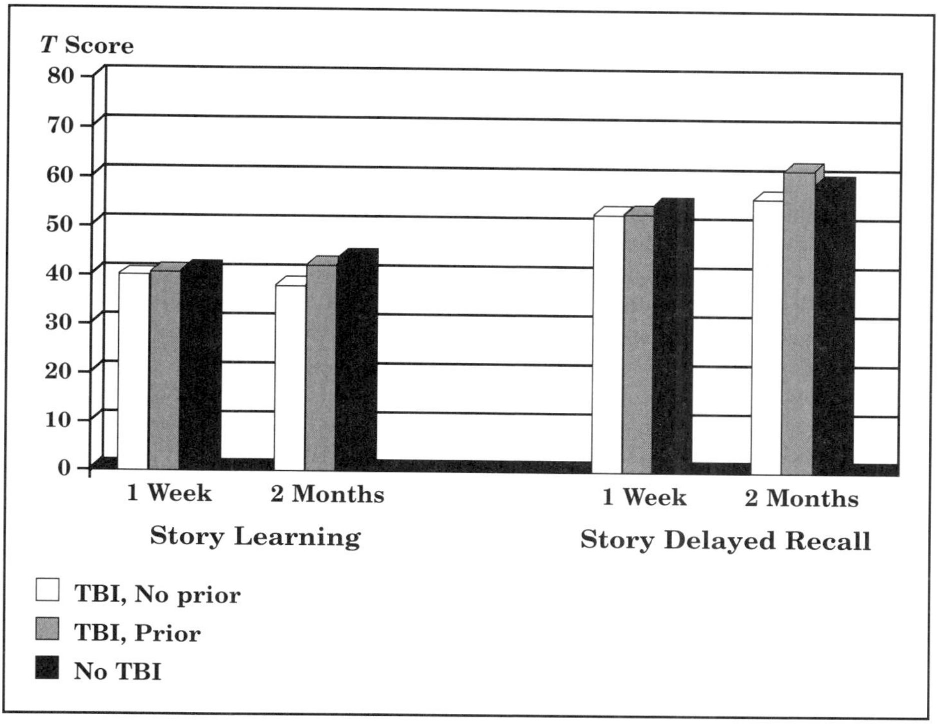

Figure 3.1. Longitudinal mean Story Learning and Story Delayed Recall scores by group.

more below the mean of the standardization sample) was four (p. 36), or 10% of all scores. Thus, any healthy individual with no history of central nervous system (CNS) risk factors can be expected to have a number of scores that fall below the "expected" level. In addition to underscoring the importance of not interpreting test results in isolation, this suggests that there is a fairly wide range of "normal" neuropsychological performance in the general population, and that this must be considered when interpreting results from TBI patients as well.

Another important point is that in the interpretation of neuropsychological test scores in the impaired range, the neuropsychologist must consider other possible causes of poor results. A common mistake is to automatically attribute deficits to the head injury that brings the patient to examination (Dikmen & Levin, 1993). As noted, prior head injuries and neurological disease may be important risk factors to consider. Furthermore, other, previously unrecognized medical and/or psychiatric conditions can influence test scores. For example, different types of learning disabilities have been identified that do not affect just academic skills, but also lower selected neuropsychological abilities (e.g., rote learning in dyslexia, abstract reasoning and visuospatial skills in nonverbal learning disability; Rourke, 1982). There is also increasing evidence that Attention-Deficit/Hyperactivity Disorder is related to an "executive function" deficit (Pennington, 1991). These are just a few examples of other risk factors for neuropsychological impairment that should be considered when examining a patient, but they highlight the complicated nature of the diagnostic process and the importance of obtaining a comprehensive history. As noted by Dikmen and Machamer (1995), outcome following TBI is a multifactorial process, and neither patient complaints nor observed neurocognitive deficiencies in an individual with a history of head injury should automatically or unquestioningly be assumed to be related to brain injury.

On the other hand, when there is a history of preexisting CNS risk factors such as previous TBI, individuals may be at higher risk for greater impairment or persistence of cognitive deficits secondary to a more recent mild TBI (e.g., see Satz, 1993). Older individuals also are at higher risk for prolonged and more serious cognitive sequelae of TBI, as well as for subsequent neurological complications (Naugle, 1991).

Recovery from Mild TBI

The precise course of recovery obviously varies, because recovery is related to a host of intraindividual factors and severity of injury issues. Interestingly, however, there are data to suggest that less severe injuries tend to be more consistent in their neurocognitive sequelae, and more severe injuries have greater variability in outcome (Dikmen et al., 1995). In general, the well known head injury recovery curve must be kept in mind, because the typical expectation following mild, uncomplicated TBI is recovery. The lowest level of neurocognitive functioning will be seen in the initial period following an uncomplicated injury, with improvement typically occurring over the ensuing days to several weeks or months, depending upon the severity of injury. When subsequent deterioration of function occurs following mild TBI, the possibility of neurological complications (e.g., hematoma, increased intracranial pressure) must be carefully evaluated. In the absence of such factors, subsequent behavioral deterioration may be explained by psychological factors such as depression and/or situational or secondary gain issues. This is also an important concept to keep in mind when cognitive symptoms arise well after TBI. Although there may be a delay in noticing symptoms due to pain, medications, and/or decreased mental demands (e.g., when someone is off work for a time), a protracted period before cognitive symptoms are reported may indicate the influence of nonneurological factors.

The course of recovery is often assessed with serial neuropsychological evaluations, which are becoming more commonplace, especially when litigation is involved. Even though adequate normative test–retest data are lacking for many measures, useful data are accruing, particularly from sports-neuropsychology applications (e.g., see Hinton-Bayre, Geffen, & McFarland, 1997; Lovell & Collins, 1998; McCrea, Kelly, Kluge, Ackley, & Randolph, 1997).

In test–retest situations, error variance is increased, and some degree of variability can be expected, depending upon the measure in question and the amount of "practice effect" inherent in a particular task. Data regarding *Wechsler Adult Intelligence Scale–Revised* (WAIS–R) test–retest effects provide a good example. Information and Vocabulary scores do not show much test–retest variability among normal subjects (e.g., usually within ± 2 scaled score points), although improvements up to 3 scaled score points can be seen on Digit Symbol, usually without any decline (adapted from Cullum, Heaton, & Grant, 1991). Similarly, certain attentional measures show little practice effect (e.g., Symbol-Digit Modalities; Barth et al., 1989; Hinton-Bayre et al., 1997), whereas some memory tests are much more sensitive to practice effect (McCaffrey, Ortega, & Haase, 1993). Unusual increases on some measures and declines on others may reflect unreliability of results and hence, invalidity (see Cullum et al., 1991; Reitan & Wolfson, 1997). Such test–retest comparisons can be particularly useful in assessing the likely effects of neurological and nonneurological factors.

Consequences of Inaccurate Diagnosis

Assessment of neuropsychological impairment due to mild TBI, and determination of the likelihood that a mild TBI occurred are clearly very complicated tasks, and are not without consequences to the patient. Much has been written in the last 10 years about the underdiagnosis of mild TBI and the lack of recognition among health professionals of the possible sequelae of such injuries. Failure to recognize that a TBI has occurred may increase the psychological and emotional sequelae of an accident, because the individual experiences increasing anxiety and concern about why he or she feels different and is experiencing increased difficulty in everyday activities. Increasing attention to this issue has clearly lowered the threshold for diagnosing TBI.

Given this, is there a danger of overdiagnosing TBI, that is, either diagnosing a TBI when none actually occurred or attributing cognitive weaknesses to a TBI when they may be due to something else? Disregarding the interests of the attorneys, this seems to be an issue worth our attention. Certainly, diagnosing brain dysfunction (possibly interpreted by the patient as brain "damage") is not innocuous, particularly if an individual is experiencing psychological distress (e.g., anxiety, depression). Further, prescribing treatment which may be time-consuming and expensive, and may continually remind the patient of his or her dysfunction may result in the patient's focusing too much on these weaknesses or thinking that he or she is "brain damaged" or even "disabled" (Alexander, 1995).

These consequences highlight the importance of being as thorough, careful, and accurate as possible in diagnosing neuropsychological problems, of recognizing our limitations in knowledge when appropriate, and of accepting the responsibility of explaining our opinions in ways that are least likely to cause further harm. Some of these issues are highlighted in the next section.

False-Positive and False-Negative Diagnostic Issues in Mild TBI

Because neuropsychological measures are so sensitive to cognitive dysfunction, some interpretive caveats must be kept in mind. To ignore any of the following questions (see Table 3.2) might at best result in faulty explanations and impressions.

These are only some examples of the questions that must be considered in evaluating the possibility of making false-positive and false-negative errors in neuropsychological interpretation. Far too often, however, some of these questions are neglected in practice. For example, serious errors can be made

Table 3.2

Key Questions To Be Addressed in the Neuropsychological Evaluation of Mild TBI

1. What likely happened to the brain of the patient in question? Is there evidence to suggest the likelihood of a brain injury in the first place, given the nature of the incident?
2. Do the reported symptoms make sense relative to the mild TBI literature?
3. Do the test results "fit" commonly reported TBI sequelae, and are they consistent within and across measures?
4. Are the observed test scores consistent with the reported nature of the injury?
5. Are the patient's complaints at all consistent with test results?
6. Are the complaints consistent with the patient's everyday functioning? Are test results consistent with current functional activities and performance?
7. In the case of test–retest situations, are the data consistent across evaluations, and does the overall profile make neuropsychological sense?
8. What other factors, aside from the TBI incident in question or specific PCS, might provide competing explanations for the observed findings and complaints?

when there is an overreliance on test scores, or an underreliance on test scores and overreliance on patient complaints. To take one extreme example, severe cognitive impairment would not be expected as a result of a single, uncomplicated, mild TBI. If test results were consistent with severe brain damage in an absolute sense, such an interpretive conclusion would be tenuous at best. In such a case, other factors (e.g., other neurocognitive causes, motivation during testing, fatigue, pain, psychological state, and/or malingering) would have to be seriously considered, lest a potentially serious false-positive error be made. Similarly, the overinterpretation of symptom complaints in the face of normal neuropsychological and other neurodiagnostic results must be done with due caution and with additional supporting information. As noted, mild TBI and PCS often present complex neurodiagnostic challenges, and neuropsychology is well positioned to continue its contributions to this charge (see Table 3.3).

Conclusions

We have attempted to identify and discuss some of the major issues in diagnosing mild TBI and the assessment of neuropsychological sequelae. These include utilizing information about likely biomechanical forces involved; consideration of base rate issues regarding both self-report and test performance; and consideration of the patient's report of the accident and subsequent symptoms, including the nature of reported symptoms, the timing of symptom onset in relation to the purported TBI, and the course of symptoms. It is also important to review other available information concerning

Table 3.3

Challenges to Neuropsychological Research on Mild TBI

1. Development of tools with greater sensitivity to subtle effects of mild TBI, keeping in mind that subtle neuropsychological impairment may have many causes
2. Development of alternative test forms and large-scale norms for more measures across ages
3. Standardization of brief cognitive screening batteries for use in sports concussion situations (e.g., see Lovell & Collins, 1998)
4. Enhanced appreciation for cross-cultural issues and appropriate test norms
5. Development of appropriate information to be routinely given to patients with mild TBI

the accident and symptoms, such as accident reports, ambulance and emergency room notes, accident witness reports, and initial physician contact notes. Information about patient functioning before and after the accident, such as reports from family and/or friends, school and job records, and previous medical records, are also useful. Accident photographs and/or information about the extent of damage to the vehicles may also provide useful information about the likely forces involved in motor vehicle accidents. The thorough examination of such information in conjunction with the neuropsychological examination provides important background data that can be used in evaluating the likelihood of TBI, the consistency of complaints with known TBI sequelae, the likelihood of a decline from presumed preinjury levels, and, importantly, the role of other factors in explaining ongoing symptoms. Clearly, mild TBI represents a complex, multifactorial issue that continues to pose many challenges for neuropsychological investigation. However, progress continues to be made, and the emerging sports-neuropsychology area may prove to be an important source of information on neuropsychological recovery following mild TBI.

References

Alexander, M. (1995). Mild traumatic brain injury: Pathophysiology, natural history, and clinical management. *Neurology, 45,* 1253–1260.

Alves, W. M., Macciocchi, S. N., & Barth, J. T. (1993). Postconcussive symptoms after uncomplicated mild head injury. *Journal of Head Trauma Rehabilitation, 8,* 48–59.

Barth, J. T., Alves, W. M., Ryan, T. V., Macciocchi, S. N, Rimel, R. W., Jane, J. A., & Nelson, W. E. (1989). Mild head injury in sports: Neuropsychological sequelae and recovery of function. In H. S. Levin, H. M. Eisenberg, & A. L. Benton (Eds.), *Mild head injury* (pp. 257–275). New York: Oxford Press.

Barth, J. T., Macciocchi, S., & Giordani, B. (1983). Neuropsychological sequelae of minor head injury. *Neurosurgery, 13,* 529–537.

Bigler, E. D., & Snyder, J. L. (1995). Neuropsychological outcome and quantitative neuroimaging in mild head injury. *Archives of Clinical Neuropsychology, 10,* 159–174.

Binder, L. M. (1986). Persisting symptoms after mild head injury: A review of the postconcussive syndrome. *Journal of Clinical and Experimental Neuropsychology, 8,* 323–346.

Bohnen, N., & Jolles, J. (1992). Neurobehavioral aspects of postconcussive symptoms after mild head injury. *Journal of Nervous and Mental Disease, 180,* 683–692.

Bohnen, N., Jolles, J., & Verhey, F. R. (1993). Persistent neuropsychological deficits in cervical whiplash patients without direct headstrike. *Acta Neurologica Belgica, 93,* 23–31.

Bohnen, N., Twijnstra, A., & Jolles, J. (1993). Persistence of postconcussional symptoms in uncomplicated, mildly head-injured patients: A prospective cohort study. *Neuropsychiatry, Neuropsychology & Behavioral Neurology, 6,* 193–200.

Cullum, C. M., Heaton, R. K., & Grant, I. (1991). Psychogenic factors influencing neuropsychological performance: Somatoform disorders, factitious disorders and malingering. In H. O. Doerr & A. Carlin (Eds.), *Forensic Neuropsychology* (pp. 141–171). New York: Guilford Press.

Dacey, R. G., Alves, W. M., Rimel, R. W., Winn, H. R., & Jane, J. A. (1986). Neurosurgical complications after apparently minor head injury: Assessment of risk in a series of 610 patients. *Journal of Neurosurgery, 65,* 203–210.

Dikmen, S., & Levin, H. S. (1993). Methodological issues in the study of mild head injury. *Journal of Head Trauma Rehabilitation, 8,* 30–37.

Dikmen, S., & Machamer, J. E. (1995). Neurobehavioral outcomes and their determinants. *Journal of Head Trauma Rehabilitation, 10,* 74–86.

Dikmen, S., Machamer, J. E., Winn, H. R., & Temkin, N. R. (1995). Neuropsychological outcome at 1-year post head injury. *Neuropsychology, 9,* 80–90.

Dikmen, S., McLean, A., & Temkin, N. (1986). Neuropsychological and psychosocial consequences of minor head injury. *Journal of Neurology, Neurosurgery, and Psychiatry, 49,* 1227–1232.

Dikmen, S., Temkin, N., & Armsden, G. (1989). Neuropsychological recovery: Relationship to psychosocial functioning and postconcussional complaints. In H. S. Levin, H. M. Eisenberg, & A. L. Benton (Eds.), *Mild head injury* (pp. 229–241). New York: Oxford Press.

Di Stefano, G., & Radanov, B. P. (1995). Course of attention and memory after common whiplash: A two-years prospective study with age, education and gender pair-matched patients. *Acta Neurologica Scandinavica, 91,* 346–352.

Ettlin, T. M., Kischka, U., Reichmann, S., Radii, E. W., Heim, S., Wengen, D., & Benson, D. F. (1992). Cerebral symptoms after whiplash injury of the neck: A prospective clinical and neuropsychological study of whiplash injury. *Journal of Neurology, Neurosurgery, and Psychiatry, 55,* 943–948.

Fox, D. D., Lees-Haley, P. R., Earnest, K., & Dolezal-Wood, S. (1995). Post-concussive symptoms: Base rates and etiology in psychiatric patients. *The Clinical Neuropsychologist, 9,* 89–92.

Gennarelli, T. A. (1986). Mechanisms and pathophysiology of cerebral concussion. *Journal of Head Trauma Rehabilitation, 1,* 23–30.

Gennarelli, T. A., Thibault, L. B., Adams, J. H., Graham, D. I., Thompson, C. J., & Marcincin, R. P. (1982). Diffuse axonal injury and traumatic coma in the primate. *Annals of Neurology, 12,* 564–574.

Gouvier, W. D., Uddo-Crane, M., & Brown, L. M. (1988). Base rates of post-concussional symptoms. *Archives of Clinical Neuropsychology, 3,* 273–278.

Gronwall, D. (1987). Advances in the assessment of attention and information processing after head injury. In H. S. Levin, J. Grafman, & H. M. Eisenberg (Eds.), *Neurobehavioral recovery from head injury* (pp. 355–371). New York: Oxford Press.

Gronwall, D., & Wrightson, P. (1980). Duration of post-traumatic amnesia after mild head injury. *Journal of Clinical Neuropsychology, 2,* 51–60.

Hall, D. F., & Loftus, E. F. (1984). The fate of memory: Discoverable or doomed? In L. R. Squire & N. Butters (Eds.), *Neuropsychology of Memory* (pp. 25–32). New York: Guilford Press.

Heaton, R. K., Grant, I., & Matthews, C. G. (1991). *Comprehensive norms for an expanded Halstead-Reitan battery.* Odessa, FL: Psychological Assessment Resources, Inc.

Hilton, D. L., Einhaus, S. L., Meric, A. L., White, R. P., Schweitzer, J. B., Park, M. R., & Robertson, J. T. (1993). Early assessment of neurologic deficits in the fluid percussion model of brain injury. *Journal of Neurotrauma, 10,* 121–133.

Hinton-Bayre, A. D., Geffen, G., & McFarland, K. (1997). Mild head injury and speed of information processing: A prospective study of professional rugby league players. *Journal of Clinical & Experimental Neuropsychology, 19*(2), 275–289.

Hirsch, A. E., Ommaya, A. K., & Mahone, R. H. (1970). Tolerance of subhuman primate brain to cerebral concussion. In E. S. Gurdjian, W. A. Lange, L. M. Patrick, & L. M. Thomas (Eds.), *Impact injury and crash protection* (pp. 352–371). Springfield, IL: Charles C. Thomas.

Jacobson, R. R. (1995). The post-concussional syndrome: Physiogenesis, psychogenesis and malingering. An integrative model. *Journal of Psychosomatic Research, 39,* 675–693.

Kay, T., Newman, B., Cavallo, M., Ezrachi, O., & Resnick, M. (1992). Toward a neuropsychological model of functional disability after mild traumatic brain injury. *Neuropsychology, 6,* 371–384.

Kelly, J. P., Nichols, J. S., Filley, C. M., Lillehei, K., Rubinstein, D., & Kleinschmidt-DeMasters, B. K. (1991). Concussion in sports. *Journal of The American Medical Association, 266,* 2867–2869.

Leininger, B. E., Gramling, S. E., Farrell, A. D., Kreutzer, J. S., & Peck, E. A. (1990). Neuropsychological deficits in symptomatic minor head injury patients after concussion and mild concussion. *Journal of Neurology, Neurosurgery, and Psychiatry, 53,* 293–296.

Levin, H. S., Eisenberg, H. M., & Benton, A. L. (Eds.). (1989). *Mild head injury.* New York: Oxford Press.

Levin, H. S., Mattis, S., Ruff, R. M., Eisenberg, H. M., Marshall, L. F., Tabaddor, K., High, W. M., & Frankowski, R. F. (1987). Neurobehavioral outcome following minor head injury: A three-center study. *Journal of Neurosurgery, 66,* 234–243.

Levin, H. S., O'Donnell, V. M., & Grossman, R. G. (1979). The Galveston Orientation and Amnesia Test. A practical scale to assess cognition after head injury. *Journal of Nervous and Mental Disease, 167,* 675–684.

Levin, H. S., Williams, D. H., Eisenberg, H. M., High, W. M., & Guinto, F. C. (1992). Serial MRI and neurobehavioral findings after mild to moderate closed head injury. *Journal of Neurology, Neurosurgery, and Psychiatry, 55,* 255–262.

Loftus, E. F. (1979). *Eyewitness testimony.* Cambridge, MA: Harvard University Press.

Loftus, E. F., Miller, D. G., & Burns, H. J. (1978). Semantic integration of verbal information into visual memory. *Journal of Experimental Psychology: Human Learning and Memory, 4,* 19–31.

Lovell, M. R., & Collins, M. W. (1998). Neuropsychological assessment of the college football player. *Journal of Head Trauma Rehabilitation, 13,* 9–26.

McCaffrey, R. J., Ortega, A., & Haase, R. F. (1993). Effects of repeated neuropsychological assessments. *Archives of Clinical Neuropsychology, 8,* 519–524.

McCrea, M., Kelly, J. P., Kluge, J., Ackley, B., & Randolph, C. (1997). Standardized assessment of concussion in football players. *Neurology, 48,* 586–588.

Melvin, J. W., Lighthall, J. W., & Ueno, K. (1993). Brain injury biomechanics. In A. M. Nahum & J. W. Melvin (Eds.), *Accidental injury: Biomechanics and prevention* (pp. 268–291). New York: Springer-Verlag.

Mild Traumatic Brain Injury Committee of the Head Injury Interdisciplinary Special Interest Group of the American Congress of Rehabilitation Medicine (1993). Definition of mild traumatic brain injury. *Journal of Head Trauma Rehabilitation, 8,* 86–87.

Mittenberg, W., DiGiulio, D. V., Perrin, S., & Bass, A. E. (1992). Symptoms following mild head injury: Expectation as etiology. *Journal of Neurology, Neurosurgery, and Psychiatry, 55,* 200–204.

Mittenberg, W., Tremont, G., Zielinski, R. E., Fichera, S., & Rayls, K. R. (1996). Cognitive-behavioral prevention of post concussion syndrome. *Archives of Clinical Neuropsychology, 11,* 139–145.

Naugle, R. I. (1991). Epidemiology of traumatic brain injury in adults. In E. D. Bigler (Ed.), *Traumatic brain injury: Mechanisms of damage, assessment, intervention, and outcome* (pp. 69–103). Austin, TX: PRO-ED.

Ommaya, A. K., & Gennarelli, T. A. (1974). Cerebral concussion and traumatic unconsciousness: Correlation of experimental and clinical observations on blunt head injuries. *Brain, 97,* 633–654.

Pennington, B. F. (1991). *Diagnosing learning disorders.* New York: Guilford Press.

Radanov, B. P., Di Stefano, G., Schnidrig, A., Sturzenegger, M., & Augustiny, K. F. (1993). Cognitive functioning after common whiplash. A controlled follow-up study. *Archives of Neurology, 50,* 87–91.

Reitan, R. M., & Wolfson, D. (1997). Consistency of neuropsychological test scores of head-injured subjects involved in litigation compared with head-injured subjects not involved in litigation: Development of the retest consistency index. *The Clinical Neuropsychologist, 11,* 69–76.

Report of the Quality Standards Subcommittee of the American Academy of Neurology. (1997). Practice parameter: The management of concussion in sports. *Neurology, 48,* 581–585.

Rimel, R. W., Giordani, B., & Barth, J. T. (1981). Disability caused by minor head injury. *Neurosurgery, 9,* 221–228.

Rourke, B. P. (1982). Central processing deficiencies in children: Toward a developmental neuropsychological model. *Journal of Clinical Neuropsychology, 4,* 1–18.

Ruff, R. M., Wylie, T., & Tennant, W. (1993). Malingering and malingering-like aspects of mild closed head injury. *Journal of Head Trauma Rehabilitation, 8,* 60–73.

Rutherford, W. H., Merrett, J. D., & McDonald, J. R. (1979). Symptoms at one year following concussion from minor head injuries. *Injury, 10,* 225–230.

Stuss, D. T. (1995). A sensible approach to mild traumatic brain injury. *Neurology, 45,* 1251–1252.

Sweeney, J. E. (1992). Nonimpact brain injury: Grounds for clinical study of the neuropsychological effects of acceleration forces. *The Clinical Neuropsychologist, 6,* 443–457.

Wells, G. L., & Loftus, E. F. (1984). *Eyewitness testimony: Psychological perspectives.* Cambridge, MA: Cambridge University Press.

Whinnery, J. E., & Whinnery, A. M. (1990). Acceleration-induced loss of consciousness. *Archives of Neurology, 47,* 764–776.

Yarnell, P. R., & Rossie, G. V. (1988). Minor whiplash injury with major debilitation. *Brain Injury, 2,* 255–258.

Youngjohn, J. R., Burrows, L., & Erdal, K. (1995). Brain damage or compensation neurosis? The controversial post-concussional syndrome. *The Clinical Neuropsychologist, 9,* 112–123.

The Influence of Age and Education on Neuropsychological Performances of Persons with Mild Traumatic Brain Injuries

4

Ralph M. Reitan
and Deborah Wolfson

The principal thrust of this chapter, and the report of original research, is the relationships of age and education to neuropsychological test scores of persons with mild head injuries. However, recent studies have reported that the effects of these variables differ strikingly in various diagnostic groups, with normals generally showing strong effects (particularly regarding education), and groups with disorders that affect brain status and function (and thus relevant to neuropsychological test scores) showing minimal, or at least reduced effects. Thus, it is important that findings on the significance of age and education be presented in the context of the more general picture. The first part of this chapter presents a general overview, describing the complex and differential significance of age and education for a number of psychological tests, for both adults and children, and for groups ranging from normals to persons with brain damage and persons with learning disabilities.

In addition, mild head injury is discussed in the context of brain impairment in general because mild brain injury does not represent a separate category, but must be considered in the context of TBI as a whole. Alves and Jane (1985) said that "mild brain injury does not form a distinct class of injury, but rather represents the end point of a continuum ranging from the most mild concussive blow to impacts which cause sudden death" (p. 255). Reitan and Wolfson (in press f) have shown that the pattern of deficits in mild and more severe brain trauma is remarkably similar, even though deficits are more pronounced in the groups with severe injuries. Finally, Williams, Levin, and Eisenberg (1990) and Reitan and Wolfson (in press f) have presented definitive evidence that mild and more severe head injuries

---

Reprinted, with changes, from "The Influence of Age and Education on Neuropsychological Performances of Persons with Mild Head Injuries," by Ralph M. Reitan and Deborah Wolfson, 1997, *Applied Neuropsychology, 4*(1), pp. 16–33. Copyright 1997 by Lawrence Erlbaum Associates, Inc.

overlap in that persons who appear initially to have very mild head injuries in some cases develop much more serious brain damage. We will therefore begin with a general review.

Interest in the effects of age and education on neuropsychological test scores of persons with brain damage has increased sharply with the realization that the effects of these variables might be diminished or even deleted when neuropsychological test scores reflect the consequences of brain damage rather than normal development. When brain damage is present, does it exert such a strong influence on neuropsychological test scores that variance normally associated with age and education is overruled? Recent research suggests that this is essentially what happens when using tests that are especially sensitive to the biological condition of the brain (Reitan & Wolfson, 1995b). In addition, even determinations of intelligence quotients and scaled subtest scores using the *Wechsler Adult Intelligence Scale* (WAIS) appear to have differing degrees of dependence on age and education among normals and persons with brain damage (Reitan & Wolfson, in press, c, g). The same differences that are found with adults also appear to hold for children, both on neuropsychological tests (Reitan & Wolfson, in press e) and on the *Wechsler Intelligence Scale for Children–Revised* (WISC–R) (Reitan & Wolfson, in press b). Considering the value our society places on education, it may be particularly significant that brain damage deletes or diminishes the significance of education.

Evidence that brain damage had such a consistent effect of delimiting the normally expected effects of age and education on psychological test scores stimulated special interest regarding children with learning disabilities. This group was particularly relevant in attempts to sort out the effects of frank neurological involvement (as seen in children with diagnosed brain damage) as compared with very subtle and largely unknown brain impairment (seen in children with learning disabilities). In fact, the results of conventional neurological diagnostic procedures are generally similar for normal children and children with learning disabilities (Gaddes & Edgell, 1994). Conversely, children with learning disabilities often demonstrate neuropsychological test results that are somewhat similar to those of children with diagnosed brain lesions (Reitan & Wolfson, 1992; Rourke, 1985). Thus, the questions are these: Do children with learning disabilities have age and education effects that are similar to normal children, considering that both groups have essentially normal brains in terms of the neurological examination? Or, do children with learning disabilities show diminished or deleted age and education effects, as appears to be true for children with brain damage, reflecting the similar types (if not degree) of neuropsychological deficits shown by both groups?

Investigation of these questions (Reitan & Wolfson, in press a, d) yielded a rather clear answer: Children ages 9 through 14 with learning disabilities demonstrated minimal relationships between age and education and raw scores on either neuropsychological tests or conventional measures of intelligence. In fact, the results raised the question of whether Wechsler IQ values could be determined accurately for either children with learning disabilities or brain damage, considering that the procedure for computing IQ is based on the relationship between age and raw scores for normal children, and the relationship was diminished or non-existent for children with learning disabilities or brain damage.

Prior studies with adults with brain damage have used subjects with definitive neurological diagnoses and unequivocal evidence of brain damage. Age and education effects are diminished among such subjects, and the effects of brain damage predominate in influencing test scores, but what are the findings in cases of mild head injury?

It seems reasonable that several factors may be influential in this situation. One set of factors concerns the differential sensitivity to brain damage of selected neuropsychological tests, as compared with education. The *General Neuropsychological Deficit Scale* (GNDS) is extremely sensitive to brain damage, so the effects of brain damage should be seen when this measure is used. The Vocabulary subtest of the Wechsler scales seems to be very sensitive to education and relatively resistant to brain damage. Considering psychological tests more generally, they might form a continuum regarding the extent to which age and education effects are disrupted by brain damage. Another set of factors would be related to the severity (and perhaps the type and location) of brain damage, the stage of the brain damage (chronic versus acute), and other indicators of the extent to which normal brain functions were disrupted. One might postulate that the greater the biological disruption of the brain, the less the effect of age and education on test results, especially if a brain-sensitive measure were used.

It is apparent that the overall circumstances are potentially quite complex, and that extensive studies will be needed to fully clarify the relationships. It is plausible, however, that if a condition limits normal brain functions, the relationships between age and education and neuropsychological measures will be diminished.

Brief Literature Review

There have been a number of studies concerning the influence of age and education in neuropsychology, but most of the information in this area has been derived from the many investigations in the fields of education and gerontology. These studies have given rise to a great respect for the significance, value, and effects of education, and have also contributed to a more complete understanding of the many psychological factors, including both strengths and weaknesses, that are associated with aging. Our present concern, however, focuses on the significance of these variables in clinical neuropsychology.

Tupper and Rosenblood (1984) reviewed many of the conceptual and statistical considerations. The presumed effect of age and education is so strong that it is routine in neuropsychological research to control their influence. For example, if a group of persons with brain damage and a group of persons without brain damage differed in age and education, it might be presumed that differences in neuropsychological test scores were due to these age and education differences rather than to brain damage. A standard requirement for published research, therefore, is that age and educational levels be controlled either through equating groups on these variables or adjusting scores to account for differences.

Such practices continue in research studies, even though the literature of clinical neuropsychology strongly suggests that age and education have far less significance for neuropsychological test scores in groups with brain damage than in normal groups. A higher level of education among normals is associated with better performances, and, among normal elderly adults, a degree of deterioration may be expected on tests that measure certain functions. When brain damage is present, however, a person may perform poorly regardless of age or level of education.

Reitan (1955a) studied the influence of age on the *Impairment Index,* a summary measure that has been shown to be very sensitive to brain damage (Reitan, 1955b; Reitan & Wolfson, 1993). Two groups were used: one in which every subject had sustained brain damage and one in which there was no evidence of brain damage. The group with brain damage did not show any relationship between the *Impairment Index* and age. The subjects were impaired as a result of brain damage, regardless of whether they were young or old. In the group with normal neurological findings, however, there was a significant relationship between age and the *Impairment Index,* with a gradual deterioration in older subjects. In their study of persons with brain damage, Vega and Parsons (1967) found no relationship between age and education and results on the *Halstead-Reitan Battery.* Prigatano and Parsons (1976) published similar negative findings for a psychiatric sample. These results suggest that the influence of age and education on neuropsychological test scores is much weaker among subjects with brain damage than among those without brain damage.

Finlayson, Johnson, and Reitan (1977) demonstrated that the educational level of persons without brain damage had a striking effect on Wechsler scale scores, but less influence on tests that are more sensitive to brain damage. In fact, all of the tests influenced by education had auditory–verbal and language requirements in common, were based on stored information, and appeared to have a minimal dependence on immediate problem-solving skills.

Conversely, studies of normal subjects, even with the same tests, reveal a strong effect of age and education. Long and Klein (1990) reported significant relationships in a group that had no evidence of neurological disorders. Heaton, Grant, and Matthews (1991), studying neurologically normal subjects, found that it was advisable to adjust scores for age and education in order to deal clinically with their effects, and published extensive tables for this purpose. Although such adjustments may be justified and potentially valuable for normal subjects, they would not be appropriate for any group (including persons with brain damage) in which age and education had no meaningful relationship.

The relationship of age and education to neuropsychological test scores is obviously an important issue, both theoretically and clinically.

Recent Studies

Age and Education as Related to Neuropsychological Status

Reitan and Wolfson (1995) investigated the influence of age and education on the GNDS, a summary measure of the neuropsychological competence of the individual. This study employed essentially the same design as the studies of mild head injury to be presented later in this chapter.

The GNDS, which is based on 42 variables from the *Halstead-Reitan Battery,* was selected as a measure of general neuropsychological adequacy because it meets several important criteria. The GNDS

1. is a comprehensive score that summarizes the results of the *Halstead-Reitan Battery;*
2. demonstrates equivalent impairment in groups with generalized, left, and right cerebral damage, thus showing broad and approximately equivalent sensitivity to brain damage across the full range of cerebral involvement;
3. is based on neuropsychological tests developed through examinations of persons with documented brain lesions of various types, locations, durations, and etiologies (i.e., a range a diversified neurological conditions);
4. differentiates between control subjects and subjects with brain damage at highly significant levels in categories of cerebrovascular disease and TBI as well as in heterogenous brain damage;
5. shows no significant gender differences; and
6. has been cross-validated regarding its sensitivity to brain damage.

Research supporting these characteristics of the GNDS are reported in Reitan and Wolfson (1988), Sherer and Adams (1993), and Wolfson and Reitan (1995).

The subjects in this study were 50 control subjects without brain damage (20 males, 30 females) and 50 subjects with brain damage (20 males, 30 females). The groups were matched for mean age and education. The brain-damaged group had a mean age of 36.64 years (SD = 14.83) and a mean education of 12.86 years (SD = 3.37). The control group had a mean age of 36.36 years (SD = 12.71) and a mean education of 12.78 years (SD = 2.28). All subjects were right-handed except for 3 subjects with brain damage and 5 control subjects.

Each potential control subject was examined neurologically, and only subjects who had no past or present evidence of brain disease or damage met the inclusion criteria for the control group. Except for 7 normally functioning subjects, individuals were selected who were hospitalized, anticipating surgery, and experiencing the stress and anxieties that often accompany a significant illness, recognizing that many subjects with brain damage have similar stresses.

Thirty-five of the control subjects were examined neuropsychologically while awaiting surgery for nonneurological disorders. The remaining 15 subjects included 8 hospitalized individuals (acute anxiety reactions, 4; depression, 1; herniated spinal disc, 1; Grave's disease, 1; labyrinthine dysfunction, 1) and 7 normally functioning individuals.

The brain-damaged group represented a diversity of types and locations of cerebral disease or damage: 12 subjects with tumors (left hemisphere, 4; right hemisphere, 4; metastatic, 4), 12 subjects with vascular lesions (left hemisphere, 4; right hemisphere, 4; generalized, 4), 12 subjects with traumatic injuries (left hemisphere, 4; right hemisphere, 4; generalized, 4), and 14 subjects with nonfocal involvement (multiple sclerosis, 3; encephalitis, 2; major motor epilepsy, 2; complex partial epilepsy, 2; cerebral palsy, 1; carbon monoxide poisoning, 1; parasagittal frontal meningioma, 1; HIV and AIDS complex, 1; tuberculous meningitis, 1). There were 20 subjects with focal lesions (left hemisphere, 10; right hemisphere, 10), 8 subjects with lateralized vascular lesions (left hemisphere, 4; right hemisphere, 4), and 22 subjects with diffuse involvement.

Pearson product-moment coefficients of correlation were computed between GNDS scores and age and education, and for subcategories of the brain-damaged and control groups subdivided at the median age and education level. Mean GNDS scores for the upper 50% and lower 50% of each distribution were compared to identify any differential effects of age and education. The brain-damaged group was subdivided by a median age of 35.50 years and a median education of 12.75 years. The control group was subdivided by a median age of 35.50 years and a median education of 13.21 years. We present these values to make it clear that the samples in this study were not sufficiently large or diversified to generalize to all cases of clinical interest.

The GNDS means were consistently much poorer (higher) for the brain-damaged group than for the control group, confirming the sensitivity of the GNDS to brain damage (Reitan & Wolfson, 1988; Wolfson & Reitan, 1995).

There were large differences (all exceeding a p of .001) between the two groups, regardless of whether the upper or lower part of the age or education distribution was considered.

Comparisons among the control group showed that the younger control subjects had significantly better GNDS scores than did the older control subjects, and those with more education performed better than did those with less education, both at significance levels exceeding .001. This finding was expected, considering the Heaton et al. (1991) norms, the findings of Long and Klein (1990), and other reports cited previously. The subjects with brain damage, however, did not demonstrate significant differences. Older subjects with brain damage actually had better mean scores than did the younger subjects with brain damage, but the difference was not significant ($p < .10$). Education had essentially no effect: the mean scores for groups with more and less education were similar ($p < .80$).

The relationships between age and education in the brain-damaged and control groups were also demonstrated by comparing coefficients of correlation. Both age and education correlated significantly with GNDS scores for the control group, as expected from the research cited previously. However, the brain-damaged group did not show significant relationships with age, and the coefficient of –.27 between education and GNDS score barely reached a significance level of .05.

In summary, the results indicated that age and education had a significant effect on the GNDS scores of control subjects. However, age and education had relatively little effect on the GNDS scores of subjects with brain damage, either in level of performance or relationships between variables. The diminished significance of age and education among subjects with brain damage indicates that neuropsychological interpretation should depend on tests that are definite indicators of brain damage or impairment, rather than on scores adjusted for attribute variables. When significant brain damage occurs, neither youth nor higher education seems to protect the individual from neuropsychological impairment. Therefore, it seems that the logical course in clinical evaluation would be to first determine whether brain damage is present. Then, if brain damage is not present, one should consider the subject's age and education to gain a complete understanding of the test scores. Identifying the effects of brain damage as shown by neuropsychological test scores requires evaluating findings beyond the subject's level of performance (Reitan, 1967; Reitan & Wolfson, 1993). If brain damage is strong enough to essentially obliterate the effects of age and education on neuropsychological test results, it seems reasonable to identify brain damage by focusing on these strong effects rather than relying on deviations from normal age and education expectancies.

As with any other single study, cross-validation of these results is required. Further work also needs to be done to extend the age and education samples, to evaluate subgroups of subjects with brain damage, and more, as pointed out in the original report.

Age and Education as Related to Verbal IQ, Performance IQ, and Full Scale IQ

Although the results reported above were obtained with the GNDS, a range of tests are generally used in clinical neuropsychological assessment, including tests that are especially sensitive to the biological condition of the brain, and other tests that may be more dependent upon variables such as age and education. For example, many studies have shown that measures of general intelligence often yield an intelligence quotient that is significantly related to educational level (Kaufman, 1990), and tables for determining IQ values often make adjustments according to age (Wechsler, 1955). How do IQ measures relate to age and education among persons with and without brain damage? Considering the evidence that years of education may be related more closely to Verbal IQ (VIQ) than to Performance IQ (PIQ) (Kaufman, 1990) and the evidence that PIQ is generally more sensitive to brain damage than is VIQ (Reitan, 1959), do VIQ and PIQ vary in their relationships to age and education? Considering that age adjustments are based solely on normative data from normal subjects, is there any justification for using the same method to compute the IQs of subjects with and without brain damage? To address these questions, Reitan and Wolfson (in press g) analyzed the WAIS results of subjects with and without brain damage. The WAIS was used instead of the WAIS–R because of the limited neuropsychological validity information on changes made in the WAIS–R (Reitan & Wolfson, 1990). Essentially the same brain-damaged and control groups were used as in the previous study, with 50 subjects per group.

This study supported a number of conclusions concerning the complex relationships between age and education and IQ variables among subjects with and without brain damage. The first point, reported previously, was that the control group performed significantly better than the brain-damaged group on VIQ, PIQ, and Full Scale IQ (FSIQ). Analyses based on subdivisions of each group at the median for age and education supported additional observations:

1. Subjects with more education consistently performed better on VIQ, PIQ, and FSIQ than did subjects with less education. However, this finding was much more consistent among control subjects than among subjects with brain damage, and was not statistically significant for PIQ in the brain-damaged group.
2. Older control subjects tended to perform better than younger control subjects, and this unexpected finding was even more pronounced and consistent among subjects with brain damage. The reason for this finding is unclear, but may reflect sampling problems in this study or possibly an overly generous age adjustment in the Wechsler norms.
3. Younger control subjects performed significantly better than younger subjects with brain damage. However, the older groups did not differ

significantly on any of the IQ variables, suggesting that among older subjects, variance may be influenced by factors other than diagnosed brain damage.

4. The correlations between education and each IQ distribution were significantly higher for the control group than for the brain-damaged group, although the correlations between age and IQ were not significantly higher for the brain-damaged group than for the control group. These findings again suggest that factors besides age and education (presumably, brain damage) are of increased influence among subjects with brain damage in determining IQ values.
5. These correlational trends were also found in the subgroups, although the brain-damaged subgroup with less education had no significant correlations with any of the IQ distributions. Because the brain-damaged subgroup with more education and the control subgroups with more and less education routinely had significant correlations between education and IQ levels, it appears that brain damage cancels the influence of education on IQ, unless a high level of education has been achieved. The younger subjects with brain damage also did not show significant correlations with the IQ variables.
6. Within the constraints imposed by T-score transformations for the combined groups, IQ values for the brain-damaged and control groups deviated significantly, and in opposite directions, with regard to both age and education.
7. Again, within the constraints of T-score transformations for the combined groups, predicted IQ means for the subjects with brain damage, based on relationships between age and education and IQ values for the control subjects, differed significantly from the actual IQ means in each case.
8. Correlations between predicted and actual IQ distributions for the brain-damaged group were statistically significant regardless of whether the predicted values were based on age or education. The predicted IQ distributions accounted for about 25% of the variance in the actual IQ distributions.

Certain significant similarities occurred in VIQ, PIQ, and FSIQ measurements for brain-damaged and control groups, but there were differences that caution against adjusting IQ values for subjects with brain damage based on normative data from normal subjects. Because many factors may influence the results of a single study, the findings of this study need to be replicated.

The results of this study should be considered with relation to the findings obtained when age and education were evaluated comparatively in control and brain-damaged groups using the GNDS. The control subjects showed significant relationships between age and education and the GNDS, in both correlation coefficients and comparison of the GNDS scores of the age and education subgroups. The brain-damaged group, however, had minimal effects of this type; the subgroup with more education had GNDS scores equivalent to those of the subgroup with less education. The brain-damaged group showed similar results for age. The effects of brain damage were dominant in determining the GNDS scores, essentially obliterating the significant age and education effects shown in the control group. Therefore, the practice of adjusting raw scores for brain-sensitive tests according to age and education appears to be invalid for subjects with brain damage, and might tend to invalidate the raw scores of neuropsychological tests. It should be noted, however, that the effects of brain damage on the GNDS should be evaluated more extensively in various categories of brain damage, including focal versus diffuse involvement, acute/progressive versus chronic/static damage, and so forth.

The somewhat mixed results of the IQ study, as compared with the results of the GNDS study, may well reflect the comparative sensitivity of the GNDS and Wechsler measures to brain damage. It might be implied that the effects of age and education are minimal when using tests that are especially sensitive to brain damage; when using tests that are less sensitive to brain damage, age and education effects may be increased. It appears that the overall relationships of age and education to psychological test scores are complex, and need much additional study.

The findings of this study should not be construed to delimit the validity of score comparisons between subjects with brain damage and any other appropriate reference group (normals, depressed persons, groups in age-restricted categories, groups that vary in socioeconomic status, etc.). Neither do the findings have implications for the use of demographic variables in predicting or estimating IQ values for normal subjects. The results should be interpreted in the frame of reference imposed by the study, namely that adjustments of the raw scores of subjects with brain damage, according to age and education relationships of normal subjects, may be in error to the extent that the age and education relationships differ for subjects with brain damage.

Age and Education as Related to WAIS Subtest Scores

An additional study by Reitan and Wolfson (in press c) evaluated the effects of age and education on each of the 11 subtests of the WAIS. Data analyses compared the influence of age and education (brain-damaged and control groups were subdivided at the median for each distribution) on WAIS subtest scores, and the correlations between these attribute values and each of the subtests.

Age appeared to have little significance in ordering the raw subtest scores. Among the older and younger brain-damaged subgroups, only Information, Arithmetic, and Vocabulary showed significant differences, and multiple individual tests were performed. There were no statistically significant differences between the older and younger control subgroups.

Among the control subjects, the subgroup with more education scored significantly better than the subgroup with less education on all subtests except Picture Completion and Object Assembly. Thus, it appears that education influences performance on a number of WAIS subtests. A rather different set of results, however, emerged in the brain-damaged group. Only 3 of the 11 subtests had statistically significant differences (Information and Comprehension at less than .05 and Vocabulary at less than .005). The remaining 8 subtests showed no significant differences between the two groups, suggesting that the effects of brain damage may mitigate the influence of education.

For the control group, none of the correlations between age and any of the subtests were significant. For the brain-damaged group, none of the Performance subtests correlated significantly with age. With the Verbal subtests, all of the correlation coefficients except Digit Span were significant in the brain-damaged group. In addition, among the subjects with brain damage, there were differences in the relationships between age and the Verbal subtests and age and the Performance subtests. Statistical comparisons of the magnitude of coefficients for age and each subtest revealed only two instances in which the control and brain-damaged groups differed significantly. Considering the differences in signs, the coefficients for age versus Similarities and age versus Digit Span were significantly higher, at probabilities of less than .05, for the brain-damaged group than for the control group.

Coefficients for education were generally larger than coefficients for age, although the brain-damaged group differed from the control group in having no significant correlations with the Performance subtests. The control group had significant correlations between education and every Performance subtest except Object Assembly. In comparing paired coefficients for the two groups, the coefficients were larger in every instance for the control group, and significantly larger for Similarities and Digit Symbol ($p < .05$).

In terms of general trends between the two groups, the brain-damaged group had a number of significant correlations between age and education and the Verbal subtests, but had no significant correlations between these variables and the Performance subtests. The overall differences in relationships for the Verbal and Performance subtests should also be noted. Considering the total number of coefficients for age plus education, 17 of 24 coefficients were significant for the Verbal subtests, whereas only 4 of 20 coefficients were significant for the Performance subtests.

The results reflected a general trend for correlations to be lower when subtests depended upon immediate problem-solving skills, and higher when subtests mainly represented stored information. To evaluate the trends quantitatively, we placed each test on a continuum from immediate problem-solving skills to stored information (with Block Design as number 1 and Information as number 11), then computed rank–difference correlations between the rank of each test on the continuum and the magnitude of each coefficient. These coefficients were quite high, especially for the brain-damaged group, and somewhat lower for education-related correlations for the control group. These results suggest that relationships between age and education and WAIS subtest scores differ systematically according to the requirements of the tests, further complicating the interpretation of the relationships between attribute variables and measures of intelligence.

In summary, the results indicate that in many ways the influence of age and education on WAIS subtests is significantly different for subjects with and without brain damage. Age did not significantly influence level of performance, but this may have been due to the age range of the subjects in the study. Higher and lower levels of education, however, had a strong effect on test scores in the control group and a lesser effect on scores in the brain-damaged group. The correlations between the attribute variables and the test scores also differed in the two groups. For the control group, there were no significant coefficients of correlation between age and subtest scores; for the brain-damaged group, the Verbal subtests were significantly correlated with age. Correlations between education and subtest scores were generally larger than the correlations between age and subtest scores, and the coefficients were larger for the control group than for the brain-damaged group. The most striking difference between the brain-damaged group and the control group was the significant correlations between education and four of the five Performance subtests among the controls. None of the corresponding coefficients were significant for the brain-damaged group.

As in our analysis of relationships of age and education to VIQ, PIQ, and FSIQ scores in subjects with and without brain damage (Reitan & Wolfson, in press g), the results were complex, and the findings were not as clear-cut as they were for the study with the GNDS (Reitan & Wolfson, 1995). In general, however, there was a tendency for WAIS subtests that are **more** sensitive to brain damage to be **less** affected by education, and subtests that are **less** sensitive to brain damage to be **more** affected by education.

Age and Education as Related to Psychological Test Scores in Children

We completed several studies on the differential effects of age and education in groups of children (normal control subjects, children with brain damage, and children with learning disabilities). As expected, age and education were significantly related to test scores among normal children, but had limited relationships among children with brain damage and learning disabilities.

First, we used children ages 9 through 14 to replicate the adult study on the influence of age and education on a neuropsychological summary score (Reitan and Wolfson, in press e). In this case we used the *Neuropsychological Deficit Scale for Older Children* (NDS) (Reitan & Wolfson, 1992). The results indicated that the older or more educated brain-damaged subgroups did not perform significantly better than the younger or less educated brain-damaged subgroups, and that there were no significant correlations between NDS scores and age and education. In the control group, however, age and education had a strong influence on test scores. These findings suggest that age and education norms developed for normal children should not be uncritically applied to children with brain damage.

We also studied the performances of older children on the WISC–R (Reitan & Wolfson, in press b). In practice, the WISC–R requires a mandatory age adjustment of raw scores to obtain the scaled scores on which IQ values are based, regardless of whether there is a condition that may diminish the relationship between age and level of performance. We evaluated the relationships between age and education and WISC–R raw and scaled scores. There were significant raw score relationships for the control group, but scarcely any effect for the brain-damaged group. In fact, there were no significant differences between the raw score performances of older and younger children with brain damage. Thus, adjusting raw scores for age is quite appropriate for normal children, but may not be justified for children with brain damage, and may lead to invalid IQ values for these children.

We also studied children with learning disabilities to determine whether they followed the pattern of the normal children or the children with brain damage (Reitan & Wolfson, in press a, d). We found no significant effects between age and education and NDS scores for the children with learning disabilities. In fact, the mean NDS scores of younger and older subgroups and more and less educated subgroups were not significantly different. Thus, the neuropsychological consequences of learning disabilities seem to override the effects of age and education in children ages 9 through 14, similar to what occurred with the children with brain damage.

These findings provide a basis for seriously questioning the mandatory scoring procedure of the WISC–R (and probably the WISC–III, as well), because an apparently unjustified adjustment, based solely on the results of normal children, is applied to the raw scores of children in whom age-related increments in performance do not exist. How many other tests may have this same problem? These results suggest that many other tests that make arbitrary adjustments of raw scores should also be investigated for the validity of their scoring procedures.

Age and Education Effects on Neuropsychological Performances in Mild Head Injury

Studies should also be extended to mild head injury. Mild head injury may be presumed to cause mild neuropsychological deficits, with relatively quick recovery; therefore, persons with mild head injury would probably perform more closely to normal control subjects than to subjects with brain damage. Obviously, however, the questions require empirical investigation. Our studies in this area are reported in this section. First, because the criteria for mild head injury varies, we will discuss the definition of mild head injury.

Definition of Mild Head Injury

Although there is some degree of consistency, few studies have used exactly the same criteria for defining mild head injury, and this has led to problems in making generalizations from research reports. Unless there is agreement on the definition of mild head injury, researchers and clinicians will be studying conditions that differ to a degree, and differences in results will be certain to occur and difficult to explain. Following are some of the definitions of mild head injury that have been used for research purposes and some that have been proposed for more general use. Variance and, in some cases, obvious inadequacies, make it quite clear that there is a significant problem concerning the definition of mild head injury, and further attention must be directed toward defining the condition to improve the prospects of meaningful communication.

If the criteria for a mild head injury included any bump or blow to the head, regardless of severity, most persons would be able to say that they have experienced a mild head injury. However, not everyone has experienced an injury to the brain, and even fewer people have sustained structural damage of the brain parenchyma, observable at surgery or with specialized diagnostic procedures. Some individuals have sustained a blow to the head that may have caused a loss of consciousness, posttraumatic amnesia (PTA), or a range of posttraumatic symptoms, even though there was no direct observation of brain tissue damage or unequivocal diagnostic evidence of brain damage. It is obviously difficult to differentiate between *head* injury and *brain* injury, particularly in mild cases. Even when there is no diagnostic evidence of brain tissue damage, there is a natural tendency to say the brain is injured based on symptoms following a blow to the head.

Alterations of consciousness often occur with a head blow, and are often presumed to reflect brain injury. Thus, many researchers have tried to correlate the duration of unconsciousness to the severity of brain damage. Jennett (1976, 1979) suggested the following classifications of brain injury:

Very Mild: loss of consciousness of less than 5 minutes
Mild: loss of consciousness of less than 1 hour
Moderate: loss of consciousness between 1 hour and 24 hours
Severe: loss of consciousness between 1 day and 7 days
Very Severe: loss of consciousness for more than 7 days
Extremely Severe: loss of consciousness for more than 4 weeks

Although loss of consciousness is undoubtedly related to severity of brain damage, the correlation is far from perfect (Reitan & Wolfson, 1986).

In addition, it is often quite difficult to determine the precise length of unconsciousness, considering the gradual and variable course of full recovery of consciousness.

PTA has been widely used as a measure of brain injury severity, and frequently is the criterion for comparative studies of head-injured groups. However, PTA, defined as the time between loss of consciousness and full recovery of continuing alertness and memory, is also extremely difficult to define precisely.

Some investigators have suggested that the Glasgow Coma Scale (GCS), which is based upon eye opening, motor response, and verbal response, provides a more refined method of evaluating level of consciousness. In addition, the GCS can be scored with a satisfactory degree of inter-rater reliability, even by observers who have been trained only briefly (Levin, Benton, & Grossman, 1982). Although there have been variations, a GCS score of 13 through 15 (on a scale of 3 to 15) represents a mild brain injury, and a score of 9 through 12 indicates a moderate brain injury.

Complications may occur following even a very mild brain injury, and sometimes these complications, such as intracranial bleeding and posttraumatic epilepsy, must be viewed as definite indications of brain pathology. In other cases, however, head injury is represented by only a broad range of subjective complaints. There is still debate about whether complaints such as dizziness, headache, and memory impairment are due to brain damage that has eluded definite identification, or to preinjury personality characteristics, psychiatric problems, pending litigation, or just a tendency to complain following an adverse advent (see Reitan & Wolfson, in press f, for a more detailed discussion). There is a need to identify reliable criteria for classifying mild brain injury (often referred to as mild head injury, despite the fact that there is an obvious difference between damage to the head and damage to the brain). Following are some of the criteria used by various investigators.

Dikmen, McLean, and Temkin (1986) studied the neuropsychological and psychosocial consequences of the condition they termed "minor head injury," admitting patients to their study based on

1. coma not exceeding 1 hour, or PTA of less than 1 hour;
2. GCS score of 12 or more on admission to the hospital;
3. no clinical evidence of cortical or brain stem contusion;
4. no prior history of traumatic brain injury, cerebral vascular disease, alcoholism, mental retardation, or significant psychiatric disorder; and
5. chronological age between 15 and 60 years.

These criteria represent both inclusionary and exclusionary conditions, and tend to identify subjects with relatively mild impairment (including the possibility of no impairment whatsoever), but would not necessarily exclude some individuals who would later manifest definite evidence of brain pathology such as posttraumatic epilepsy. It clearly is a difficult task to propose criteria that exclude persons who have sustained no brain injury and persons who have sustained injuries that will have relatively serious and continuing clinical consequences. Nevertheless, if degree of severity of brain injury is to be studied, some attempt must be made to identify the degree of severity; the criteria used by Dikmen et al. (1986) are objective and explicit, and can be met by other investigators.

It is interesting to review the definitions of mild or minor head injury in *Mild Head Injury,* edited by Levin, Eisenberg, and Benton (1989). Kraus and Nourjah (1989) reviewed four population-based studies of mild head injury, but warned that because of "vast differences" in study designs and definitions, conclusions based on these four studies must be "guarded." They pointed out that among the four studies, the criteria for defining mild head injury varied, selection processes appeared to differ, and other factors also were not constant. In one of these studies, Annegers, Grabow, Kurland, and Laws (1980) used criteria of loss of consciousness or PTA of less than 30 minutes and no evidence of a skull fracture. A second group of studies (Jagger, Levine, Jane, & Rimel, 1984; Rimel, 1981; Rimel, Giordani, Barth, Boll, & Jane, 1981) used criteria of hospital admission for at least overnight and a GCS score of 12 or greater. Kraus et al. (1984) used hospital admission and a GCS score of 13 or more as their criteria. Whitman, Coonley-Hoganson, and Desai (1984) used criteria of hospital admission and loss of consciousness of less than 30 minutes.

Using these somewhat variable criteria to select subjects raises a question about the comparability of research results, and justifies Jennett's (1989) comment that "a further problem is the lack of uniformity in the definitions (of mild head injuries) used in different reports" (p. 28).

For their study, Eisenberg and Levin (1989) defined mild and moderate head injuries as GCS scores of 9 through 15 when the subject was admitted to the hospital. Because a GCS score of 15 represents a perfectly normal performance, any subject who had sustained a head blow, even if it was very mild and there was no evidence implicating the brain, would be included if he or she was admitted to the hospital.

In reporting on attention and cognition in patients who had suffered concussion, Gronwall (1989) offered no criteria, either to define mild head injury or for selection of the subjects. In another study, Gentilini, Nichelli, and Schoenhuber (1989) included subjects who had lost consciousness for less than 20 minutes, had an initial GCS score of 13 through 15, were hospitalized less than 3 days, and had a negative neurological examination on admission and at discharge.

Ruff et al. (1989) reported the results of a three-center study. The inclusion criteria were loss of consciousness of 20 minutes or less (including no loss of consciousness), a GCS score of 13 through 15 upon admission and 15 at 48 hours after admission, no focal neurological deficits or evidence of a massive brain lesion, no hemiparesis or impaired movements, and an age between 15 and 50 years.

From a review of the criteria used by various investigators, it is apparent that there is no uniform definition of mild head injury. In fact, the majority of studies included in the volume edited by Levin et al. (1989) might well have selected subjects who had sustained a head blow but had no evidence of loss of consciousness, PTA, or other impairment (as presumed from perfectly normal results on the GCS). This would be consistent with the title of the book, *Mild Head Injury,* instead of a title that would imply investigation of mild brain injury. It is clear that the criteria for selecting subjects with mild head injury do not necessarily include any symptoms of brain injury. The criteria proposed for mild head injury raises the question of whether every person who has sustained any head blow, regardless of severity, would be presumed to sustain some degree of neuropsychological deficit.

Even casual information and personal experience suggest that mild head injuries are often followed by no continuing symptoms, complaints, or neuropsychological deficits. Over the last several years we have done informal surveys of attendees at our workshops in clinical neuropsychology. We find that at least 30%—and sometimes up to 50%—of the practicing psychologists in the audience respond that they have lost consciousness at least briefly from a blow to the head. If we include loss of consciousness due to anesthetic (although one would have to question whether any continuing deficits result from general anesthesia), the frequency is generally 50% or more. The number of psychologists who say they had no lasting effects whatsoever is essentially equivalent to the number of psychologists who meet the criteria for mild head injury.

One of the authors (RMR) was motivated to conduct this informal survey because of the contrast between the professional interest in mild head injury and his personal experiences with head injuries and loss of consciousness. This author has sustained multiple head blows over the years, with loss of consciousness on a few occasions. In one instance, following a series of head blows, he performed complex activities over several hours (including discussions with others, showering and changing clothes, using public transportation over fairly extended distances, etc.), but later had amnesia for these events.

Similar reports have been made by athletes who have sustained head injuries. For example, some baseball players report being struck in the head by the ball, then playing the rest of the game without error, although they later have no memory for the game. Although head injuries, including brain injuries, can certainly have lasting adverse consequences, it would appear that in some instances the brain can be insulted without long-term adverse consequences.

A formal definition of mild traumatic brain injury was offered by the Mild Traumatic Brain Injury Committee of the Head Injury Interdisciplinary

Special Interest Group of the American Congress of Rehabilitation Medicine (1993), with Thomas Kay, PhD as the senior contributor. According to this definition, a patient with mild traumatic brain injury is a person who has had a traumatically induced physiological disruption of brain function, as manifested by *at least* one of the following:

1. any period of loss of consciousness
2. any loss of memory for events immediately before or after the accident
3. any alteration in mental state at the time of the accident (e.g., feeling dazed, disoriented, or confused)
4. focal neurological deficit(s) that may or may not be transient; but where the severity of the injury does not exceed (a) loss of consciousness of approximately 30 minutes or less; (b) after 30 minutes, an initial GCS score of 13 through 15; and (c) PTA not greater than 24 hours

If individuals can suffer definite but temporary adverse effects of head blows without any residual complaints or deficits, and if up to 50% of practicing psychologists meet the criteria for the category of mild head injury (despite having no residual problems or complaints), one must wonder whether "mild head injury," in a clinical sense, is a legitimate classification. On the other hand, some people who experience a mild blow to the head do, in fact, have very real and continuing brain-related defects and problems (even though they may represent a minor fraction of the population).

It is apparent that mild head injury means different things to different people, and that many cases that initially appear quite mild do, in fact, result in permanent brain impairment. Until we develop more exacting methods for describing structural and functional pathology following mild head blows, it seems unlikely that it will be possible to identify criteria for mild head injury without including some persons with no brain injury at all and/or including some persons with significant and permanent cerebral dysfunction.

Research Findings

In our current investigation of the effects of age and education on neuropsychological performances of persons with mild head injuries (Reitan & Wolfson, in press f), we elected to use three groups for comparison:

1. a group of persons with significant head injuries and definite damage of the brain tissue, for reference regarding the effects of diagnosed and identified brain damage and for comparison with groups having mild head injury
2. a research group of persons with mild head injuries, included regardless of whether they had any clinical complaints

3. a group of persons with mild head injuries who initially seemed similar to the members of the research group, but who later had continuing symptoms and complaints that were severe enough that they sought additional medical attention

These groups will be described in more detail in the next section. None of the cases was involved in litigation.

Although references are frequently made to the fact that some persons who meet criteria for mild head injury do actually develop indications that their head injuries are more severe, most research studies are based on subjects who meet specified criteria and recover over a fairly short time. We know of no prior study specifically of subjects with mild head injuries who later return with significant problems, but these persons are obviously of clinical interest, in contrast to the majority of subjects with mild head injury, who recover without noticeable deficits or complaints. A report by Williams et al. (1990) made it quite clear that outcome is poorer in some cases of mild head injury than in others, especially when complications occur; they suggest a "revision of mild head injury classification." Our decision to compare two groups initially judged to have mild head injuries is based on research reports that patients who return with clinically significant complaints have, in fact, suffered more severe neuropsychological impairment than subjects routinely used in research studies.

It is generally presumed that consecutive cases who meet specified criteria for inclusion make a more representative, and perhaps less biased, sample than cases who are selected after the fact and for specific reasons. For our purposes, however, the differentiation stems from the fact that consecutive cases of mild head injury usually recover quite well with minimal, if any, residual deficits, whereas the "selected" cases represent individuals of clinical neuropsychological interest. Although such cases are included in research studies, their numbers are small and represent a small proportion of consecutive-case samples. Thus, a group composed of consecutive cases tends to greatly diminish, and effectively "wash out," the deficits shown by the cases of clinical interest.

Dikmen and Reitan (1976), Dikmen, Reitan, and Temkin (1983), and Reitan and Wolfson (1993) reported evidence of only mild impairment in subjects who had mild head injury and were tested shortly after the injuries were sustained. A number of researchers have studied patients at varying intervals following the mild head injury to identify recovery trends (Dikmen et al., 1986; Dikmen & Reitan, 1976; Gentilini et al., 1989; Gronwall, 1976, 1977, 1989; Gronwall & Sampson, 1974; Gronwall & Wrightson, 1974; McLean, Temkin, Dikmen, & Wyler, 1983; Ruff et al., 1989). The consensus is that a mild degree of impairment is present shortly after the injury, but that performance curves show no symptoms 1 to 3 months postinjury, and appear to represent essentially full recovery.

Because subjects who have no clinical problems or complaints are of limited interest clinically, one might be tempted to conclude from consecutive-case studies that mild head injury is of limited import. Recognizing that some patients with mild head injury do have significant clinical problems, we composed such a group for study (Reitan & Wolfson, in press f). As will be shown, this group (Group 3) demonstrated significantly more neuropsychological impairment than did the consecutive research cases (Group 2), and actually more closely resembled cases of definite brain damage (Group 1).

Group 1 included 14 males and 4 females who had a mean age of 31.22 years (*SD* = 13.09) and a mean education of 12.28 years (*SD* = 2.30). Of these 18 subjects, 16 had evidence of cerebral contusions, and 2 had penetrating head injuries. The contusions were limited to cerebral areas in 9 cases and were multiple and widespread in 7 cases. A penetrating missile injury caused brain tissue damage in two cases. Neurological examination revealed hemiparesis, hemiplegia, and dysphasia as the most common focal signs; 7 subjects had motor deficits, and 7 subjects had dysphasia. Eleven of the subjects showed evidence of focal signs; the remaining 7 subjects did not. None of these patients had seizures during the time of hospitalization. Fifteen of the subjects lost consciousness from the head blow, and the durations varied. Loss of consciousness ranged from less than 15 minutes for 2 subjects, to 1 to 5 hours for 6 subjects, 20 hours to 2 days for 2 subjects, 20 to 30 days for 3 subjects, 60 days for 1 subject, and 120 days for 1 subject. It is apparent that these subjects all sustained traumatic brain tissue damage and had relatively significant injuries.

To select subjects for Group 2, we applied the following criteria:

1. evidence of a physical blow to the head that caused at least a dazed or confused state for a minimum of 10 minutes
2. loss of consciousness for 25 minutes or less (if at all)
3. a GCS score of at least 13 at the time of hospital admission
4. normal neurological examination at the time of hospital admission
5. no prior history or evidence of brain disease or injury
6. a decision that the injury was sufficiently severe to require hospitalization for observation

Application of this last may vary among examiners, but it was included to ensure the availability of patients for extended evaluation.

Group 2 included 17 males and 1 female. The mean age was 27.44 years (*SD* = 11.98), and the mean education was 13.06 years (*SD* = 2.31). Of these 18 subjects, 17 had closed head injuries with a diagnosis of concussion. The remaining subject had a right frontal depressed skull fracture that was elevated surgically. The surgeon reported that the cerebral cortex underlying the minimally depressed bone appeared to be normal. Three subjects did not lose consciousness, and 5 subjects were unconscious for 2 minutes or less. Two subjects were unconscious for approximately 5 minutes, 2 for 10 minutes, 1 for 15 minutes, 4 for approximately 20 minutes, and 1 for 25 minutes. Thirteen subjects had at least a brief period of amnesia for events before or after the injury, with anterograde amnesia occurring in 7 cases, retrograde amnesia in 3 cases, and both in 3 cases. Defining PTA as the interval from the time of injury to consciousness with continuing memory for events in the environment, 3 subjects had no PTA, 3 subjects had no PTA beyond the period of loss of consciousness, 1 subject had PTA between 1 and 2 minutes, 4 subjects had PTA between 15 and 30 minutes, 5 subjects had PTA between 1 and 2 hours, and 2 subjects had PTA between 6 and 7 hours. None of these subjects had any evidence of focal signs, and none experienced a seizure during hospitalization. Subjects in Group 2 were all examined within 30 days following their head injuries.

Group 3 included 17 males and 3 females who had a mean age of 31.80 years (SD = 15.09) and a mean education of 11.35 years (SD = 3.51). These subjects initially appeared to have sustained relatively mild closed head injuries. For 7 of the 20 subjects there was no loss of consciousness. Among the remaining 13 subjects, 8 lost consciousness for less than 1 minute, 3 for less than 5 minutes, 1 for approximately 20 minutes, and 1 for approximately 25 minutes. These subjects were all examined in the emergency room, but only 11 were hospitalized. The remaining 9 subjects were judged not to require hospitalization. Although none of the 20 subjects was felt to have sustained serious brain damage, and definitive diagnostic tests were not considered necessary, each of these subjects returned to the hospital with various complaints. The principal complaints were as follows (some subjects had more than one): posttraumatic epilepsy, 5; memory loss, 6; mental slowing, 5; headaches, 4; emotional problems, 3; dizziness, 1; academic problems, 1; and pain, 1. These complaints all began after the head injury. Comprehensive neurological evaluations were performed at this time. The times between head injury and neuropsychological testing varied as follows: less than 1 month, 2 subjects; 1 to 3 months, 5 subjects; 4 to 6 months, 2 subjects; 7 to 8 months, 4 subjects; 9 to 11 months, 1 subject; 12 to 14 months, 1 subject; and 2 years and more, 5 subjects. Five subjects had small areas of subdural bleeding, 3 were believed to have sustained cerebral contusions, and 1 had evidence of a small intracerebral hematoma. It is thus quite clear that some patients, initially thought to have only mild head injuries, have more serious brain involvement.

The 20 subjects in Group 3 initially appeared to be even less severely injured than the subjects in Group 2. However, the subjects in Group 2 were consecutive research cases and may have been representative of mild head injury cases rather generally. As noted, research suggests that such individuals recover in a relatively short time. The subjects in Group 3, even though judged to have sustained mild injuries, had significant and persisting problems. The development of posttraumatic epilepsy in five of these cases must have been associated with more serious cerebral impairment than generally occurs among patients with mild head injuries. The important point, however, is that many persons who sustain a mild head injury have more serious involvement of the brain, which may become more apparent at a later time. This point has been well made in the literature (McAlister, 1992; Williams, Levin, & Eisenberg, 1990; Yarnell & Rossie, 1988). Even in children, injuries that initially appear mild may give rise to significant neurological symptoms. Roberts, Manshadi, Bushnell, and Hines (1995) have recently described a child who was normal before a mild whiplash type of injury. Her symptoms increased over a 2-year period even though EEG tracings and CT of the head were normal. Because staring spells continued 4 years after the accident, a positron emission tomography (PET) scan was done and showed evidence of marked hypometabolism in both temporal lobes. Treatment with antiepileptic medications greatly improved the child's staring episodes.

Group 3 would appear to represent a meaningful subset of patients with mild head injuries, although we have no information to estimate the proportion of patients with mild head injury who later have significant and persisting complaints. Stein and Spettell (1995) reported the incidence of complications in patients with minimal head injury at 8.1%, and in patients with mild head injury at 11.4%, but they considered complications to be present if for any reason (e.g., observation at home was not available) hospitalization was advisable, not just if neurological abnormalities (e.g., seizures) occurred. Thus, their report is of limited relevance to the present study.

The methods of data collection and analyses were the same as we have used in our previous studies of age and education influences on neuropsychological status. The GNDS was used to assess overall neuropsychological status because it has been shown to be very sensitive to the effects of mild head injury (Reitan & Wolfson, in press f; Rojas & Bennett, 1995).

Means and standard deviations were computed for age, education, and GNDS scores. In addition, coefficients of correlation were computed between age, education, and GNDS scores. The next step was to subdivide each group at the median age and compare the mean GNDS scores of the younger and older subgroups. As previously noted, we had found that control subjects with more education had better GNDS scores and that older subjects performed more poorly than younger subjects (Reitan & Wolfson, 1995b). Among the brain-damaged subgroups, however, there were no significant differences.

Although age and education distributions were not significantly different among the three groups, there were statistically significant differences in mean GNDS scores (see Table 4.1). Group 2 earned the best GNDS scores, Group 3 had significantly poorer scores than Group 2, and Group 1 showed significantly more impairment than either Group 3 or Group 2.

Table 4.2 presents coefficients of correlation between age, education, and GNDS scores among the three groups, and comparisons of mean GNDS scores for age and education subgroups. We might expect no significant correlations

Table 4.1
Means, Standard Deviations, and t Ratios
for Three Groups with Traumatic Head Injuries

Group	N	Age (years) M	Age (years) SD	Education (years) M	Education (years) SD	GNDS score M	GNDS score SD
1. Definite TBI (research cases)	18	31.22	13.09	12.28	2.30	52.11	19.39
2. Mild head injury (research cases)	18	27.44	11.98	13.06	2.31	26.56	13.34
3. Mild head injury (clinical cases)	20	31.80	15.09	11.35	3.51	38.00	17.56

Group comparisons

	Age t	Age p	Education t	Education p	GNDS t	GNDS p
Group 1 vs. Group 2	0.90	.40	1.03	.40	4.60	.001
Group 1 vs. Group 3	0.01	1.00	0.96	.40	2.44	.025
Group 2 vs. Group 3	0.98	.40	1.76	.10	2.45	.025

Note. GNDS = *General Neuropsychological Deficit Scale.*

between age and education and GNDS scores in Group 1, according to the postulate that brain damage assumes an overpowering role in determining the variance on the GNDS, essentially eliminating the influence of age and education. As noted in Table 4.2, the coefficients of correlation for Group 1 were not statistically significant, which contrasts with results previously reported for subjects without brain damage.

The more critical question in this study, however, concerned persons with mild head injury. Correlations with age and education were not statistically significant in any of our groups, indicating no basis for concluding that either age or education had a systematic relationship to GNDS scores in either of the groups with mild head injuries. Thus, the findings for subjects with mild head injuries were essentially similar to those reported for subjects with definite traumatic brain tissue damage, rather than to those reported for subjects without brain damage. It is interesting to note that these findings classify subjects with traumatic head injuries into a single group regardless of the severity of neuropsychological deficits, much in the same manner noted for the nature, if not the degree, of neuropathological findings (Oppenheimer, 1968).

Table 4.2

Coefficients of Correlation Between Age, Education, and GNDS Scores; and Comparisons of Mean GNDS Scores for Subdivisions of Head-Injured Groups

Group	Age		Education	
	r with GNDS	GNDS *t* ratios: younger vs. older[a]	*r* with GNDS	GNDS *t* ratios: more vs. less education[b]
1. Definite TBI (research cases)	0.32	0.92	0.00	0.50
2. Mild head injury (research cases)	0.16	0.27	– 0.24	0.21
3. Mild head injury (clinical cases)	0.32	2.43*	– 0.34	0.06

[a] Groups were subdivided into a group younger than the median age and a group older than the median age.

[b] Groups were subdivided into a group with more than the median years of education and a group with fewer than the median years of education.

$^*p < .05$.

Finally, mean GNDS scores were compared for the age and education subgroups (see Table 4.2). None of the comparisons based on education showed significant differences. In other words, the less educated subgroups earned GNDS scores equivalent to those earned by the more educated subgroups. However, in comparisons based on age, the differences were statistically insignificant in only two of the three comparisons. The older subjects in Group 3 had poorer GNDS scores than the younger subjects in this group, although the probability level exceeded only .05.

This study clearly suggests that the effects of age and education on neuropsychological status are diminished in cases of mild head injury in much the same way as in cases of more severe head injury, or as shown previously, in groups with diversified brain lesions. Neuropsychological impairment, presumably resulting from brain involvement even in cases of mild head injury, would seem to be the common factor that diminishes or largely deletes the significance of age and education in determining GNDS scores. This finding contrasts with the significant effects of age and education previously reported for subjects without brain damage.

It must be emphasized that cross-validation of these findings is required, and further research is needed. The samples of persons with mild head injuries were small, and included an insufficient range and representation of either the age or education distributions. Brain damage is susceptible to many subdivisions beyond the degree of severity, such as lateralization and localization, diffuse involvement, recent and remote injuries, acute and chronic status, and so on. These various categories, as well as possible differences in age and education effects for persons with psychiatric and emotional disturbances, should be studied in relation to control subjects. Subjects in any of these categories may demonstrate results that caution against adjusting raw scores according to relationships that apply for normal persons but maybe not for persons in other categories.

Conclusions

The advantages of education are widely recognized in our society. The results of the studies reviewed in this chapter strongly suggest that brain injury, even mild head injury, sharply diminishes the advantages of education, at least in terms of neuropsychological and intellectual test performances.

References

Alves, W. M., & Jane, J. A. (1985). Mild brain injury: Damage and outcome. In D. P. Becker and J. T. Povlishock (Eds.), *Central nervous system trauma research status report—1985.* Bethesda, MD: National Institutes of Health.

Annegers, J. R., Grabow, J. D., Kurland, L. T., & Laws, E. R., Jr. (1980). The incidence, causes, and secular trends of head trauma in Olmsted County, Minnesota, 1935–1974. *Neurology, 30,* 912–919.

Dikmen, S., McLean, A., & Temkin, N. (1986). Neuropsychological and psychosocial consequences of minor head injury. *Journal of Neurology, Neurosurgery, and Psychiatry, 49,* 1227–1232.

Dikmen, S., & Reitan, R. M. (1976). Psychological deficits and recovery of functions after head injury. *Transactions of the American Neurological Association, 101,* 72–77.

Dikmen, S., Reitan, R. M., & Temkin, N. R. (1983). Neuropsychological recovery in head injury. *Archives of Neurology, 40,* 333–338.

Eisenberg, H. M., & Levin, H. S. (1989). Computed tomography and magnetic resonance imaging in mild to moderate head injury. In H. S. Levin, H. M. Eisenberg, & A. L. Benton (Eds.), *Mild head injury* (pp. 133–141). New York: Oxford University Press.

Finlayson, M. A. J., Johnson, K. A., & Reitan, R. M. (1977). Relationship of level of education to neuropsychological measures in brain-damaged and non-brain-damaged adults. *Journal of Consulting and Clinical Psychology, 45,* 536–542.

Gaddes, W. H., & Edgell, D. (1994). *Learning disabilities and brain functions. A neuropsychological approach* (3rd ed.). New York: Springer-Verlag.

Gentilini, M., Nichelli, P., & Schoenhuber, R. (1989). Assessment of attention in mild head injury. In H. S. Levin, H. M. Eisenberg, & A. L. Benton (Eds.), *Mild head injury* (pp. 163–175). New York: Oxford University Press.

Gronwall, D. (1976). Performance changes during recovery from closed head injury. *Proceedings of the Australian Association of Neurology, 13,* 143–147.

Gronwall, D. (1977). Paced auditory serial addition task: A measure of recovery from concussion. *Perceptual and Motor Skills, 44,* 367–373.

Gronwall, D. (1989). Cumulative and persisting effects of concussion on attention and cognition. In H. S. Levin, H. M. Eisenberg, & A. L. Benton (Eds.), *Mild head injury* (pp. 153–162). New York: Oxford University Press.

Gronwall, D., & Sampson, H. (1974). *The psychological effects of concussion.* Auckland, New Zealand: Auckland University Press.

Gronwall, D., & Wrightson, P. (1974). Delayed recovery after minor head injury. *Lancet, 2,* 605–609.

Heaton, R. K., Grant, I., & Matthews, C. G. (1991). *Comprehensive norms for an expanded Halstead-Reitan Battery.* Odessa, FL: Psychological Assessment Resources.

Jagger, J., Levine, J. I., Jane, J. A., & Rimel, R. W. (1984). Epidemiologic features of head injury in a predominantly rural population. *Journal of Trauma, 24,* 40–44.

Jennett, B. (1976). Assessment of the severity of head injury. *Journal of Neurology, Neurosurgery, and Psychiatry, 39,* 647–655.

Jennett, B. (1979). Severity of brain damage: Altered consciousness and other indicators. In G. L. Odom (Ed.), *Central nervous system trauma research status report* (pp. 204–219). Washington, DC: National Institute of Neurological and Communicative Disorders and Stroke.

Jennett, B. (1989). Some international comparisons. In H. S. Levin, M. N. Eisenberg, & A. L. Benton (Eds.), *Mild head injury* (pp. 23–34). New York: Oxford University Press.

Kaufman, A. S. (1990). *Assessing adolescent and adult intelligence.* Boston: Allyn & Bacon.

Kraus, J. F., Black, M. A., Hessol, N., Ley, P., Rokaw, W., Sullivan, C., Bowers, S., Knowlton, S., & Marshall, L. (1984). The incidence of acute brain injury and serious impairment in a defined population. *American Journal of Epidemiology, 119,* 186–201.

Kraus, J. F., & Nourjah, P. (1989). The epidemiology of mild head injury. In H. S. Levin, H. M. Eisenberg, & A. L. Benton (Eds.), *Mild head injury* (pp. 8–22). New York: Oxford University Press.

Levin, H. S., Benton, A. L., & Grossman, R. G. (1982). *Neurobehavioral consequences of closed head injury.* New York: Oxford University Press.

Levin, H. S., Eisenberg, H. M., & Benton, A. L. (Eds.). (1989). *Mild head injury.* New York: Oxford University Press.

Long, C. J., & Klein, K. (1990). Decision strategies in neuropsychology II. Determination of age effects on neuropsychological performance. *Archives of Clinical Neuropsychology, 5,* 335–345.

McAlister, T. W. (1992). Neuropsychiatric sequelae of head injuries. *Psychiatric Clinics of North America, 15,* 395–413.

McLean, A., Temkin, N. R., Dikmen, S., & Wyler, A. R. (1983). The behavioral sequelae of head injury. *Journal of Clinical Neuropsychology, 5,* 361–376.

Mild Traumatic Brain Injury Committee of the Head Injury Interdisciplinary Special Interest Group of the American Congress of Rehabilitation Medicine. (1993). Definition of mild traumatic brain injury. *Journal of Head Trauma Rehabilitation, 8,* 86–87.

Oppenheimer, D. R. (1968). Microscopic lesions in the brain following head injury. *Journal of Neurology, Neurosurgery, and Psychiatry, 31,* 299–306.

Prigatano, G. P., & Parsons, O. A. (1976). Relationship of age and education to Halstead test performance in different patient populations. *Journal of Consulting and Clinical Psychology, 44,* 527–533.

Reitan, R. M. (1955a). The distribution according to age of a psychologic measure dependent upon organic brain functions. *Journal of Gerontology, 10,* 338–340.

Reitan, R. M. (1955b). An investigation of the validity of Halstead's measures of biological intelligence. *Archives of Neurology and Psychiatry, 73,* 28–35.

Reitan, R. M. (1959). The comparative effects of brain damage on the Halstead Impairment Index and the Wechsler-Bellevue Scale. *Journal of Clinical Psychology, 15,* 281–285.

Reitan, R. M. (1967). Psychological assessment of deficits associated with brain lesions in subjects with normal and subnormal intelligence. In J. L. Khanna (Ed.), *Brain damage and mental retardation: A psychological evaluation.* Springfield, IL: Charles C. Thomas.

Reitan, R. M., & Wolfson, D. (1986). *Traumatic brain injury: Vol. I. Pathophysiology and neuropsychological evaluation.* Tucson, AZ: Neuropsychology Press.

Reitan, R. M., & Wolfson, D. (1988). *Traumatic brain injury: Vol. II. Recovery and rehabilitation.* Tucson, AZ: Neuropsychology Press.

Reitan, R. M., & Wolfson, D. (1990). A consideration of the comparability of the WAIS and WAIS–R. *The Clinical Neuropsychologist, 4,* 80–85.

Reitan, R. M., & Wolfson, D. (1992). *Neuropsychological evaluation of older children.* Tucson, AZ: Neuropsychology Press.

Reitan, R. M., & Wolfson, D. (1993). *The Halstead-Reitan Neuropsychological Test Battery: Theory and clinical interpretation* (2nd ed.). Tucson: Neuropsychology Press.

Reitan, R. M., & Wolfson, D. (1995). Influence of age and education on neuropsychological test results. *The Clinical Neuropsychologist, 9,* 151–158.

Reitan, R. M., & Wolfson, D. (in press a). Can WISC–R IQ values be computed validly for learning-disabled children? *Applied Neuropsychology.*

Reitan, R. M., & Wolfson, D. (in press b). Differences in age-related improvement in WISC–R performances for brain-damaged and control groups: Implications for computing intelligence quotients. *Child Neuropsychology.*

Reitan, R. M., & Wolfson, D. (in press c). Differential relationships of age and education to WAIS subtest scores among brain-damaged and control groups. *Archives of Clinical Neuropsychology.*

Reitan, R. M., & Wolfson, D. (in press d). The diminished effect of age and education on neuropsychological performances of learning-disabled children. *Child Neuropsychology.*

Reitan, R. M., & Wolfson, D. (in press e). Influence of age and education on neuropsychological test performances of older children. *Child Neuropsychology.*

Reitan, R. M., & Wolfson, D. (in press f). *Mild head injury. Intellectual, cognitive, and emotional consequences.* Tucson: Neuropsychology Press.

Reitan, R. M., & Wolfson, D. (in press g). Relationships of age and education to Wechsler Adult Intelligence Scale IQ values in brain-damaged and non-brain-damaged groups. *The Clinical Neuropsychologist.*

Rimel, R. W. (1981). A prospective study of patients with central nervous system trauma. *Journal of Neurology, Neurosurgery, and Psychiatry, 21,* 132–141.

Rimel, R. W., Giordani, B., Barth, J. T., Boll, T. J., & Jane, J. A. (1981). Disability caused by minor head injury. *Neurosurgery, 9,* 221–228.

Roberts, M. A., Manshadi, F. F., Bushnell, D. L., & Hines, M. E. (1995). Neurobehavioural dysfunction following mild traumatic brain injury in childhood: A case report with positive findings in positron emission tomography (PET). *Brain Injury, 9,* 427–436.

Rojas, D. C., & Bennett, T. L. (1995). Single versus composite score discriminative validity with the Halstead-Reitan Battery and the Stroop Test in mild head injury. *Archives of Clinical Neuropsychology, 2,* 101–110.

Rourke, B. R. (Ed.). (1985). *Neuropsychology of learning disabilities.* New York: Guilford.

Ruff, R. M., Levin, H. S., Mattis, S., High, W. M., Marshall, L. F., Eisenberg, H. M., & Tabaddor, K. (1989). Recovery of memory after mild head injury: A three-center study. In H. S. Levin, H. M. Eisenberg, & A. L. Benton (Eds.), *Mild head injury* (pp. 176–188). New York: Oxford University Press.

Sherer, M., & Adams, R. L. (1993). Cross-validation of Reitan and Wolfson's Neuropsychological Deficit Scales. *Archives of Clinical Neuropsychology, 8,* 429–435.

Stein, S. C., & Spettell, C. (1995). The Head Injury Severity Scale (HISS): A practical classification of closed head injury. *Brain Injury, 9,* 437–444.

Tupper, D. E., & Rosenblood, L. K. (1984). Methodological considerations in the use of attribute variables in neuropsychological research. *Journal of Clinical Neuropsychology, 6,* 441–453.

Vega, A., & Parsons, O. A. (1967). Cross-validation of the Halstead-Reitan tests for brain damage. *Journal of Consulting Psychology, 31,* 619–625.

Wechsler, D. (1955). *The measurement and appraisal of adult intelligence* (4th ed.). Baltimore: Williams & Wilkins.

Whitman, S., Coonley-Hoganson, R., & Desai, B. T. (1984). Comparative head trauma experiences in two socioeconomically different Chicago-area communities—A population study. *American Journal of Epidemiology, 119,* 570–580.

Williams, D. H., Levin, H. S., & Eisenberg, H. M. (1990). Mild head injury classification. *Neurosurgery, 27,* 422–428.

Wolfson, D., & Reitan, R. M. (1995). Cross-validation of the General Neuropsychological Deficit Scale (GNDS). *Archives of Clinical Neuropsychology, 10,* 125–131.

Yarnell, P. R., & Rossie, G. V. (1988). Minor whiplash head injury with major debilitation. *Brain Injury, 2,* 255–258.

Assessment of Mild Traumatic Brain Injury in Children for Neuropsychological Rehabilitation

5

Cynthia A. Riccio
and Cecil R. Reynolds

Neuropsychological assessment is often recommended for a variety of disorders with an identified neurological basis (e.g., seizure disorder) as well as for disorders with a presumed neurological basis (e.g., learning disabilities). For children with TBI, neuropsychological assessment is particularly important because a comprehensive evaluation of brain integrity is needed. The research literature supports the use of neuropsychological assessment to understand short- and long-term problems associated with TBI in childhood (Bigler, 1990; Snow & Hooper, 1994). Children and youth with TBI comprise a heterogeneous group with regard to neurocognitive functioning, prognosis, and outcome (Haak & Livingston, 1997). Boll (1983) asserted that the consequences of TBI in children are often underappreciated, and they cannot be predicted well with a standard neurological examination or even advanced imaging techniques. Ylvisaker (1985) also suggested that deficits associated with TBI are often not recognized. Children are less likely than adults to undergo neuropsychological assessment following head injury (Boll, 1983). This would seem particularly true of children with mild head injuries. Research further suggests that head injuries in children are much more likely to be closed head injuries than penetrating injuries (Boll & Barth, 1981; Spreen, Tupper, Risser, Tuokko, & Edgell, 1984), further decreasing the likelihood of a thorough evaluation following the injury. Neuropsychological tests are sensitive to the subtle deficits that persist with TBI (Ryan, LaMarche, Barth, & Boll, 1996), and thus can be of assistance in rehabilitation planning.

For children with neurologically based disorders such as TBI, clinical child neuropsychology provides a theoretical framework for understanding identified patterns of strengths and weaknesses, the relationships between strengths and weaknesses, and the extent to which these patterns remain stable or are subject to change over the course of development (Fletcher & Taylor, 1984; Temple, 1997). Understanding of the child's strengths and weaknesses can help identify areas that may be difficult for the child in the future, and strategies or methods to circumvent these difficulties. It has been suggested that neuropsychological assessment of children provides a better understanding of the ways in which neurological conditions affect behavior, and translation of this knowledge into educationally relevant information (Allen, 1989).

The major premise of neuropsychological assessment is that different behaviors, including higher order cognitive skills, involve differing neurological structures or functional systems (Luria, 1980). As such, this approach involves assessment of various behavioral domains believed to be related to functional neurological systems, and making inferences about brain integrity based on the individual's performance. Neuropsychological assessment samples behaviors that depend on the integrity of the central nervous system, using measures that correlate with cognitive, sensorimotor, and emotional functioning (Dean & Gray, 1990).

TBI can affect the central nervous system (CNS) through discrete impairment and more diffuse impairment (Ryan et al., 1996). Discrete impairment is less subtle, and is more likely to be evidenced through assessment of cognition and achievement. The extent of discrete impairment and the chronicity of the impaired functions are related directly to severity, and are therefore less likely to be seen in mild TBI. Diffuse impairment such as may occur with mild TBI is less likely to be seen on neuroradiological measures like CT and MRI scans. When neuroradiological evaluations do not show structural damage, its absence may be misinterpreted as indicating that no damage has occurred, and therefore no further assessment is needed. This assumption may be incorrect because neurocognitive deficits can result from the shearing, tearing, and compression frequently associated with mild closed head injuries, even when there is no neuroradiological evidence of structural damage (Levin, Benton, & Grossman, 1982). The movement of the brain within the skull may cause a twisting or shearing of nerve fibers, creating microscopic lesions that are not detected by a CT scan. Even in minor head injury, permanent damage in the form of microscopic lesions can occur, but may be seen on a CT scan in only 5% of the cases. In contrast, studies with MRI show that a majority of individuals with mild head injuries may have microscopic lesions (e.g., Levin et al., 1988). Diffuse impairment is also less likely to be seen on standard measures of cognitive ability or achievement, but may affect more complex cognitive functions (e.g., problem solving of novel situations), as well as processing speed, ability to concentrate, and overall cognitive efficiency. Although more subtle than discrete deficits, these generalized deficits affect not only the child's immediate functioning level, but perhaps later development and the acquisition of new skills (Ryan et al., 1996).

With serial neuropsychological assessment, progress can be monitored, intervention methods can be evaluated, and changes in the pattern of symptomatology can be detected. The same methods can be used through adolescence to monitor the appropriate development of skills and abilities based on the typical curve. Both the diffuse and generalized effects of TBI vary in number, nature, and severity. This variability precludes the use of a single measure for assessment or a single method for treatment. The interaction of the child's neuropsychological profile and his or her environment may also affect symptom presentation and chronicity. Thus, there are multiple roles for neuropsychological assessment of children with TBI: a) the identification of strengths and weaknesses at a given point in development; b) the short-term assessment of treatment effects through careful psychometric monitoring of changes in neurocognition and behavior; and c) the long-term monitoring of expected neurodevelopmental progression and development of subsequent skills.

The influences of child psychology, school psychology, and education are evident in the composition of neuropsychological assessment batteries, procedures, and measures used with children (Batchelor, 1996a). The emergence of clinical neuropsychology as a specialty has been led by advances in neuroscience, clinical evidence specific to brain behavior relationships based on localized brain damage in children and youth, advances in technology (e.g., functional imaging), and continued research efforts specific to children's problems that are adding to knowledge on brain development and function. There are several positive outcomes of the application of neuropsychology to children and adolescents: an extended range of diagnostic techniques, providing for better integration of behavioral data (Dean, 1986; Gray & Dean, 1990; Obrzut & Hynd, 1983); an increased ability to deal adequately with the multidimensionality of observed behavior, creating a unified picture of a student's functioning (Rothlisberg & D'Amato, 1988); and documentation of changes in behavior and development over time (Hynd & Willis, 1988). As a result of this growing interest in clinical child neuropsychology, knowledge about the developing brain has increased dramatically in the past two decades, including advanced understanding of the typical development of neuropsychological functions (e.g., Ardila & Roselli, 1994; Halperin, McKay, Matier, & Sharma, 1994; Miller & Vernon, 1996; Molfese, 1995).

Although more research has focused on educational problems, increased risk for psychiatric disorder and long-term adjustment problems is associated with brain injury in adults and children (e.g., Breslau & Marshall, 1985; Rutter, Graham, & Yule, 1970; Seidel, Chadwick, & Rutter, 1975). Research consistently demonstrates that adjustment and behavioral problems are associated with children who have neurodevelopmental deficits (e.g., Hooper & Tramontana, 1997; Tramontana & Hooper, 1997). Children with neurological impairment are 6 times more likely to develop emotional/behavioral/motivational problems secondary to, if not as a direct result of, the neurological impairment (Dean, 1986). It was believed that specific relationships between brain dysfunction and child psychopathology would be found; it is now believed that the relationships between brain integrity and psychopathology are nonspecific and affected by secondary influences including failure, frustration, social stigma, family reaction, and so on (Tramontana & Hooper). Various models (e.g., Gray, 1982; Kinsbourne, 1989; Nussbaum et al., 1988; Rourke, 1989; Tucker, 1989) have been proposed to explain the relationships between brain function and behaviors associated with childhood psychopathology.

This chapter provides a framework for the neuropsychological assessment of TBI, and the translation of the assessment to the development and monitoring of treatment plans. Although the problems associated with mild TBI are often more subtle than with moderate to severe TBI, the framework is intended to address the range of problems that may be associated with various severity levels of TBI. Thus, this chapter will include an overview of the necessary components of neuropsychological assessment in general, the assessment process, and neurodevelopmental issues that need to be considered, with an emphasis on the complexity of these issues with TBI. In addition, the assessment of various behavioral domains will be discussed. The chapter will provide information on the relevance of neuropsychological results to educational needs, remediation techniques, educational placement, and parental expectations.

Neuropsychological Assessment Process

Neuropsychological assessment of children needs to focus more directly on the symptoms that accompany and follow injury, as opposed to identification of neurological disorder (Riccio & Reynolds, 1998). This is particularly true for children with TBI. Neuropsychological assessment generally consists of a number of functional domains that are, based on clinical evidence, associated with functional systems of the brain. This is important for the development of hypotheses and potential interventions (Hartlage & Telzrow, 1986; Whitten, D'Amato, & Chitooran, 1992). The assessment itself should be organized so that the majority of functional domains and the various contexts in which the child is expected to function are considered. Riccio and Reynolds identified a number of features key to the organization of neuropsychological assessment of children; these are presented in Table 5.1. These points are highlighted and discussed further throughout the remainder of this chapter.

As pointed out by Ryan et al. (1996), the actual instruments used and the timing of the assessment need to be considered in interpretation and treatment planning. The neuropsychological assessment should optimally be conducted prior to the child's return to school, to assess strengths and identify areas of immediate need. For children with mild TBI who return to school, even a standard psychoeducational evaluation may not be completed in a timely manner due to the nature of the special education process. The general practice in many school districts is to wait until a child is failing or in

Table 5.1
Organizational Features for Neuropsychological Assessment of Children with TBI

1. Coordinate assessment efforts with school personnel for efficiency.
2. Obtain a comprehensive history.
3. Assess relevant cognitive skills and higher order processes.
4. Sample right and left hemispheric functions.
5. Sample anterior versus posterior functions.
6. Assess affect, personality, and behavior.
7. Determine specific deficits.
8. Locate intact complex functional systems.
9. Determine acuteness versus chronicity of deficits.
10. Assess contextual variables that may contribute to or hinder rehabilitation.
11. Present results for use in home and school rehabilitation settings.

danger of failing, or until the child's behavior has been problematic over time, to begin the referral process. The school district is then required to document interventions within the regular program. It is only after various interventions have been unsuccessful that a child is referred for assessment. This can delay the assessment process for a child with TBI for an extended time and, with the length of time between the injury and the assessment, there may be misinterpretation of the results. For example, a number of children with TBI are subsequently classified as having a learning disability or other disorder (Ewing-Cobbs, Fletcher, & Levin, 1986).

For these reasons, whenever possible, it is recommended that the neuropsychological assessment be conducted efficiently and coordinated with the child's school district. It may be appropriate, for example, for school personnel (e.g., school psychologist, speech/language pathologist) to participate in the evaluation process, thus reducing the financial strain on the school system. This type of collaborative effort can facilitate school program planning for the child. Early notification to the school district of the child's projected discharge date and timely assessment also allow the school district to make necessary arrangements for any direct or indirect service delivery.

After TBI, children generally rapidly recover function for the first 3 to 6 months, with a plateau at about 18 to 24 months postinjury and continuing recovery for 3 to 5 years postinjury (Klonoff, Low, & Clark, 1977; Ryan et al., 1996). This requires monitoring of neurocognitive function over time with standardized and non-standardized measures. There is also evidence that although children with TBI demonstrate improved neurocognitive functioning over 2 to 3 years, increased behavioral and psychiatric problems emerge at 1 to 2 years postinjury (Tramontana & Hooper, 1997). The fluctuation or variability in symptom presentation with TBI does not occur in most other disorders. Thus, for children with TBI, the primary issue is not one of differential diagnosis or classification, but one of establishing postinjury baseline data and monitoring strengths and weaknesses in neurocognitive and behavioral/emotional areas, to most appropriately address the child's changing profile. The rehabilitation plan or individualized educational plan (IEP) for a child with TBI needs to be re-assessed more frequently due to repeated assessments (formal or informal) of the child's progress in previously identified deficit areas and identification of additional areas of concern (Ball & Zinner, 1994; Ewing-Cobbs et al., 1986; Hynd & Obrzut, 1981; Rothlisberg & D'Amato, 1996). Re-assessment should occur at least every 6 to 12 months (Boll & Stanford, 1997). Children change too rapidly to advise otherwise, and the brain continues to mature physically and functionally into adulthood. Damaged or injured brains may well develop in ways that are unique, and there is no time that the brain changes more rapidly, barring disease, than in childhood.

In general, behavioral domains will include cognition, achievement, and behavior/affect as would be assessed as part of a general psychological evaluation. A neuropsychological evaluation covers a wider array of functions, however, than is addressed in a typical psychological or psychoeducational evaluation (Dean, 1985, 1986; Obrzut, 1981; Reynolds & Mayfield, in press). In general, the neuropsychological evaluation is more thorough and also assesses perceptual, motor, and sensory areas; attention; executive function (planning, organization, problem solving); and learning and memory (e.g., Dean & Gray, 1990; Obrzut, 1981; Shurtleff, Fay, Abbott, & Berninger, 1988). Because of the more subtle deficits associated with TBI, measures of attention, executive function, and learning and memory take on increased importance.

The neurodevelopment of Luria's functional systems and the child's experiences are reciprocal (Spreen, Risser, & Edgell, 1995), and there is potential for adjustment/behavioral difficulties. Therefore, many have advocated a transactional/reciprocal model that considers the reciprocal interactions of the child, home and family members, classroom (teacher and peers), and other social environments (Batchelor, 1996b; D'Amato & Rothlisberg, 1996; D'Amato, Rothlisberg, & Leu, in press; Teeter, 1997; Teeter & Semrud-Clikeman, 1997). This model should incorporate information from a variety of sources (e.g., parents, teachers, physicians, medical records, school records, etc.) to enable cross-comparison (Batchelor, 1996b). In addition, motivational factors (Batchelor, 1996b) and the child's ability to cope with the injury and any resulting impairment need to be determined (Dean, 1986). Thus, the neuropsychological assessment process not only incorporates a thorough review of information regarding the child, but attempts to integrate this information with an understanding of brain behavior relations and environmental factors (Taylor & Fletcher, 1990). With TBI, the assessment must be multifaceted and consider the preinjury and postinjury development of the child as well as the location, severity, chronicity, and psychosocial/environmental factors that may affect rehabilitation efforts (Ryan et al., 1996).

Given these caveats, a neuropsychological assessment should involve a wide range of tasks focused on the child, as well as measures/observations of the various contexts in which the child functions and the associated expectations. Assessment of a wider range of higher cortical functions is supported by research findings that neurological disorders are seldom expressed as a single dysfunction (Dean & Gray, 1990). The child's cumulative performances on neuropsychological measures are seen as behavioral indicators of brain function (Fennell & Bauer, 1997). The additional areas of functioning included in the neuropsychological assessment are needed to support inferences about the integrity of various functional systems of the brain (Shurtleff et al., 1988). For this reason, the neuropsychological assessment should be organized to ensure (a) evaluation of a majority of cognitive and higher order processes that relate to educational functioning and (b) evaluation of all four quadrants (right/left hemispheres, anterior/posterior regions) of the cortex. In particular, the nature and extent of deficits in the anterior/posterior regions will affect treatment choices. Damage in one region of the brain may affect function in other regions, and a review of all major functional systems—intellectual, emotional, and behavioral—is required.

Deriving hypotheses for intervention planning is a complex process that requires a comprehensive assessment battery coupled with neuropsychological foundations and familiarity with the contexts and task demands of the child (Gaddes, 1983; Rourke, 1994). The neuropsychological perspective leads to better understanding of the underlying causes of learning and behavior problems; this in turn results in an increased ability to develop appropriate interventions or circumvent future problems (Boll & Stanford, 1997; D'Amato, Rothlisberg, & Rhodes, 1997). This is particularly important for children with TBI, due to the potential subtlety of deficits, particularly with mild to moderate injury.

Based on the data from the evaluation process, hypotheses are generated about how and why a child processes information (D'Amato, 1990; Dean, 1986; Leu & D'Amato, 1994; Whitten et al., 1992). Inferences are then made based on the child's performance and the clinician's theoretical perspective. There are a variety of paradigms for understanding and interpreting neuropsychological data (e.g., Ayers, 1974; Batchelor, 1996a; Das, Kirby, & Jarman, 1979; Luria, 1966; Nussbaum & Bigler, 1997; Reynolds, 1981b). Interpretation is further affected by the neuropsychologist's clinical skills and acumen (D'Amato et al., 1997). Interpretation may be based on overall performance level across tasks (e.g., Reitan, 1986, 1987), performance patterns across tasks (e.g., Mattarazzo, 1972; Reitan, 1986, 1987), asymmetry of function (e.g., Hartlage, 1982; Reitan, 1986, 1987), the presence of pathognomonic signs (e.g., Kaplan, 1988; Lezak, 1995; Reitan, 1986, 1987), or some combination of these features (Boll, 1981; Reitan, 1986, 1987; Riccio & Reynolds, 1998). Whichever model is used, it should allow the neuropsychologist to make predictions about the child's ability to perform in a variety of contexts and provide information about the efficacy of the rehabilitation plan (Reynolds, Kamphaus, Rosenthal, & Hiemenz, 1997).

With information about how various skills correlate in the developmental process, one can use neuropsychological assessment to make inferences not only about the skills measured, but also about skills that have not been evaluated. Ultimately, data generated from the neuropsychological assessment process are used to develop recommendations on whether the individual would profit from compensatory strategies, remedial instruction, or a combination (Gaddes & Edgell, 1994). Further, by understanding the neurological correlates of these skills and of instructional methods, neuropsychological assessment can assist in the formulation of hypotheses regarding potential instructional methods/materials for a particular child (Reynolds, Kamphaus, et al., 1997).

Thus, one organizational component of the neuropsychological assessment process is the identification of the child's specific deficits and any intact complex functional systems. It may not be plausible or effective to address all areas of deficit simultaneously. Once deficits are identified, depending on the number and severity, it may be necessary to prioritize them according to the settings in which the child is expected to function (home and school). For example, those behaviors necessary for reintegration or maintenance in the regular classroom may be of priority in the educational arena. The specific goals and objectives also should relate to the home and school settings, the expectations for the child in these settings, and the supports/resources available for the child.

There is often a tendency to focus on deficits; however, it is imperative to the development of treatment programs that the child's strengths and intact systems also be identified. The brain functions as a series of interdependent systems (see Luria, 1966), and although multiple systems may be affected by the TBI, it is likely that some systems have been spared, except in more severe cases. Identification of intact systems seems more positive to parents and teachers, and makes it more likely that the child will have support. With the potential for rapid recovery of function following TBI, this is of particular importance. Reynolds (1981a) pointed out that research based on deficits focuses on areas of the brain that are damaged or dysfunctional. With a focus on intact functional systems, rehabilitation and remediation programs based on strengths can be implemented (see Reynolds, 1986b; Reynolds & Hickman, 1987). At the same time, the intact systems can be used to develop compensatory behaviors. The fact that some children and adults with TBI have residual impairments, however subtle, suggests the need for development of compensatory behaviors.

It has been suggested that interventions must be multidimensional and incorporate not only academic, behavioral, and psychotherapeutic techniques, but also motivational, metacognitive, medical, and classroom management techniques (Batchelor, 1996b; Teeter & Semrud-Clikeman, 1997). Although "treatment" in education generally consists of eligibility, placement decisions, and the development of an educational plan, effective interventions for children with TBI also need to consider the myriad psychosocial contexts in which the child functions, adjustment and coping issues, and environmental modifications that can ameliorate or reduce the behavioral effects of brain dysfunction (Batchelor, 1996b; Teeter & Semrud-Clikeman, 1997). For children with TBI, the supports/services available to the family can affect outcome (Satz & Fletcher, 1981). For this reason, the families of children with TBI or chronic illness may also be a target for intervention (Boll & Stanford, 1997). Comprehensive assessment and early implementation of effective treatment strategies are cost-effective in dollars and in quality of a child's life (Reynolds, Wilen, & Stone, 1997). Children with TBI can dramatically improve with appropriate intervention (Bigler, 1987; McMillan & Glucksman, 1987; Telzrow, 1987). Because the most rapid recovery from TBI is evident within the first 6 months postinjury, the earlier the interventions are in place, the more effective they are likely to be.

Consideration of Neurodevelopmental Issues

In the development of clinical child neuropsychology, the assessment measures and processes used have historically been modifications of neuropsychological batteries and other measures made for adults (Hartlage & Long, 1997). In some cases, tasks were modified or added. Alternatively, normative data was collected on children, using existing tasks. Both of these strategies were based on the clinical efficacy of the measures with adults and the assumption that the tasks measure the same thing for adults and children. Similarly, it is tempting to assume that neuropsychological findings from adults will be useful with children, but this assumption has not been proven.

When applied to children and adolescents, the premise that behavior can be used to make inferences about brain function and integrity has to be expanded to consider neurodevelopmental differences that exist because of the child's age. To directly apply adult hypotheses to children ignores what is known about changes in the functional organization of the brain as children grow (Cohen, Branch, Willis, Weyandt, & Hynd, 1992; Fletcher & Taylor, 1984). Because of the neurodevelopmental changes, it is also not possible to view brain dysfunction on a continuum based on behavioral deficits, as these may change over time (Fletcher & Taylor).

Neurodevelopment follows an ontogenetic course, with primary cortical zones generally mature by birth (Luria, 1980). Secondary and tertiary areas continue to develop postnatally. These include the integrative systems involved in higher order functions of learning, memory, attention, emotion, cognition, and language, and the association areas. The association areas are the last of these areas to develop and myelinate (Goldman & Lewis, 1978; Goldman-Rakic, 1987). Vygotsky (1980) suggested that not only is there continued development of secondary and tertiary areas, but that the interaction of primary, secondary, and tertiary areas is likely to change with age (Merola & Leiderman, 1985; Rutter, 1981). Although the developmental sequence for the formation of neural pathways and myelination of specific locations corresponding to specific behaviors have been identified, these do not correspond directly to models of cognitive development (Spreen, Risser, & Edgell, 1995).

Knowledge of typical neurodevelopmental progress has increased over the past two decades; however, most of current theory and practice is based on observations and informal assessment of individuals with identified brain damage (Reynolds, 1997b). Extensive research on typical neurodevelopment, particularly related to higher order cognitive skills, is limited, and the changing organization over time of children's brain function is only beginning to be understood (Hynd & Willis, 1988). Thus, there are still many unanswered questions about the developmental progression of functional systems, particularly at the associative and integrative levels, and about how the neurodevelopmental progression maps onto the cognitive functioning observed.

Not only do neurodevelopmental courses need to be considered, but there are complex differences between children and adults in the mechanisms of brain pathology that lead to neuropsychological and behavioral/affective problems; these mechanisms do not necessarily follow a similar progression in children and adults (Fennell & Bauer, 1997; Fletcher & Taylor, 1984). Research suggests that TBI can disrupt the neurodevelopmental process, particularly in younger children (Kriel, Krach, & Panser, 1989). The impact of neurological insult is influenced by age as well as by location and nature of injury, gender, socioeconomic status, level of emotional adjustment and coping, and the individual's own adaptive skills (Bolter & Long, 1985). For this reason, age at the time of injury is an important factor to consider in assessment for rehabilitation planning (Fletcher-Janzen & Kade, 1997).

Historically, the theory of neural plasticity (Harris, 1957) has been used to explain the potential for recovery of function in children that is not seen in adults. It has since been suggested that what is termed "recovery" may, in fact, reflect "reorganization" of brain function (Satz & Fletcher, 1981). Although there is minimal empirical data to hypothesize how children regain skills initially depressed by TBI, it is known that this "recovery" or "reorganization" is more likely to occur following a focal lesion as opposed to more diffuse injury or injury in more neurodevelopmentally mature children (Brink, Garrett, Hale, Woo-Sam, & Nickel, 1970). Brink and colleagues as well as others (e.g., Kriel et al., 1989) found that children over 10 years old were likely to have a better prognosis than those under age 6, regardless of the injury's severity. This may be due to the difference in neurodevelopmental status of children in these age ranges. An alternative explanation is that older children have spent more time in school, and many of the functions assessed by standard measures correlate with the number of years of formal school experience (Ryan et al., 1996). This is not to suggest that children with TBI do not have long-term impairment. One of the more comprehensive longitudinal studies of pediatric TBI (Klonoff et al., 1977) indicated that by the 5th year of the study, the majority of children showed good recovery; however, 23.7% demonstrated impaired neurocognitive performance.

With both the neurodevelopmental and recovery trajectories to consider, there is a need for long-term follow-up through adolescence, parallel to the normal neurodevelopmental progression. The full extent of neurocognitive deficits resulting from TBI may not be identified until much later, when higher order processes fail to develop (Lehr, 1990). Functions or behaviors that have not yet developed at the time of injury cannot be assessed until the child has reached the age at which these functions should have developed (Ryan et al., 1996), or, as in the case of substance abuse, are likely to be a concern (Boll & Stanford, 1997). With both the neurodevelopmental and recovery sequences to be assessed over time, it is therefore important that normative test data that are developmentally referenced be used with children with brain injury.

It is evident that assessment of TBI in children is even more complex than in adults, due to the neurodevelopmental nature of skills and abilities. The age-dependent variability of development not only affects assessment of abilities and skills that should already be in place, but also requires long-term assessment to evaluate how well later developing skills and abilities do in fact develop; the injury might disrupt the development of subsequent cognitive, physical, and psychological skills and abilities (Ryan et al., 1996).

Evaluation of children with TBI, therefore, is complex because of the rapidly changing nature and extent of the child's needs. Research suggests that children with TBI undergo significant and rapid cognitive and emotional changes over time, with the majority of these changes occurring within the first 2 years postinjury (Shaw & Yingst, 1992). This is further complicated by the normally rapid rate of neurodevelopment through adolescence.

Test Selection and Behavioral Domains in TBI Assessment

There is no single method for selecting neuropsychological assessment measures. Many neuropsychologists continue to include observation and informal assessment, whereas others have adopted more statistical approaches and still others combine observation, informal methods, and statistical approaches (Reynolds, 1997b). A more qualitative approach using experimental/informal measures may provide additional information or insight into how the child approaches and processes tasks (e.g., the Boston Approach; see Kaplan, 1988, 1990). A strictly qualitative approach, however, does not allow for verification of diagnostic accuracy, is not easily replicated, and does not allow for formal evaluation of treatment methods; as a result, most clinicians prefer a combination of quantitative and qualitative measures (Rourke, 1994). In addition to standardized measures that may require substantial improvement to demonstrate change over time, it may be necessary to include some measures that are not norm-referenced (i.e., curriculum based or criterion referenced), in order to document small changes in behavior.

In practice, many clinicians use a predetermined battery of tests for neuropsychological assessment of children; this is often referred to as the "fixed battery" approach. To address rehabilitation efforts of children with TBI and consider the potential for rapid changes in functioning, it may be necessary to supplement the "fixed battery" with additional measures. Other neuropsychologists adopt a more individual approach and select measures based on the presenting problems. Regardless of the selection approach, a number of behavioral domains should be addressed; the more idiographic approach may fail to assess important domains and subsequently affect rehabilitation efforts.

Psychometric Issues

In selecting standardized measures for the assessment, a number of factors need to be considered. Research methods and statistical tools have greatly improved since the early 1970s; however, clinical child neuropsychology is often criticized for its failure to attend to basic principles of research and to incorporate psychometric advances (e.g., Cicchetti, 1994; Parsons & Prigatano, 1978; Reschly & Gresham, 1989; Ris & Noll, 1994; Sandoval, 1981; Willson & Reynolds, 1982). One major concern relates to the extent and nature of normative data for many measures used in the neuropsychological assessment of children. Sound normative data provides a backdrop against which to evaluate clinical insight (Reynolds, 1997b) and to appropriately assess change (e.g., Reynolds & Mayfield, in press). Insufficient attention has been given to the systematic development and presentation of normative data for many neuropsychological assessments (Reynolds, 1986a). A second concern is that all too frequently, neuropsychologists rely on the "clinical" nature of tests and overlook the psychometric concepts of reliability and validity. The need for neuropsychological test scores and interpretation to be reliable and valid is a frequent issue in the literature (e.g., Parsons & Prigatano, 1978; Reynolds, 1982). Reliability of test scores is critical, as it relates to the amount of variance that is systematic and related to true interindividual differences; as such, reliability influences the likelihood that effects will be detected. Reliability is also the foundation of a measure's validity (Reynolds, 1986a).

A third concern relates to the sensitivity and appropriateness of measures for children. Neuropsychological assessment of children and adolescents requires not only measures that are age appropriate and have sufficient empirical support for the inferences made between neurological substrates and the behavioral performance of the child, but developmental issues must also be considered (Cohen et al., 1992). Further, it is important to document the measures' sensitivity to neurobehavioral and neurodevelopmental functioning in children (Fletcher & Taylor, 1984). Although child neuropsychology is derived predominantly from neuropsychological study and clinical evidence of adults with known brain injury, a developmental perspective needs to be maintained (Hooper & Tramontana, 1997). Unfortunately, many of the measures used with adults are not sensitive enough to reflect developmental issues; as a result, using adult procedures in the neuropsychological assessment of children has multiple pitfalls and has been questioned (e.g., Cohen et al.; Fletcher & Taylor). Thus, in choosing measures for the neuropsychological assessment of children with TBI, it is important to attend to the psychometric properties and limitations of available measures. In addition to selecting tests based on psychometric properties, neuropsychologists should select measures that vary along a continuum of difficulty, include both rote and novel tasks, and include variations with regard to processing and response requirements within modalities (Rourke, 1994). With the need for serial assessments of children with TBI, measures that can be readministered frequently and in a short amount of time should also be considered.

Domains for Assessment

In the evaluation of children with TBI, it is important to estimate preinjury functioning in cognitive, adaptive, and emotional/behavioral areas. It is also important to assess current functioning in a variety of domains, so that the efficacy of rehabilitation can be measured against this baseline data (Rothlisberg & D'Amato, 1996). Domains of current functioning include (a) assessment of cognitive functioning including language; (b) assessment of sensory and motor functioning; (c) assessment of academic achievement; (d) assessment of learning, memory, attention, and executive function; (e) assessment of emotional/behavioral status, and (f) assessment of environmental variables (home and school) that may affect the outcome. Each of these domains will be discussed in more detail.

Preinjury Status

A comprehensive history is an important component of neuropsychological assessment. A complete history provides useful information for differentiating chronic deficits or neurodevelopmental disorders from new, acute problems that are the direct or indirect result of TBI. This in turn may affect the selection of rehabilitation approaches. For children with TBI this history may be used to estimate preinjury status. One of the questions asked in cases of TBI is the extent to which any identified deficits are the result of the injury. Estimation of preinjury status is also important for setting realistic expectations for rehabilitation, in that prognosis is best predicted by preinjury IQ (Reynolds, 1981b; Reynolds & Stanton, in press). Psychosocial factors that may have increased the predisposition for TBI should also be assessed, as these factors may affect the outcome of rehabilitation (Boll & Stanford, 1997).

In estimating preinjury status, it is necessary to obtain a complete educational and developmental history. A number of forms exist for this purpose. The Structured Developmental History (SDH) of the *Behavior Assessment System for Children* (BASC; Reynolds and Kamphaus, 1992) is one example of a developmental history form. Most of these forms, including the SDH, can be completed by interview or independently by the parents. The SDH solicits information specific to the prenatal, perinatal, and postnatal early childhood development, medical problems and concerns, exposure to formal education, progress in school, and so on. It also asks for information specific to the family situation, living quarters, leisure activities of the child, preferred activities, and so on. Estimation of preinjury ability is best obtained from previous, individualized, standardized cognitive or achievement tests or if this is unavailable, from school records of group-administered, standardized tests, with some consideration for potential regression effects (Reynolds, 1997c). If the school district used a screening measure prior to or at the time of school entry, review of this may also be helpful, particularly for the younger child who has not yet taken group-administered tests. For school-age children, the educational history can also be supplemented with a complete review of educational records, including portfolios or work folders, report cards, attendance records, school health records, and discipline records.

Because preinjury personality and behavior may be predisposing factors for children and adults with TBI (Chadwick, Rutter, Brown, Shaffer, & Traub, 1981; Rutter, 1981; Rutter, Chadwick, & Shaffer, 1983), it is important to assess these areas. It is particularly important to identify any maladaptive behaviors that may interfere with rehabilitation (Chadwick et al.). It may therefore be helpful to have the child's parents and current teacher complete a behavior rating scale (e.g., the Parent Rating Scale and the Teacher Rating Scale of the BASC) based on the child's behavior for the 6 months prior to the injury. Depending on the severity of the injury and the presence of discrete deficits that affect adaptive behavior, it may be appropriate to also complete an interview-format adaptive behavior scale (e.g., *Vineland Adaptive Behavior Scales;* Sparrow, Balla, & Cicchetti, 1984) with the parents, specific to preinjury functioning. Clearly, retrospective ratings of behavior and adaptive skills are best completed prior to the child's return to home or school, so that the ratings are not biased by postinjury functioning.

In estimating preinjury functioning, it is important to keep a few things in mind. With the continuous and rapid development of the child, it is often difficult to obtain sufficient consistency from the preinjury history (Batchelor, 1996a). For very young children, standardized information (individual or group) is not generally available. Prenatal, perinatal, and postnatal developmental histories may be inaccurate, incomplete, or unknown (Batchelor, Gray, Dean, & Lowery, 1988; Gray, Dean, & Rattan, 1987). Even in school-age children, teacher reports, grades, and so on may result in inaccurate estimations of preinjury ability (Reynolds, 1997c). These concerns, however, do not preclude obtaining a comprehensive picture of the child's preinjury functioning.

Cognitive Functioning

Assessment should include measures of the child's cognitive skills. This will generally include an assessment of general intellectual ability (*g*) using a comprehensive IQ test. Assessment of cognition with a strong measure of *g* is essential in providing a baseline for the interpretation of other aspects of the assessment process. Although any of the major intelligence tests may serve this purpose, only the *Kaufman Assessment Battery for Children* (K-ABC; Kaufman & Kaufman, 1983a, 1983b) was specifically developed with current neuropsychological models of higher order thinking (Reynolds & Kamphaus, 1997). The K-ABC is based on the Luria-Das model of successive/simultaneous processing (Das et al., 1979), in conjunction with the cerebral lateralization research by Sperry (1968, 1974), Kinsbourne (1975), and others. Rather than basing lateralization on content or method of presentation, as is done on the Wechsler scales, the lateralization component of the K-ABC is based on how the information is processed. Within each scale, mode of presentation and response varies, allowing for further evaluation of complex functional systems (Reynolds & Kamphaus, 1997).

The K-ABC is a good complement to other neuropsychological tests, providing information useful in differential diagnosis of right hemisphere dysfunction that is consistent with physical evidence (Morris & Bigler, 1985; Shapiro & Dotan, 1985). It is also sensitive to TBI in specific cortical regions (Donders, 1992). K-ABC interpretation is intended to identify not only the neuropsychological strengths of the child, but also the related instructional methods and activities that will capitalize on these strengths and circumvent deficit areas (Riccio & Reynolds, 1998). The variation in content and method of presentation allows the neuropsychologist to tease out any modality or content effects for a specific child. For children under age 5, the K-ABC may well be the test of choice (Reynolds, Kamphaus, et al., 1997). The use of sample and teaching items adds to the likelihood that a neurological substrate is being assessed, as opposed to language, experience, or culture (Reynolds & Kamphaus, 1997). The K-ABC has strong validity and reliability (Kamphaus, 1993), is sensitive to developmental changes in information processing (Reynolds & Kamphaus, 1997), and is considered an appropriate instrument for use with ethnic minorities (e.g., Fan, Willson, & Reynolds, 1995; Kamphaus & Reynolds, 1987).

Regardless of the measure used for assessment of cognitive functioning (*g*), it may also be appropriate to supplement with additional language measures. Difficulties in language areas are not infrequent among children or adults with TBI and are often subtle (Williams & Boll, 1997). Additionally, measures of language provide for assessment of anterior (expressive language) and posterior (receptive language) brain function. The major neuropsychological batteries include some language components, as do the majority of measures of general cognitive ability.

Sensory and Motor Functioning

As previously noted, assessment should sample the relative efficiency of the right and left hemispheres of the brain, as well as anterior and posterior regions of cortical function. When results of sensory and motor tasks are combined with the cognitive assessment, the four major quadrants of the neocortex can be evaluated. This is important because differing brain systems are involved to some extent in each hemisphere, and asymmetry of function can have implications for treatment. Similarly, the anterior of the brain is generally viewed as subserving differing functions (e.g., regulatory), as opposed to the posterior region of the brain (receptivity). Even in a diffuse injury, it is possible to find greater impact to one area of the brain than to others. Specific neuropsychological batteries such as the *Halstead-Reitan Neuropsychological Battery* (HRNB; Reitan & Davison, 1974), the *Reitan-Indiana Neuropsychological Battery* (RINB; Reitan, 1969), and the *Luria Nebraska Neuropsychological Battery–Children's Revision* (LNNB–CR; Golden, 1984) are often used with intelligence tests in neuropsychological assessment; they provide a sampling of sensory and motor functions and additional information relating to hemisphere and anterior–posterior differences.

The HRNB and RINB are both downward extensions of the original adult version of the battery and are considered to be the most widely used in clinical practice (Howieson & Lezak, 1992; Nussbaum & Bigler, 1997). These batteries contain numerous measures necessary for understanding brain behavior relationships. Areas of functioning tapped by these batteries include concept formation, sensory abilities, attention/concentration, motor speed and dexterity, verbal abilities, and memory. Both the HRNB and RINB incorporate a multiple inferential approach to interpretation. This includes examination of level of performance, pathognomonic signs, patterns of performance, and right–left differences (Reitan, 1986, 1987). A brief description of the functional domains covered by the HRNB is provided in Table 5.2. (For a more detailed description of tasks, see Reitan & Wolfson, 1985, 1988; Riccio & Reynolds, 1998.)

The neurodevelopmental stages of the child provide the basis for the LNNB–CR (Golden, 1981, 1997). The various tasks provide information

Table 5.2

Functional Domains of the *Halstead-Reitan Neuropsychological Battery for Children* (Ages 9–14 Years)

Subtest	Function assessed
Category Test	Assesses general abstraction and concept formation as well as general neuropsychological functioning.
Tactual Performance Test	Measures tactual discrimination, sensory recognition, and spatial memory. The drawing component is a measure of incidental learning/memory.
Speech Sounds Perception	Measures alertness, attention, concentration, and verbal ability.
Seashore Rhythm Test	Is an indicator of generalized cerebral function and a measure of alertness and attention/concentration.
Trail Making Test	Measures conceptual flexibility, symbolic recognition, and visual tracking under time constraints. It is also used as a measure of overall functioning.
Finger Oscillation Test	Measures motor speed, manual dexterity, and lateral dominance.
Aphasia Screening Test	Measures verbal ability and the verbal-to-motor process.
Sensory Perceptual Examination	All measure receptive sensory function.
Tactile Perception	
Auditory Perception	
Visual Perception	
Tactile Form Recognition	Measures tactile perception and attention.
Finger-Tip Number Writing	Measures sensory perceptual functioning.
Grip Strength Test	Measures motor functioning and lateral dominance.

Note. Functions identified are based on Nussbaum & Bigler, 1997; Reitan & Wolfson, 1985, 1988; Selz, 1981.

specific to motor, rhythm, tactile, visual, verbal (receptive and expressive), and memory functions. Interpretation of the LNNB–CR focuses predominantly on scale patterns (intraindividual differences), as opposed to levels of performance or pathognomonic signs. The LNNB–CR is sensitive to deficits in language and rhythm (Geary & Gilger, 1984). It is also more sensitive than either cognitive or achievement measures to improvement in functioning following medical intervention (e.g., shunt placement) (Torkelson, Leibrook, Gustavson, & Sundell, 1985). This sensitivity to changes in functioning may make the LNNB–CR the preferred measure for following up on rehabilitation efforts for children with TBI. A brief description of the functional domains assessed with the LNNB–CR is provided in Table 5.3. (For a more detailed description, see Golden, 1997; Riccio & Reynolds, in press.)

Academic Achievement

Assessment of basic academic skills including reading, written language, and mathematics is also important in determining the need for classroom modifications or remediation efforts. In general, the most recently acquired skills will be the most affected by TBI (Golden, Zillmer, & Spiers, 1992). A standardized battery such as the *Woodcock-Johnson Psychoeducational Battery–Revised–Tests of Achievement* (Woodcock & Johnson, 1989) can provide information on the child's current functioning in major academic areas. Standardized measures of achievement, however, are generally untimed, and children with mild TBI show impairment on timed measures, although they do not demonstrate specific cognitive or academic deficits (Chadwick et al., 1981). Chadwick and colleagues suggested that standardized measures of reading may be less sensitive to the effects of TBI, as compared to timed measures.

Due to the potential for more subtle deficits with TBI, as well as the need for repeated, serial assessment, curriculum-based measurement (CBM) is recommended as a component of academic assessment (Shaw & Yingst, 1992). CBM is a fluency-based model for academic assessment; results are based on the amount of work completed in a specific time frame, usually 1 minute (Deno, 1989; Shinn, Nolet, & Knutson, 1990). The use of a fluency-based measure is important given the findings of Chadwick et al. (1981) and other indications that children with TBI are often slow in processing or retrieving needed information (Shaw & Yingst). This reduced rate of processing can have cumulative effects on long-term educational progress (Chadwick et al.). Fluency-based measures such as CBM are also more sensitive to changes over time (Fuchs & Shinn, 1989). Because CBM is time limited, it can be repeated frequently, thus providing ongoing feedback on the efficacy of the rehabilitation process. It should be noted that CBM is included primarily for monitoring intraindividual change. If local norms are available, they may give some indication of how the child's fluency compares to that of peers, but they will not necessarily have the reliability and validity of other norm-referenced measures.

Table 5.3

Functional Domains of the *Luria Nebraska Neuropsychological Battery–Children's Revision*

Scale	Function assessed
C1 (Motor)	Measures motor domains but is sensitive to many types of problems.
C2 (Rhythm)	Is most sensitive to attention and concentration.
C3 (Tactile)	Measures the extent of cutaneous sensation and stereognostic perception.
C4 (Visual)	Measures visuospatial organization and perception as well as right hemisphere function.
C5 (Receptive Speech)	Measures receptive language and auditory skills as well as left hemisphere function.
C6 (Expressive Speech)	Measures expressive language and left hemisphere function. Results may be affected by reading ability.
C7 (Writing)	Measures visual motor and auditory motor abilities, and is believed to measure functioning of the temporal-parietal-occipital area.
C8 (Reading)	Measures reading ability and left hemisphere function.
C9 (Arithmetic)	Measures arithmetic skills, but is most sensitive to educational deficits and dysfunction.
C10 (Memory)	Measures short-term memory functions and is most sensitive to verbal dysfunction.
C11 (Intellectual)	Is reflective of general neuropsychological function, concept formation, and reasoning.

Note. Functions are based on "The Nebraska neuropsychological children's battery," by C. J. Golden, 1997, in C. R. Reynolds and E. Fletcher-Janzen (Eds.), *Handbook of Clinical Child Neuropsychology* (2nd ed., pp. 237–251), New York: Grune & Stratton.

Learning, Memory, Attention, and Executive Function

Neither standardized achievement tests nor CBM directly tap into many of the behaviors and abilities necessary for success in the classroom. As a result, areas of learning and memory, attention, and executive function should also be assessed. Problems with memory, learning new information, and attention are the most common complaints following any type of CNS compromise, and are often subtle (Gillberg, 1995; Reynolds & Bigler, 1997a). Children with mild to moderate TBI are likely to demonstrate adequate levels of academic achievement. This does not, however, mean that there are no long-term or residual deficits that might interfere with learning new information.

Learning and memory. Although able to demonstrate expected levels of achievement, children with TBI may have difficulty in storing and retrieving information that is necessary for future learning (Ewing-Cobbs, Fletcher, & Levin, 1985; Lezak, 1986; Ryan et al., 1996). For example, children with TBI frequently show impaired storage and retrieval processes, with the degree of impairment related to the severity of the head injury (Levin & Eisenberg, 1979). Research across neurological disorders points to the importance of assessing memory to effectively evaluate brain integrity (Reynolds & Bigler, 1997a). Because memory involves a number of interconnections throughout the brain, damage to one or more of the structures involved in memory can affect the formation or retrieval process. The assessment of learning and memory can also provide useful information and have direct implications for treatment planning (Wasserman, 1995).

Historically, the assessment of memory in children was derived from specific subtests of the various cognitive batteries (e.g., Branch, Cohen, & Hynd, 1995; Nussbaum et al., 1988), particularly Digit Span subtests from the Wechsler scales. A number of concerns with the reliance on Digit Span or similar subtests can be found in the literature (e.g., Reynolds, 1997a; Talley, 1986), particularly concern about combining forward and backward digits (Ramsey & Reynolds, 1995; Reynolds, 1997a). In the past 5 to 10 years, three comprehensive measures for the assessment of memory and learning have been developed specifically for children; the various components or subtests of these measures are provided in Table 5.4.

The first of the measures developed for the assessment of memory in children was the *Wide Range Assessment of Memory and Learning* (WRAML; Sheslow & Adams, 1990). As indicated in Table 5.4, the WRAML consists of 12 subtests and yields verbal memory, visual memory, and learning scores. Delayed recall trials can be given for four of the subtests. The WRAML is a substantial improvement over previous methods of assessing memory in children. Some concern, however, has been raised about the overlap of attention and memory in the WRAML tasks, and about the absence of a factor associated specifically with attention/concentration (Haut, Haut, Callahan, & Franzen, 1992). The WRAML visual memory scale is also contaminated heavily by verbal mediation.

The *Test of Memory and Learning* (TOMAL; Reynolds & Bigler, 1994) consists of 10 core subtests that yield verbal memory, nonverbal memory, and composite scores. As with the WRAML, the TOMAL includes a delayed recall procedure that yields a delayed recall index. In addition, the TOMAL provides a number of supplemental indices (e.g., sequential recall, free recall, attention/concentration, and learning) that may provide additional insight

Table 5.4

Subtests of Memory Scales used with Children

WRAML	TOMAL	CMS
Core subtests:		
Number/Letter Memory	Memory for Stories[a]	Dot Location[a]
Sentence Memory	Word Selective Reminding[a]	Stories[a, b]
Story Memory[a]	Object Recall	Faces[a]
Verbal Learning[a]	Digits Forward	Word Pairs[a, b]
Finger Windows	Paired Recall	Numbers
Design Memory	Facial Memory[a]	Sequences
Picture Memory	Visual Selective Reminding[a]	
Visual Learning[a]	Abstract Visual Memory	
Sound Symbol[a]	Visual Sequential Memory	
	Memory for Location	
Supplementary subtests:		
None	Letters Forward	Family Pictures
	Digits Backward	Word Lists
	Letters Backward	Picture Locations
	Manual Imitation	
Summary scores:		
Verbal Memory Scale	Verbal Memory Index	Verbal Immediate
Visual Memory Scale	Nonverbal Memory Index	Visual Immediate
Learning Scale	Composite Memory Index	General Memory
Delayed Recall	Delayed Recall Index	Learning
		Verbal Delayed
		Visual Delayed
		Attention/Concentration
		Delayed Recognition
Supplementary indexes:		
None	Sequential Recall Index	None
		Free Recall Index
		Associative Recall Index
		Learning Index
		Attention/Concentration Index
Factor scores (empirically derived):		
None	Complex Memory Factor	None
	Sequential Recall Factor	
	Backwards Recall Factor	
	Spatial Memory Factor	

Note. WRAML = *Wide Range Assessment of Learning and Memory;* TOMAL = *Test of Memory and Learning;* CMS = *Children's Memory Scale.*

[a]Subtests used for Delayed Recall

[b]Subtests used for Delayed Recognition

into the child's specific deficits. Unlike many neuropsychological measures (Reynolds, 1997b), the TOMAL included studies of ethnic and gender bias during standardization, and items showing cultural bias were eliminated. The TOMAL has been described as "the most comprehensive of its kind" and "will undoubtedly be a useful tool for assessing memory function" (Ferris & Kamphaus, 1996, p. 254). The variety of well normed and reliable subtests, as well as the capability to group subtests in a variety of ways, provides increased flexibility in the assessment of memory function (Reynolds & Bigler, 1997b). Further, the inclusion of multiple trials to criterion (e.g., on selective reminding) enables the neuropsychologist to derive learning or acquisition curves. The TOMAL Nonverbal Memory Index subtests are also truly nonverbal and difficult to reconstruct through verbal mediation.

The most recent addition to comprehensive measures of memory available for children is the *Children's Memory Scale* (CMS; Cohen, 1997). The composition of the CMS was based on extensive clinical practice with children with neurologically based disorders. The CMS consists of six core subtests that represent verbal memory, attention/concentration, and visual/nonverbal memory. As with the TOMAL, the CMS provides for evaluation of immediate and delayed recall. Seven index scores can be calculated to examine differences between immediate and delayed verbal and visual memory, learning, recognition, and attention/concentration (Cohen). As such, the CMS can provide important information regarding specific deficits and information relevant to intervention planning; however, extensive research on using the CMS with children with TBI has not been completed yet.

Attention. The most frequent symptoms associated with childhood neuropsychological disorder are attention/concentration, self-regulation, and emotional/behavioral problems (Nussbaum & Bigler, 1990). This is also true for children with TBI (Lezak, 1986; Marlowe, 1992; Mateer & Williams, 1991), and the symptoms are most often associated with frontal lobe damage (e.g., Mateer & Williams). Not only can attention/concentration affect self-regulation and emotional/behavioral problems, but it is the neural traces left by attention that are likely the root of memory. As such, the measurement of attentional processes is important in the initial assessment and throughout the rehabilitation process. The TOMAL has an Attention and Concentration Index that is designed to assist in differentiating memory from attention.

Attention has been described as "the most difficult cognitive construct to compartmentalize and quantify" (Williams & Boll, 1997, p. 248). It is a multidimensional construct including alertness, selective attention, sustained attention or vigilance, and more (Barkley, 1988). Children with TBI often have the most difficulty with selective and sustained attention (Williams & Boll). A number of measures have been developed for the assessment of selective and sustained attention. These include a variety of cancellation tasks, reaction-time tasks, the *Children's Embedded Figures Test* (CEFT; Witkin, Oltman,

Raskin, & Karp, 1971), the *Matching Familiar Figures Task* (MFFT; Kagan, Rosman, Day, Albert, & Phillips, 1964), and continuous performance tasks.

One of the most frequently employed measures of attention is some version of the continuous performance test (CPT) (Halperin, 1991). The initial CPT was developed in the 1950s (Rosvold, Mirsky, Sarason, Bransome, & Beck, 1956). Currently, there are a variety of CPTs available with variations in modality, type of stimuli, and nature of the task (Halperin). The basic paradigm for all CPTs is selective attention or vigilance for an infrequently occurring stimulus (Eliason & Richman, 1987). CPTs are characterized by the rapid presentation of changing stimuli, with a "target" stimulus or pattern. In one variation, the response is inhibited when the target is presented (e.g., Conners, 1995). Studies of CPTs dating from Rosvold and colleagues to the present provide evidence that CPTs are sensitive to brain damage or dysfunction (e.g., Chadwick et al., 1981; Timmermans & Christenson, 1991). CPTs can also provide information specific to attentional deficits associated with TBI or other neurological disorders (Timmermans & Christensen), and despite problems with specificity, are considered better measures of sustained attention than simple reaction-time tasks (Williams & Boll, 1997). There is not sufficient comparative research with the various CPTs available to suggest that one is best. Consistent with the idea of multimodal assessment, it may be best to ensure that assessment of attentional processes includes both auditory and visual modalities.

CPTs can be helpful not only in the initial assessment of attentional processes, but also throughout the rehabilitation process. CPTs are useful in monitoring both intentional and unintentional effects of medications (e.g., Aman, Kern, McGhee, & Arnold, 1993; Aman & Turbott, 1991; Conners et al., 1996), as well as the effects of other treatments including cognitive training (e.g., Benedict et al., 1994). It is not unusual for children with TBI to be prescribed medication to prevent postinjury seizures (Bigler, 1987). At least some anti-seizure medications negatively affect processing skills including attention (Skilbeck, 1984), and the impact of these medications on attention and on learning and memory needs to be monitored. The BASC ADHD Monitor (Kamphaus & Reynolds, 1998) may also be useful in monitoring attentional processes and impulsivity during rehabilitation. Although specific to Attention-Deficit/Hyperactivity Disorder, this system allows the clinician to graph changes in behavior and document intervention effectiveness over time.

Executive function. Even though a child with TBI may demonstrate IQ and achievement consistent with preinjury status, higher order processes associated with planning, organization, and problem solving (judgment) may be impaired. More precisely, those behaviors believed to constitute executive function include the ability to maintain an appropriate problem-solving set for attainment of a goal (Luria, 1966; Zelazo, Carter, Reznick, & Frye, 1997), mental representation of a task (Luria, 1966), planning and self-monitoring of behavior (e.g., Zelazo et al.), and the ability to use environmental cues effectively (Passler, Isaac, & Hynd, 1985). From a brain–behavior relationship perspective, executive processes are related to the frontal and prefrontal areas. When TBI damage is discrete and localized to the frontal area, assessment of executive function has increased importance. Diffuse damage resulting from TBI can also affect executive function, as the frontal lobes constitute a complex neurological and functional system (Luria, 1966; Welsh & Pennington, 1988). Case studies of children with damage to the frontal lobe (focal and nonfocal) as a result of TBI found that these children had difficulty with self-regulation and ability to carry out a plan or strategy (Marlowe, 1992; Mateer & Williams, 1991). Developmentally, because the frontal and prefrontal areas continue to mature through adolescence, age at the time of injury may have a significant impact on executive functioning. At the same time, due to the developmental nature of executive function, the ability to assess it in children will be limited; for some aspects (those that normally develop later), assessment immediately postinjury will not be feasible.

The domain of executive function may incorporate a variety of constructs (e.g., attention, self-regulation, working memory), but the "executive" processes focus on effortful and flexible organization, strategic planning, and proactive reasoning (Denckla, 1994). The measurement of executive function in children is made exceptionally difficult due to the ongoing development and maturation of the frontal lobes through adolescence. Factor analytic study of executive function tasks (Welsh, Pennington, & Grossier, 1991) yielded factors that appeared to be based on developmentally related constructs rather than theoretical ones (Denckla, 1994). The majority of executive function measures used with children are downward extensions of adult measures, and many lack sufficient normative data and psychometric study. Those most frequently used include the *Wisconsin Card Sorting Test* (WCST; Heaton, 1981) and the *Children's Category Test* (CCT; Boll, 1993). Measures of executive function have also been found to be related to intelligence (Chelune & Thompson, 1987; Riccio et al., 1994) as well as internalized language (Denckla, 1996). In addition, the emphasis on the use of novel tasks in assessment of executive function places significant limitations on the evaluation of interventions in the area of executive processes. Torgesen (1994) stated that there is a need to include assessment of tasks that are ecologically based and require executive function in order to enhance evaluation of treatment programs designed to remediate executive processes. Certainly, child-centered, developmentally sensitive measures of executive processing that are more directly linked to real life activities for the development of interventions, and have sufficient flexibility to allow for pre- and post-evaluation, are needed.

Emotional/Behavioral Status

Any type of CNS compromise is likely to change personality and behavior and affect neurocognitive functioning. In addition to potential difficulties in learning and memory, attention, and other executive processes, children with TBI sometimes demonstrate increased irritability and fatigue, which can compound academic difficulties and lead to decreased self-esteem (Ryan et al., 1996). This increase in irritability and fatigue, along with possible impulsivity, forgetfulness, and distractibility, strains interpersonal relations (Boll, 1983; Boll & Stanford, 1997; Martin, 1988). Brooks and McKinlay (1983) found that in 50% of cases, family members complained of mood changes, temper, irritability, and so on following TBI. Conduct disorder (Haak, 1989), anger control, social problems, and adjustment disorders (Hynd & Willis, 1988) are also frequent in children and youth with TBI. For children who are aware of loss of skills and status, frustration and despair may impede the rehabilitation process (Kraus, Fife, & Conroy, 1987). Alternatively, children with TBI may have an impaired self-awareness (Boll & Stanford). Depending on the mechanism of injury (e.g., child abuse), children may also experience various symptoms associated with posttraumatic stress disorder (Bijur, Haslum, & Golding, 1990). Prigatano (1992) provided a review of postinjury behavioral/emotional problems associated with TBI.

The most common approach to emotional/behavioral assessment relies on published rating scales, of which there are many. A multifaceted approach that includes parent and teacher rating scales, self-report measures, direct observation, and clinical interviews provides the most comprehensive, broad-based view of the child's emotional and behavioral status (Semrud-Clikeman, Kamphaus, Teeter, & Vaughn, 1997). The BASC includes not only teacher and parent forms, but also a structured observation system (SOS), and for children over age 9, a self-report measure that can effectively assess emotional and behavioral status. Particularly over the short term, direct observation may be more appropriate for monitoring smaller and gradual changes. Direct observation also provides an objective measure without the potential bias of raters, and can be especially useful when raters (e.g., parent and teacher) disagree in their portrayal of the child. Another advantage to the BASC (rating scales and SOS) is the inclusion of positive adaptive behaviors (e.g., social skills, adaptability to change in the environment) in addition to the more common maladaptive skills included on many rating scales. Where adaptive behavior is an identified concern, completion of an adaptive behavior scale (e.g., *Vineland Adaptive Behavior Scales*), using both the parent interview and classroom edition, may be particularly helpful for intervention planning.

Environmental Variables

For children, the nature and persistence of learning problems are dependent not only on the developmental status of various brain structures, effects of the injury, and interactions between functional and dysfunctional neurological systems, but also on environmental influences (Teeter & Semrud-Clikeman, 1997). For this reason, a more transactional approach (see Teeter

& Semrud-Clikeman) to neuropsychological assessment is needed. Rutter (1981) found that adverse psychosocial factors affected the eventual psychiatric outcome of children with TBI; 20% to 25% of children from adverse environments had higher frequency of psychiatric or behavioral disorders. Adverse environmental factors include crowded living conditions and marital or familial dysfunction (Klonoff, 1971). Socioeconomic status has been a confounding factor in some studies (e.g., Klonoff, 1971; Rutter, Chadwick, Shaffer, & Brown, 1980), but not in others (Chadwick et al., 1981). As already noted, comprehensive assessment needs to include the contexts in which the child is expected to function, and the supports and services available through these contexts. These contexts include both home and school.

Family/home setting. As noted, the behavioral and functional changes that may accompany TBI can produce additional stress on the family. The family is often disrupted as a result of TBI, with the extent of disruption directly related to the severity of the injury (Brooks & McKinlay, 1983; McLaughlin & Schaffer, 1985; Zarski, Hall, & DePompei, 1987). There is little empirical data on family adjustment or the effectiveness of family-based interventions (Waaland & Kreutzer, 1988). The family may react with denial or may avoid dealing with necessary issues (Ryan et al., 1996). Professionals who work with the parents may find that the parents' hopes are unrealistic (McGuire & Rothenberg, 1986). When the head injury is mild and medical professionals assure that there is no structural damage, there may be an increased likelihood of denial of more subtle problems and inappropriate reactions to behavioral changes in the child. Families need support and concrete information about their child's status and prognosis (Rosenthal & Young, 1988), but medical professionals may not realize or effectively address parental concerns (Casey, Ludwig, & McCormick, 1987). The importance of the family to long-term recovery and adjustment following TBI has been recognized for some time (Kreutzer, Marwitz, & Kepler, 1992; Williams & Kay, 1991). It has been suggested, in fact, that the ability of the family to provide support is a significant predictor of recovery (Rosenthal, 1984). Thus, some type of assessment (quantitative or qualitative) is needed to determine the impact of the child's TBI on the family, and the extent to which family-based intervention should be included as part of the rehabilitation program. At the same time, the supports and services available through the family need to be identified.

School setting. Schools are the second major environment in which children must function. Eventually, the child with TBI will return to school or another educational setting. Schools in many ways have the greatest long-term effect on outcome, as the resources and support available from the school district will be with the child through graduation. In addition to the contribution of factors related to the child and family, the resources of the school system also affect the realization of the goal of graduation, as well as optimal recovery. For children, rehabilitation efforts focus on the goal of reintegration into school, preferably the regular education classroom (Ryan et al., 1996). To be successful, rehabilitation needs to be coordinated with the school system. It may be appropriate to assess resources available in the schools and arrange inservice training for educators and administrators as needed. A majority of educators may not be well prepared for the variability in functioning of children with TBI (Lehr, 1990). As a result, school personnel may have inaccurate expectations (either too high or too low) and inaccurate perceptions of the child with TBI (Rothlisberg & D'Amato, 1996). It is particularly important that educators understand the variability of intraindividual deficits and strengths and the potential for recovery at varying rates (Ryan et al., 1996).

Translating Assessment Information to Rehabilitation

As previously discussed, the data generated from assessments are used to make inferences about the integrity of various functional systems of the brain, and to identify specific deficits and intact functional systems. Inferences are made about specific behaviors that were assessed and about skills that were not assessed. However, neuropsychological assessment has been criticized (e.g., Little & Stavrou, 1993; Reschley & Gresham, 1989) for not providing information directly related to rehabilitation or intervention planning. In contrast, the comprehensive nature of the neuropsychological evaluation is necessary to support inferences that lead to recommendations for rehabilitation programming. The impression that neuropsychological assessment does not transfer to rehabilitation programming may be partly due to the fact that neuropsychological reports are often written expressly for medical personnel or acute care facilities from a biomedical model (Fletcher-Janzen & Kade, 1997).

Test results need to be presented so that parents and educators can understand both the abilities and problems facing the child postinjury. The immediate goal of rehabilitation for children with TBI, and therefore a focus of the assessment process, is the return to school. Teachers and parents look to the neuropsychological assessment for information on current status and some indication of prognosis. As noted by others (e.g., Kamphaus, 1993; Reynolds & Mayfield, in press), reports should be written in language that is easily understood by nonmedical persons; where jargon is unavoidable, concrete examples or explanations should be provided. The purpose of the report is to communicate the results to the parent, teacher, and others and to provide information needed for the development of an appropriate program. The focus of the report should be on the child and the child's level of functioning, as opposed to tests. Results need to clearly address any academic, learning, or behavioral concerns and reflect the instructional level of the child. The report should provide a summation and integration of all the data presented and include any diagnostic conclusions. Finally, treatment implications should be provided by the neuropsychologist.

Based on both quantitative and qualitative data, inferences are made regarding rehabilitation. This inferential process needs to take into consideration not only the type and number of systems impaired, but also the nature, extent, and characteristics of the impairments (Reynolds & Mayfield, in press; Riccio & Reynolds, in press). This information is then taken together with information on the type, number, and nature and characteristics of the functional systems that remain intact. The quality of the neuropsychological strengths, as evidenced by intraindividual (ipsative) comparison, is also important. Intraindividual strengths or weaknesses in planning and concept formation skills, as well as in other areas, will have an important effect on the long-term prognosis and the selection of rehabilitation options (Reynolds & Mayfield).

It has been suggested that a neurodevelopmental rather than a biomedical approach be used in explaining the impact of TBI in children, to facilitate translation into rehabilitation planning (Fletcher-Janzen & Kade, 1997). The neurodevelopmental perspective incorporates the neuropsychological model (emphasis on dysfunction and potential growth) rather than the biomedical model (emphasis on treatment). The neuropsychological model is nonlinear, has proven heuristic value, and presumes that learning occurs (Fletcher-Janzen & Kade). This orientation may help parents and educators understand the tenuousness of results obtained immediately postinjury, and the potential for recovery of function. This is extremely important so that "brain injury" is not interpreted as a hopeless situation. The changing nature of symptoms and the need for frequent re-assessment of the child can also be presented from the neurodevelopmental perspective. As assessment for most disorders occurs only every 3 years, it is important to ensure that parents and school personnel understand why more frequent assessment occurs with TBI.

Recommendations need to include information about whether the child would most likely benefit from remediation, compensatory training, or some combination, and make clear that this may vary from one deficit area to another. Potential instructional materials or methods that may be best suited to the child should also be indicated (Reynolds et al., 1997). Neuropsychological results provide information about the appropriateness of using specific types of interventions, such as neurocognitive therapy, or a specific group of interventions, such as cognitive behavioral therapy (Reynolds & Mayfield, in press). From a neuropsychological and neurodevelopmental perspective, treatment needs to be flexible and have a broad scope that is efficient and integrated and promotes growth (Fletcher-Janzen & Kade, 1997). Based on assessment of environmental factors and expectations, any environmental modifications that may facilitate the child's academic reintegration need to be identified. These may include variations in the child's daily schedule if fatigue is an issue, more time allowed for tasks if slowed processing is evident, or the use of educational support materials (e.g., computers, calculators, tape recorders). With the current emphasis on cost containment, involvement of school personnel and family members in service delivery and on the treatment team can help ensure necessary and broad-based services (Fletcher-Janzen & Kade, 1997; Haak & Livingston, 1997). Although the recommendations on rehabilitation programming that are provided in the neuropsychological report may not be exhaustive, there should be enough information to assist in developing an appropriate intervention that meets the child's needs.

Conclusions

Neuropsychological assessment and clinical child neuropsychology in general have much to offer toward an understanding of the functional systems of the brain and the mechanisms involved in learning and self-regulation. Child neuropsychology provides a theoretical framework for understanding identified patterns of strengths and weaknesses, the relationships between strengths and weaknesses, and the extent to which these patterns may remain stable or change over time (Fletcher & Taylor, 1984; Temple, 1997). Increased understanding of the child's strengths and weaknesses can be used to identify areas that may later provide difficulty for the child, as well as compensatory strategies or methods to circumvent these difficulties. This is particularly important for children with TBI where one or more of the functional systems has been disrupted, and there is potential for disruption of the neurodevelopmental trajectory that will affect long-term and current functioning. For the child with mild TBI whose difficulties may be more subtle due to diffuse damage, disruption of functional systems may not be seen immediately postinjury, but may have long-term effects on the child's outcome.

Neuropsychological assessment can be translated into information that is relevant to the development of rehabilitation programs and the identification of needed accommodations in various contexts. Comprehensive neuropsychological assessment can identify the subtle deficits associated with mild TBI, which may be missed in a more traditional psychological evaluation, help predict how these deficits may affect long-term outcome, and help identify appropriate remediation or compensation strategies. For all children with TBI, neuropsychological assessment that examines the contexts in which the child is expected to function, and incorporates the potential resources of these environments, can make a positive outcome from rehabilitation more likely.

There are, however, some continued problems in the practice of child neuropsychology. Historically, neuropsychological assessment of children has taken its lead from research and practice with adults. Issues relating to neurodevelopment, task appropriateness, varying contexts for children, progression following brain injury with children, and so on render a continuation of this approach inappropriate. A variety of theoretical models exist; however, many of these are adult-based and do not consider developmental issues. Continued methodological and measurement problems in the research that serves as a foundation for interpretation of neuropsychological data impede progress in the field of clinical child neuropsychology, and affect the accuracy of diagnosis and appropriateness of treatment planning. Lack of attention to standard psychometric methods within the field of clinical neuropsychology is all too rampant and poses serious limitations to research; intuitive appeal, clinical acumen, and perceived utility are not sufficient, but must be combined with sound empirical research (Reynolds, 1986a, 1997b).

References

Allen, C. (1989). Why use neuropsychology in the schools? *The Neuro-Transmitter, 1,* 1–2.

Aman, M. G., Kern, R. A., McGhee, D. E., & Arnold, L. E. (1993). Fenfluramine and methylphenidate in children with mental retardation and attention deficit hyperactivity disorder: Laboratory effects. *Journal of Autism and Developmental Disorders, 23,* 491–506.

Aman, M. G., & Turbott, S. H. (1991). Prediction of clinical response in children taking methylphenidate. *Journal of Autism and Developmental Disorders, 21,* 211–228.

Ardila, A., & Roselli, M. (1994). Development of language, memory, and visuospatial abilities in 5- to 12-year old children using a neuropsychological battery. *Developmental Neuropsychology, 10,* 97–120.

Ayers, A. J. (1974). *Sensory integration and learning disorders.* Los Angeles: Western Psychological Services.

Ball, J. D., & Zinner, E. S. (1994). Pediatric brain injury: Psychoeducation for parents and teachers. *Advances in Medical Psychotherapy, 7,* 39–50.

Barkley, R. A. (1988). The effects of methylphenidate on interactions of preschool ADHD children with their mothers. *Journal of the American Academy of Child and Adolescent Psychiatry, 27,* 336–341.

Batchelor, E. S. (1996a). Introduction. In E. S. Batchelor, Jr. & R. S. Dean (Eds.), *Pediatric neuropsychology: Interfacing assessment and treatment for rehabilitation* (pp. 1–8). Boston: Allyn & Bacon.

Batchelor, E. S. (1996b). Neuropsychological assessment of children. In E. S. Batchelor, Jr. & R. S. Dean (Eds.), *Pediatric neuropsychology: Interfacing assessment and treatment for rehabilitation* (pp. 9–26). Boston: Allyn & Bacon.

Batchelor, E. S., Gray, J. W., Dean, R. S., & Lowery, R. (1988). Interactive effects of socioeconomic factors and perinatal complications. *NASA Program Abstracts, F-169,* 115–116.

Benedict, R. H. B., Harris, A. E., Markow, T., McCormick, J. A., Nuechterlein, K. H., & Asarnow, R. F. (1994). The effects of attention training on information processing in schizophrenia. *Schizophrenia Bulletin, 20,* 537–546.

Bigler, E. R. (1987). Acquired cerebral trauma: Epidemiology, neuropsychological assessment, and academic/educational deficits. *Journal of Learning Disabilities, 20,* 516–517.

Bigler, E. R. (1990). *Traumatic brain injury: Mechanisms of damage, assessment, intervention and outcome.* Austin, TX: PRO-ED.

Bijur, P. E., Haslum, M., & Golding, J. (1990). Cognitive and behavioral sequelae of mild head injury in children. *Pediatrics, 86,* 337–344.

Boll, T. J. (1981). The Halstead-Reitan Neuropsychological Battery. In S. Filkov & T. J. Boll (Eds.), *Handbook of clinical neuropsychology* (pp. 577–607). New York: Wiley-Interscience.

Boll, T. J. (1983). Minor head injury in children—out of sight, but not out of mind. *Journal of Clinical Child Psychology, 12,* 74–80.

Boll, T. J. (1993). *The Children's Category Test.* New York: The Psychological Corporation.

Boll, T. J., & Barth, J. T. (1981). Neuropsychology of brain damage in children. In S. B. Filskov and T. J. Boll (Eds.), *Handbook of clinical neuropsychology* (pp. 418–452). New York: Wiley.

Boll, T. J., & Stanford, L. D. (1997). Pediatric brain injury: Brain mechanisms and amelioration. In C. R. Reynolds and E. Fletcher-Janzen (Eds.), *Handbook of clinical child neuropsychology* (2nd ed., pp. 140–156). New York: Plenum.

Bolter, J. F., & Long, C. J. (1985). Methodological issues in research in developmental neuropsychology. In L. Hartlage and C. Telzrow (Eds.), *The neuropsychology of individual differences* (pp. 42–60). New York: Plenum.

Branch, W. B., Cohen, M. J., & Hynd, G. W. (1995). Academic achievement and attention-deficit/hyperactivity disorder in children with left- or right-hemisphere dysfunction. *Journal of Learning Disabilities, 28,* 35–43.

Breslau, N., & Marshall, I. A. (1985). Psychological disturbance in children with physical disabilities: Continuity and change in a 5-year follow-up. *Journal of Abnormal Child Psychology, 13,* 199–216.

Brink, J. D., Garrett, A. L., Hale, W. R., Woo-Sam, J., & Nickel, V. C. (1970). Recovery of motor and intellectual function in children sustaining severe head injuries. *Developmental Medicine and Child Neurology, 12,* 545–571.

Brooks, D. N., & McKinlay, W. (1983). Personality and behavior change after severe blunt head injury: A relative's view. *Journal of Neurology, Neurosurgery, and Psychiatry, 46,* 333–334.

Casey, R., Ludwig, S., & McCormick, M. (1987). Minor head trauma in children: An intervention to decrease functional morbidity. *Pediatrics, 80,* 159–164.

Chadwick, O., Rutter, M., Brown, G., Shaffer, D., & Traub, M. (1981). A prospective study of children with head injuries: II. Cognitive sequelae. *Psychological Medicine, 11,* 49–61.

Chelune, G. J., & Thompson, L. L. (1987). Evaluation of the general sensitivity of the Wisconsin Card Sorting Test among younger and older children. *Developmental Neuropsychology, 3,* 81–89.

Cicchetti, D. V. (1994). Multiple comparison methods: Establishing guidelines for their valid application in neuropsychological research. *Journal of Clinical and Experimental Neuropsychology, 16,* 155–161.

Cohen, M. J. (1997). *The Children's Memory Scale.* San Antonio, TX: The Psychological Corporation.

Cohen, M. J., Branch, W. B., Willis, W. G., Weyandt, L. L., & Hynd, G. W. (1992). Childhood. In A. E. Puente & R. J. McCaffrey (Eds.), *Handbook of neuropsychological assessment* (pp. 49–79). New York: Plenum.

Conners, C. (1995). *Continuous performance test computer program 3.0: User's manual.* Toronto: Multi-Health Systems.

Conners, C. K., Casat, C. D., Gualtieri, T., Weller, E., Reader, M., Reiss, A., Weller, R. A., Khayrallah, M., & Ascher, J. (1996). Bupropion hydrochloride in attention deficit disorder with hyperactivity. *Journal of the American Academy of Child and Adolescent Psychiatry, 34,* 1314–1321.

D'Amato, R. C. (1990). A neuropsychological approach to school psychology. *School Psychology Quarterly, 5,* 141–160.

D'Amato, R. C., & Rothlisberg, B. A. (1996). How education should respond to students with traumatic brain injuries. *Journal of Learning Disabilities, 29,* 670–683.

D'Amato, R. C., Rothlisberg, B. A., & Leu, P. W. (in press). Neuropsychological assessment for intervention. In C. R. Reynolds & T. B. Gutkin (Eds.), *The handbook of school psychology* (3rd ed.). New York: Wiley.

D'Amato, R. C., Rothlisberg, B. A., & Rhodes, R. L. (1997). Utilizing neuropsychological paradigms for understanding common educational and psychological tests. In C. R. Reynolds & E. Fletcher-Janzen (Eds.), *Handbook of clinical child neuropsychology* (2nd ed., pp. 270–295). New York: Plenum.

Das, J. P., Kirby, J. R., & Jarman, R. F. (1979). *Simultaneous and successive cognitive processes.* New York: Academic Press.

Dean, R. S. (1985). Foundation and rationale for neuropsychological bases of individual differences. In L. D. Hartlage & C. F. Telzrow (Eds.), *The neuropsychology of individual differences: A developmental perspective* (pp. 203–244). New York: Plenum.

Dean, R. S. (1986). Lateralization of cerebral functions. In D. Wedding, A. M. Horton, & J. S. Webster (Eds.), *The neuropsychology handbook: Behavioral and clinical perspectives* (pp. 80–102). Berlin: Springer-Verlag.

Dean, R. S., & Gray, J. W. (1990). Traditional approaches to neuropsychological assessment. In C. R. Reynolds & R. W. Kamphaus (Eds.), *Handbook of psychological and educational assessment of children* (pp. 317–388). New York: Guilford.

Denckla, M. B. (1994). Measurement of executive function. In G. R. Lyon (Ed.), *Frames of reference of the assessment of learning disabilities: New views on measurement issues* (pp. 117–142). Baltimore: Brookes.

Denckla, M. B. (1996). A theory and model of executive function: A neuropsychological approach. In G. R. Lyon & N. A. Krasnegor (Eds.), *Attention, memory and executive function* (pp. 263–295). Baltimore: Brookes.

Deno, S. L. (1989). Curriculum based measurement and special education services: A fundamental and direct relationship. In M. R. Shinn (Ed.), *Curriculum-based measurement: Assessing special children* (pp. 1–17). New York: Guilford.

Donders, J. (1992). Validity of the Kaufman Assessment Battery for Children when employed with children with traumatic brain injury. *Journal of Clinical Psychology, 48,* 225–229.

Eliason, M. J., & Richman, L. C. (1987). The continuous performance test in learning disabled and nondisabled children. *Journal of Learning Disabilities, 20,* 614–619.

Ewing–Cobbs, L., Fletcher, J. M., & Levin, H. S. (1985). Neuropsychological sequelae following pediatric head injury. In M. Ylvisaker (Ed.), *Head injury rehabilitation: Children and adolescents* (pp. 71–89). Boston: College Hill.

Ewing-Cobbs, L., Fletcher, J. M., & Levin, H. S. (1986). Neurobehavioral sequelae following head injury in children: Educational implications. *Journal of Head Trauma Rehabilitation, 1*(4), 57–65.

Fan, X., Willson, V. L., & Reynolds, C. R. (1995). Assessing the similarity of the construct structure of the KABC for black and white children from 7 to 12½ years in age. *Journal of Psychoeducational Assessment, 13,* 120–131.

Fennell, E. B., & Bauer, R. M. (1997). Models of inference in evaluating brain-behavior relationships in children. In C. R. Reynolds & E. Fletcher-Janzen (Eds.), *Handbook of clinical child neuropsychology* (2nd ed., pp. 204–215). New York: Plenum.

Ferris, L. M., & Kamphaus, R. W. (1996). Review: Test of Memory and Learning. *Archives of Clinical Neuropsychology, 11,* 251–255.

Fletcher, J. M., & Taylor, H. G. (1984). Neuropsychological approaches to children: Toward a developmental neuropsychology. *Journal of Clinical Neuropsychology, 6,* 139–156.

Fletcher-Janzen, E., & Kade, H. D. (1997). Pediatric brain injury rehabilitation in a neurodevelopmental milieu. In C. R. Reynolds & E. Fletcher-Janzen (Eds.), *Handbook of clinical child neuropsychology* (pp. 452–481). New York: Plenum.

Fuchs, L. S., & Shinn, M. R. (1989). Writing CBM IEP Objectives. In M. R. Shinn (Ed.), *Curriculum-based measurement: Assessing special children* (pp. 130–152). New York: Guilford.

Gaddes, W. H. (1983). Applied educational neuropsychology: Theories and problems. *Journal of Learning Disabilities, 16,* 511–514.

Gaddes, W. H., & Edgell, D. (1994). *Learning disabilities and brain function: A neurodevelopmental approach.* New York: Springer-Verlag.

Geary, D. C., & Gilger, J. W. (1984). The Luria-Nebraska Neuropsychological Battery—Children's Revision: Comparison of learning disabled and normal children matched on full scale IQ. *Perceptual and Motor Skills, 58,* 115–118.

Gillberg, C. (1995). *Clinical child neuropsychiatry.* London: Cambridge University Press.

Golden, C. J. (1981). The Luria-Nebraska children's battery: Theory and formulation. In G. W. Hynd & J. E. Obrzut (Eds.), *Neuropsychological assessment and the school-age child: Issues and procedures* (pp. 277–302). New York: Grune & Stratton.

Golden, C. J. (1984). *Luria-Nebraska Neuropsychological Battery: Children's Revision.* Los Angeles: Western Psychological Services.

Golden, C. J. (1997). The Nebraska neuropsychological children's battery. In C. R. Reynolds & E. Fletcher-Janzen (Eds.), *Handbook of clinical child neuropsychology* (2nd ed., pp. 237–251). New York: Plenum.

Golden, C. J., Zillmer, E., & Spiers, M. (1992). *Neuropsychological assessment and intervention.* Springfield, IL: Charles C. Thomas.

Goldman, P. S., & Lewis, M. E. (1978). Developmental biology of brain damage and experience. In C. W. Cotman (Ed.), *Neuronal plasticity* (pp. 151–185). New York: Raven.

Goldman-Rakic, P. S. (1987). Development of cortical circuitry and cognitive function. *Child Development, 58,* 601.

Gray, J. A. (1982). *The neuropsychology of anxiety: An enquiry into the functions of the septo-hippocampal system.* Oxford, England: Oxford University Press.

Gray, J. W., & Dean, R. S. (1990). Implications of neuropsychological research for school psychology. In T. B. Gutkin & C. R. Reynolds (Eds.), *The handbook of school psychology* (pp. 269–288). New York: Wiley.

Gray, J. W., Dean, R. S., & Rattan, G. (1987). Assessment of perinatal risk factors. *Psychology in the Schools, 24,* 15–21.

Haak, R. A. (1989). Establishing neuropsychology in a school setting: Organization, problems and benefits. In C. R. Reynolds and E. Fletcher-Janzen (Eds.), *Handbook of clinical child neuropsychology* (pp. 489–502). New York: Plenum.

Haak, R. A., & Livingston, R. B. (1997). Treating traumatic brain injury in the schools: Mandates and methods. In C. R. Reynolds and E. Fletcher-Janzen (Eds.), *Handbook of clinical child neuropsychology* (2nd ed., pp. 482–505). New York: Plenum.

Halperin, J. M. (1991). The clinical assessment of attention. *International Journal of Neuroscience, 58,* 171–182.

Halperin, J. M., McKay, K. E., Matier, K., & Sharma, V. (1994). Attention, response inhibition, and activity level in children: Developmental neuropsychological perspectives. In M. G. Tramontana and S. R. Hooper, *Advances in child neuropsychology* (Vol. 2, pp. 1–54). New York: Springer-Verlag.

Harris, P. (1957). Head injuries in childhood. *Archives of Diseases in Childhood, 6,* 488–491.

Hartlage, L. C. (1982). Neuropsychological assessment techniques. In C. R. Reynolds & T. B. Gutkin (Eds.), *The handbook of school psychology* (pp. 296–313). New York: Wiley.

Hartlage, L. C., & Long, C. J. (1997). Development of neuropsychology as a professional specialty: History, training, and credentialing. In C. R. Reynolds & E. Fletcher-Janzen (Eds.), *Handbook of clinical child neuropsychology* (2nd. ed., pp. 3–16). New York: Plenum.

Hartlage, L. C., & Telzrow, C. F. (1986). *Neuropsychological assessment and intervention with children and adolescents.* Sarasota, FL: Professional Resource Exchange.

Haut, J. S., Haut, M. W., Callahan, T. S., & Franzen, M. D. (1992, November). *Factor analysis of the Wide Range Assessment of Memory and Learning (WRAML) scores in a clinical sample.* Paper presented at the 12th annual meeting of the National Academy of Neuropsychology, Pittsburgh, PA.

Heaton, R. K. (1981). *A manual for the Wisconsin Card Sorting Test.* Odessa, FL: Psychological Assessment Resources.

Hooper, S. R., & Tramontana, M. G. (1997). Advances in neuropsychological bases of child and adolescent psychopathology: Proposed models, findings, and on-going issues. *Advances in Clinical Child Psychology, 19,* 133–175.

Howieson, D. B., & Lezak, M. D. (1992). The neuropsychological evaluation. In S. C. Yudofsky & R. E. Hales (Eds.), *The American Psychiatric Press textbook of neuropsychiatry* (2nd ed., pp. 127–150). Washington, DC: American Psychiatric Press.

Hynd, G. W., & Obrzut, J. E. (1981). *Neuropsychological assessment and the school-aged child.* New York: Grune & Stratton.

Hynd, G. W., & Willis, W. G. (1988). *Pediatric neuropsychology.* New York: Grune & Stratton.

Kagan, J., Rosman, B. L., Day, D., Albert, J., & Phillips, W. (1964). Information processing in the child: Significance of analytic and reflective attitudes. *Psychological Monographs, 78,* 1–37.

Kamphaus, R. W. (1993). *Clinical assessment of children's intelligence.* Boston: Allyn & Bacon.

Kamphaus, R. W., & Reynolds, C. R. (1987). *Clinical and research applications of the K-ABC.* Circle Pines, MN: American Guidance Service.

Kamphaus, R. W., & Reynolds, C. R. (1998). *BASC ADHD Monitor.* Circle Pines, MN: American Guidance Services.

Kaplan, E. (1988). A process approach to neuropsychological assessment. In T. Boll & B. K. Bryant (Eds.), *Clinical neuropsychology and brain function* (pp. 125–167). Washington, DC: American Psychological Association.

Kaplan, E. (1990). The process approach to neuropsychological assessment of psychiatric patients. *Journal of Neuropsychiatry, 2*(1), 72–87.

Kaufman, A. S., & Kaufman, N. L. (1983a). *Kaufman Assessment Battery for Children (K-ABC) administration and scoring manual.* Circle Pines, MN: American Guidance Services.

Kaufman, A. S., & Kaufman, N. L. (1983b). *Kaufman Assessment Battery for Children (K-ABC) interpretative manual.* Circle Pines, MN: American Guidance Services.

Kinsbourne, M. (1975). Cerebral dominance, learning, and cognition. In H. R. Myklebust (Ed.), *Progress in learning disabilities.* New York: Grune & Stratton.

Kinsbourne, M. (1989). A model of adaptive behavior related to cerebral participation in emotional control. In G. Gainotti and C. Caltagirone (Eds.), *Emotions and the dual brain* (pp. 248–260). New York: Springer-Verlag.

Klonoff, H. (1971). Head injuries in children: Predisposing factors, accident conditions, accident proneness, and sequelae. *American Journal of Public Health, 61,* 2405–2417.

Klonoff, H., Low, M. D., & Clark, L. (1977). Head injuries in children: A prospective five year follow up. *Journal of Neurology, Neurosurgery, and Psychiatry, 40,* 1211–1219.

Kraus, J. F., Fife, D., & Conroy, C. (1987). Pediatric brain injuries: The nature, clinical course, and early outcomes in a defined United States population. *Pediatrics, 79,* 501–507.

Kreutzer, J. S., Marwitz, J. H., & Kepler, K. (1992). Traumatic brain injury: Family response and outcome. *Archives of Physical Medicine and Rehabilitation, 73,* 771–778.

Kriel, R., Krach, L., & Panser, L. (1989). Closed head injury: comparison of children younger and older than six years of age. *Pediatric Neurology, 5*(5), 296–300.

Lehr, E. (1990). *Psychological management of traumatic brain injuries in children and adolescents.* Rockville, MD: Aspen.

Leu, P. W., & D'Amato, R. C. (1994, April). *Right children, wrong teachers? Using an ecological assessment for placement decisions.* Paper presented at the 26th annual convention of the National Association of School Psychologists, Seattle, WA.

Levin, H. S., Benton, A. L., & Grossman, R. G. (1982). *Neurobehavioral consequences of closed head injury.* London: Oxford University Press.

Levin, H. S., & Eisenberg, H. M. (1979). Neuropsychological impairment after closed head injury in children and adolescents. *Journal of Pediatric Psychology, 4,* 389–402.

Levin, H. S., High, W. M., Ewing-Cobbs, L., Fletcher, J. M., Eisenberg, H. M., Minor, M. E., & Goldstein, F. C. (1988). Memory functioning during the first year after closed head injury in children and adolescents. *Neurosurgery, 22,* 1043–1052.

Lezak, M. D. (1986). Psychological implications of traumatic brain damage for the patient's family. *Rehabilitation Psychology, 31,* 241–250.

Lezak, M. D. (1995). *Neuropsychological assessment* (4th ed.). New York: Oxford University Press.

Little, S. G., & Stavrou, E. (1993). The utility of neuropsychological approaches with children. *The Behavior Therapist, 16,* 104–106.

Luria, A. R. (1966). *Higher cortical functions in man.* New York: Basic Books.

Luria, A. R. (1980). *Higher cortical functions in man* (2nd ed.). New York: Basic Books.

Marlowe, W. (1992). The impact of a right frontal lesion on the developing brain. *Brain and Cognition, 20,* 205–213.

Martin, R. P. (1988). *Personality and behavior assessment.* New York: Guilford.

Mateer, C. A., & Williams, D. (1991). Effects of frontal lobe injury in childhood. *Developmental Neuropsychology, 7,* 359–379.

Mattarazzo, J. D. (1972). *Wechsler's measurement and appraisal of adult intelligence.* Baltimore: Williams & Wilkins.

McGuire, T. L., & Rothenberg, M. B. (1986). Behavioral and psychosocial sequelae of pediatric head injury. *Journal of Head Trauma and Rehabilitation, 1*(4), 1–6.

McLaughlin, A. M., & Schaffer, V. (1985). Rehabilitation or remold? Family involvement in head trauma recovery. *Cognitive Rehabilitation, 3,* 14–17.

McMillan, T. M., & Glucksman, C. E. (1987). The neuropsychology of moderate head injury. *Journal of Neurology, Neurosurgery, and Psychiatry, 50,* 393–397.

Merola, J. L., & Leiderman, J. (1985). The effect of task difficulty upon the extent to which performance benefits from between hemisphere division of inputs. *International Journal of Neuroscience, 51,* 35–44.

Miller, L. T., & Vernon, P. A. (1996). Intelligence, reaction time, and working memory in 4- to 6-year-old children. *Intelligence, 22,* 155–190.

Molfese, D. L. (1995). Electrophysiological responses obtained during infancy and their relation to later language development: Further findings. In M. G. Tramontana & S. R. Hooper (Eds.), *Advances in Child Neuropsychology* (Vol. 3, pp. 1–11). New York: Springer-Verlag.

Morris, J. M., & Bigler, E. (1985, January). *An investigation of the Kaufman Assessment Battery for Children (K-ABC) with neurologically impaired children.* Paper presented at the annual meeting of the International Neuropsychological Society, San Diego, CA.

Nussbaum, N. L., & Bigler, E. D. (1990). *Identification and treatment of attention deficit disorder.* Austin, TX: PRO-ED.

Nussbaum, N. L., & Bigler, E. D. (1997). Halstead-Reitan neuropsychological test batteries for children. In C. R. Reynolds & E. Fletcher-Janzen (Eds.), *Handbook of clinical child neuropsychology* (2nd ed., pp. 219–236). New York: Plenum.

Nussbaum, N. L., Bigler, E. D., Koch, W. R., Ingram, J. W., Rosa, L., & Massman, P. (1988). Personality/behavioral characteristics in children: Differential effects of putative anterior versus posterior cerebral asymmetry. *Archives of Clinical Neuropsychology, 3,* 127–135.

Obrzut, J. E. (1981). Neuropsychological procedures with school-age children. In G. W. Hynd & J. E. Obrzut (Eds.), *Neuropsychological assessment and the school-age child: Issues and procedures* (pp. 237–275). New York: Grune & Stratton.

Obrzut, J. E., & Hynd, G. W. (1983). The neurobiological and neuropsychological foundations of learning disabilities. *Journal of Learning Disabilities, 16,* 515–520.

Parsons, O. A., & Prigatano, G. P. (1978). Methodological considerations in clinical neuropsychological research. *Journal of Consulting and Clinical Psychology, 46,* 608–619.

Passler, M., Isaac, W., & Hynd, G. W. (1985). Neuropsychological development of behavior attributed to frontal lobe functioning in children. *Developmental Neuropsychology, 1,* 349–370.

Prigatano, G. P. (1992). Personality disturbances associated with traumatic brain injury. *Journal of Consulting and Clinical Psychology, 60,* 360–368.

Ramsey, M. C., & Reynolds, C. R. (1995). Separate digits tests: A brief history, a literature review, and re-examination of the factor structure of the Test of Memory and Learning (TOMAL). *Neuropsychology Review, 5,* 151–171.

Reitan, R. M. (1969). *Manual for the administration of neuropsychological test batteries for adults and children.* Indianapolis, IN: Author.

Reitan, R. M. (1986). *Theoretical and methodological bases of the Halstead-Reitan Neuropsychological Test Battery.* Tucson, AZ: Neuropsychological Press.

Reitan, R. M. (1987). *Neuropsychological evaluation of children.* Tucson, AZ: Neuropsychological Press.

Reitan, R. M., & Davison, L. A. (1974). *Clinical neuropsychology: Current status and applications.* Washington, DC: Winston.

Reitan, R. M., & Wolfson, D. (1985). *The Halstead-Reitan Neuropsychological Battery: Theory and clinical interpretation.* Tucson, AZ: Neuropsychological Press.

Reitan, R. M., & Wolfson, D. (1988). The Halstead-Reitan neuropsychological test batteries and REHABIT: A model for integrating evaluation and remediation of cognitive impairment. *Cognitive Rehabilitation, 10,* 10–17.

Reschley, D., & Gresham, F. M. (1989). Current neuropsychological diagnosis of learning problems: A leap of faith. In C. R. Reynolds & E. Fletcher-Janzen (Eds.), *Handbook of clinical child neuropsychology* (pp. 503–520). New York: Plenum.

Reynolds, C. R. (1981a). Neuropsychological assessment and the habilitation of learning: Considerations in the search for the aptitude X treatment interaction. *School Psychology Review, 10,* 343–349.

Reynolds, C. R. (1981b). The neuropsychological basis of intelligence. In G. W. Hynd & J. E. Obrzut (Eds.), *Neuropsychological assessment and the school-aged child: Issues and procedures* (pp. 87–124). New York: Grune & Stratton.

Reynolds, C. R. (1982). The importance of norms and other traditional psychometric concepts to assessment in clinical neuropsychology. In R. N. Malathesha & L. C. Hartlage (Eds.), *Neuropsychology and cognition* (Vol. III, pp. 55–76). The Hague: Nijhoff.

Reynolds, C. R. (1986a). Clinical acumen but psychometric naivete in neuropsychological assessment of educational disorders. *Archives of Clinical Neuropsychology, 1*(2), 121–137.

Reynolds, C. R. (1986b). Transactional models of intellectual development, yes. Deficit models of process remediation, no. *School Psychology Review, 15,* 256–260.

Reynolds, C. R. (1997a). Forward and backward memory span should not be combined for clinical analysis. *Archives of Clinical Neuropsychology, 12,* 29–40.

Reynolds, C. R. (1997b). Measurement and statistical problems in neuropsychological assessment of children. In C. R. Reynolds & E. Fletcher-Janzen (Eds.), *Handbook of clinical child neuropsychology* (2nd ed., pp. 180–203). New York: Plenum.

Reynolds, C. R. (1997c). Postscripts on premorbid ability estimation: Conceptual addenda and a few words on alternative and conditional approaches. *Archives of Clinical Neuropsychology, 12,* 769–778.

Reynolds, C. R., & Bigler, E. D. (1994). *Manual for the Test of Memory and Learning.* Austin, TX: PRO-ED.

Reynolds, C. R., & Bigler, E. D. (1997a). Clinical neuropsychological assessment of child and adolescent memory with the Test of Memory and Learning. In C. R. Reynolds & E. Fletcher-Janzen (Eds.), *Handbook of clinical child neuropsychology* (2nd ed., pp. 296–319). New York: Plenum.

Reynolds, C. R., & Bigler, E. D. (1997b). Factor structure, factor indexes, and other useful statistics for interpretation of the Test of Memory and Learning (TOMAL). *Archives of Clinical Neuropsychology, 11,* 29–43.

Reynolds, C. R., & Hickman, J. A. (1987). Remediation, deficit-centered models. In C. R. Reynolds and L. Mann (Eds.), *Encyclopedia of Special Education* (pp. 1339–1342). New York: Wiley-Interscience.

Reynolds, C. R., & Kamphaus, R. W. (1992). *Behavior Assessment System for Children.* Circle Pines, MN: American Guidance Services.

Reynolds, C. R., & Kamphaus, R. W. (1997). The Kaufman Assessment Battery for Children: Development, structure and applications in neuropsychology. In A. M. Horton, D. Wedding, & J. Webster (Eds.), *The neuropsychology handbook* (Vol. 1, pp. 291–330). New York: Springer.

Reynolds, C. R., Kamphaus, R. W., Rosenthal, B. L., & Hiemenz, J. R. (1997). Application of the Kaufman Assessment Battery for Children (K-ABC) in neuropsychological assessment. In C. R. Reynolds & E. Fletcher-Janzen (Eds.), *Handbook of clinical child neuropsychology* (2nd. ed., pp. 252–269). New York: Plenum.

Reynolds, C. R., & Mayfield, J. W. (in press). Neuropsychological assessment in genetically linked neurodevelopmental disorders. In S. Goldstein & C. R. Reynolds (Eds.), *Handbook of neurodevelopmental and genetic disorders in children.* New York: Guilford.

Reynolds, C. R., & Stanton, H. C. (in press). *Premorbid ability estimator.* Los Angeles: Psychological Services.

Reynolds, C. R., Wilen, S., & Stone, B. (1997, November). *The economy of neuropsychological evaluations.* Paper presented at the annual meeting of the National Academy of Neuropsychology, Las Vegas, NV.

Riccio, C. A., Hall, J., Morgan, A., Hynd, G. W., Gonzalez, J. J., & Marshall, R. M. (1994). Executive function and the Wisconsin Card Sorting Test: Relationship with behavioral ratings and cognitive ability. *Developmental Neuropsychology, 10,* 215–229.

Riccio, C. A., & Reynolds, C. R. (1998). Neuropsychological assessment of children. In M. Hersen & A. Bellack (Series Eds.) & C. R. Reynolds (Vol. Ed.), *Comprehensive clinical psychology: Vol. 4. Assessment* (pp. 267–301). New York: Elsevier.

Ris, M. D., & Noll, R. B. (1994). Long-term neurobehavioral outcome in pediatric brain tumor patients: Review and methodological critique. *Journal of Clinical and Experimental Neuropsychology, 16,* 21.

Rosenthal, M. (1984). Strategies for intervention with families of brain injured. In B. A. Edelstein and E. T. Coutoure (Eds.), *Behavioral assessment and rehabilitation of the traumatically brain damaged* (pp. 227–246). New York: Plenum.

Rosenthal, M., & Young, T. (1988). Effective family intervention after traumatic brain injury: Theory and practice. *Journal of Head Trauma Rehabilitation, 3,* 42–50.

Rosvold, H. E., Mirsky, A. F., Sarason, I., Bransome, E. D., & Beck, L. H. (1956). A continuous performance test of brain damage. *Journal of Consulting Psychology, 20,* 343–350.

Rothlisberg, B. A., & D'Amato, R. C. (1996, April). *Programming for students with traumatic brain injury: An S. O. S. approach to intervention.* Paper presented at the National Association of School Psychologists, Atlanta, GA.

Rothlisberg, B. A., & D'Amato, R. C. (1988). Increased neuropsychological understanding seen as important for school psychologists. *Communique, 17*(2), 4–5.

Rourke, B. P. (1989). *Nonverbal learning disabilities: The syndrome and the model.* New York: Guilford.

Rourke, B. P. (1994). Neuropsychological assessment of children with learning disabilities: Measurement issues. In G. R. Lyon (Ed.), *Frames of reference for the assessment of learning disabilities: New views on measurement issues* (pp. 475–514). Baltimore: Brookes.

Rutter, M. (1981). Psychological sequelae of brain damage in children. *American Journal of Clinical Neuropsychology, 138,* 1533–1544.

Rutter, M., Chadwick, O., & Shaffer, D. (1983). Head injury. In M. Rutter (Ed.), *Developmental neuropsychiatry* (pp. 83–111). New York: Guilford.

Rutter, M., Chadwick, O., Shaffer, D., & Brown, G. (1980). A prospective study of children with head injuries: I. Design and methods. *Psychological Medicine, 10,* 633–646.

Rutter, M., Graham, P., & Yule, W. (1970). *A neuropsychiatric study in childhood.* London: Lavenham Press.

Ryan, T. V., LaMarche, J. A., Barth, J. T., & Boll, T. J. (1996). Neuropsychological consequences and treatment of pediatric head trauma. In E. S. Batchelor & R. S. Dean (Eds.), *Pediatric neuropsychology* (pp. 117–137). New York: Pergamon.

Sandoval, J. (1981, August). *Can neuropsychology contribute to rehabilitation in educational settings? No.* Paper presented at the annual meeting of the American Psychological Association, Los Angeles, CA.

Satz, P., & Fletcher, J. M. (1981). Emergent trends in neuropsychology: An overview. *Journal of Consulting and Clinical Psychology, 49,* 851–865.

Seidel, U. P., Chadwick, O., & Rutter, M. (1975). Psychological disorders in crippled children: A comparative study of children with and without brain damage. *Developmental Medicine and Child Neurology, 17,* 563.

Selz, M. (1981). Halstead-Reitan neuropsychological test batteries for children. In G. W. Hynd & J. E. Obrzut (Eds.), *Neuropsychological assessment of the school-aged child* (pp. 195–235). New York: Grune & Stratton.

Semrud-Clikeman, M., Kamphaus, R. W., Teeter, P. A., & Vaughn, M. (1997). Assessment of behavior and personality in neuropsychological diagnosis of children. In C. R. Reynolds and E. Fletcher-Janzen (Eds.), *Handbook of clinical child neuropsychology* (pp. 320–341). New York: Plenum.

Shapiro, E. G., & Dotan, N. (1985, October). *Neurological findings and the Kaufman Assessment Battery for Children.* Paper presented at the annual meeting of the National Association of Neuropsychologists, Philadelphia, PA.

Shaw, S. R., & Yingst, C. A. (1992). Assessing children with traumatic brain injuries: Integrating educational and medical issues. *Diagnostique, 17,* 255–265.

Sheslow, D., & Adams, W. (1990). *Wide Range Assessment of Memory and Learning.* Wilmington, DE: Jastak Associates.

Shinn, M. R., Nolet, V., & Knutson, N. (1990). Best practices in curriculum-based measurement. In A. Thomas & J. Grimes (Eds.), *Best practices in school psychology* (pp. 287–300). Washington, DC: National Association of School Psychologists.

Shurtleff, H. A., Fay, G. E., Abbott, R. D., & Berninger, V. W. (1988). Cognitive and neuropsychological correlates of academic achievement: A levels of analysis assessment model. *Journal of Psychoeducational Assessment, 6,* 298–308.

Skilbeck, C. (1984). Computer assistance in the management of memory and cognitive impairment. In B. Wilson and N. Moffat (Eds.)., *Clinical management of memory problems* (pp. 112–131). New York: Aspen.

Snow, J. H., & Hooper, S. R. (1994). *Pediatric traumatic brain injury.* Thousand Oaks, CA: Sage.

Sparrow, S. S., Balla, D. A., & Cicchetti, D. V. (1984). *Vineland Adaptive Behavior Scales.* Circle Pines, MN: American Guidance Services.

Sperry, R. W. (1968). Hemisphere deconnection and unity in conscious awareness. *American Psychologist, 23,* 723–733.

Sperry, R. W. (1974). Lateral specialization in the surgically separated hemispheres. In F. O. Schmitt & F. G. Worden (Eds.), *The neurosciences: Third study program.* Cambridge, MA: MIT Press.

Spreen, O., Risser, A. H., & Edgell, D. (1995). *Developmental neuropsychology.* London: Oxford University Press.

Spreen, O., Tupper, D., Risser, A., Tuokko, H., & Edgell, P. (1984). *Human developmental neuropsychology.* New York: Oxford University Press.

Talley, J. L. (1986). Memory in learning disabled children: Digit span and the Rey Auditory Verbal Learning Test. *Archives of Clinical Neuropsychology, 1,* 315–322.

Taylor, H. G., & Fletcher, J. M. (1990). Neuropsychological assessment of children. In G. Goldstein & M. Hersen (Eds.), *Handbook of neuropsychological assessment* (pp. 228–255). New York: Plenum.

Teeter, P. A. (1997). Neurocognitive interventions for childhood and adolescent disorders: A transactional model. In C. R. Reynolds & E. Fletcher-Janzen (Eds.), *Handbook of clinical child neuropsychology* (2nd ed., pp. 387–417). New York: Plenum.

Teeter, P. A., & Semrud-Clikeman, M. (1997). *Child neuropsychology: Assessment and interventions for neurodevelopmental disorders.* Boston: Allyn & Bacon.

Telzrow, C. F. (1987). Management of academic and educational problems in head injury. *Journal of Learning Disabilities, 20,* 536–545.

Temple, C. M. (1997). Cognitive neuropsychology and its application to children. *Journal of Child Psychology, Psychiatry, and Allied Disciplines, 38,* 27–52.

Timmermans, S. R., & Christensen, B. (1991). The measurement of attention deficit in TBI children and adolescents. *Cognitive Rehabilitation, 9,* 26.

Torgesen, J. K. (1994). Issues in the assessment of executive function: An information processing perspective. In G. R. Lyon (Ed.), *Frames of reference for the assessment of learning disabilities: New views on measurement issues* (pp. 143–162). Baltimore: Brookes.

Torkelson, R. D., Leibrook, L. G., Gustavson, J. L., & Sundell, R. R. (1985). Neurological and neuropsychological effects of cerebral spinal fluid shunting in children with assumed arrested ("normal pressure") hydrocephalus. *Journal of Neurology, Neurosurgery, and Psychiatry, 48,* 799–806.

Tramontana, M., & Hooper, S. (1997). Neuropsychology of child psychopathology. In C. R. Reynolds & E. Fletcher-Janzen (Eds.), *Handbook of clinical child neuropsychology* (2nd ed., pp. 120–139). New York: Plenum.

Tucker, D. M. (1989). Neural substrates of thought and affective disorders. In G. Gainotti & C. Caltagirone (Eds.), *Emotions and the dual brain* (pp. 225–234). New York: Springer-Verlag.

Vygotsky, L. S. (1980). *Mind in society: The development of higher psychological process.* Cambridge, MA: Harvard University Press.

Waaland, P. K., & Kreutzer, J. S. (1988). Family response to childhood traumatic brain injury. *Journal of Head Trauma and Rehabilitation, 3,* 51–63.

Wasserman, J. (1995, February). *Assessment and remediation of memory deficits in children.* Paper presented at the meeting of the Supervisors of School Psychologists for the New York Board of Education, New York.

Welsh, M. C., & Pennington, B. F. (1988). Assessing frontal lobe functioning in children: Views from developmental psychology. *Developmental Neuropsychology, 4,* 199–230.

Welsh, M. C., Pennington, B. F., & Grossier, D. B. (1991). A normative developmental study of executive function: A window on prefrontal function in children. *Developmental Neuropsychology, 7,* 131–139.

Whitten, C. J., D'Amato, R. C., & Chitooran, M. M. (1992). The neuropsychological approach to interventions. In R. C. D'Amato & B. A Rothlisberg (Eds.), *Psychological perspectives on intervention: A case study approach to prescriptions for change* (pp. 112–136). New York: Longman.

Williams, J. M., & Kay, T. (1991). *Head injury: A family matter.* Baltimore: Paul H. Brookes.

Williams, M. A., & Boll, T. J. (1997). Recent advances in neuropsychological assessment of children. In G. Goldstein & T. M. Incagnoli (Eds.), *Contemporary approaches to neuropsychological assessment* (pp. 231–267). New York: Plenum.

Willson, V. L., & Reynolds, C. R. (1982). Methodological and statistical problems in determining membership in clinical populations. *Clinical Neuropsychology, 4,* 134–138.

Witkin, H. A., Oltman, P., Raskin, E., & Karp, S. (1971). *Manual for the Children's Embedded Figures Test.* Palo Alto, CA: Consulting Psychologists Press.

Woodcock, R. W., & Johnson, M. B. (1989). *Woodcock Johnson Psychoeducational Battery–Revised: Tests of Achievement.* Allen, TX: DLM Teaching Resources.

Ylvisaker, M. (1985). *Head injury rehabilitation: Children and adolescents.* San Diego: College Hill.

Zarksi, J. J., Hall, D. E., & DePompei, R. (1987). Close head injury patients: A family therapy approach to the rehabilitation process. *The American Journal of Family Therapy, 15,* 62–68.

Zelazo, P. D., Carter, A., Reznick, J. S., & Frye, D. (1997). Early development of executive functions: A problem-solving framework. *Review of General Psychology, 1*(2), 198–226.

Mild Traumatic Brain Injury in Sports

6

Robert A. Ruchinskas,
Joseph P. Francis, and Jeffrey T. Barth

Introduction

The rise of sports as entertainment and big business during the 1990s has focused society's attention, for better or worse, on issues relating to the athlete who once played just a game. Besides defining new antitrust rules and who is or is not a "role model," the media has focused on the problems of high profile athletes, rekindling interest in sports-related head injuries. A defining moment occurred during the 1993 National Football League's conference playoffs. During the games played that day, two starting quarterbacks, Joe Montana and Troy Aikmen, sustained what were termed "concussions." Given the perception of violence in modern football, the likelihood of two starting quarterbacks sustaining mild head injuries with short losses of consciousness (concussion) on the same day is actually relatively low. Among reported injuries, the chances of any athlete incurring mild head trauma are generally between 2% and 10%, but range as high as 91% for equestrian accidents. Although head injuries can occur in virtually any sport or recreational activity, Table 6.1 lists the sports for which head injury rates are described in the literature.

Along with the low probability of injury, rapid and full recovery from a mild head injury is expected (as was seen in Aikmen's performance in the Super Bowl 2 weeks later). However, complicated recoveries from concussions have been reported where cognitive and emotional sequelae are potentially long-lasting (e.g., Barth et al., 1983; Rimel, Giordani, Barth, Boll, &

Reprinted, with changes, from "Mild Head Injury in Sports," by Robert A. Ruchinskas, Joseph P. Francis, and Jeffrey T. Barth, 1997, *Applied Neuropsychology, 4*(1), pp. 43–49. Copyright 1997 by Lawrence Erlbaum Associates, Inc.

Table 6.1

Estimated Rate of Concussion/Mild Head Trauma Among Sports Injuries

Sport	% Range
Auto racing	0–10.5
Bicycling	0–13.8
Boxing	1–70
Equestrian	3–91
Football	2–20
Ice hockey	3–7.5
Martial arts	0–11
Rugby	2–25
Soccer	4–22

Note. Percentages were obtained from literature cited in text.

Jane, 1981). In addition, there has been much publicity surrounding football and hockey athletes who prematurely retire after suffering multiple mild head injuries. Hence, there is a small but growing body of literature devoted to examining mild head injury in athletes, particularly in boxing, football, and more recently, soccer. The goals of this research are threefold:

1. to increase safety for the athletes
2. to aid in understanding the mechanisms of and recovery from uncomplicated and complicated mild head injuries that occur in more common settings (automobile accidents, falls, etc.)
3. to broaden limited scientific knowledge on effects of repeated mild TBI

Professional and amateur athletes tend to be good research subjects, as they do not have many of the risks or complicating factors for spontaneous cognitive decline (age, poor health, substance abuse, etc.). Unfortunately, athletes tend to underreport head injuries, and injuries in general, for fear of letting down the team, being seen as weak, or reducing their probability of playing in the next game (Gerberich, Priest, Boen, Staub, & Maxwell, 1983). Team trainers and physicians historically have also downplayed the possible effects of concussions, yet with important new scientific data, both have become strong advocates for a cautious approach to return-to-play decisions.

What Is Mild Head Injury?

The theory and study of mild TBI is still in its infancy. Over the last two decades, scientists have been examining the mechanisms of mild head injury and one possible negative outcome, the "postconcussive syndrome." Mild head trauma or mild TBI (used interchangeably in this chapter) refer to brief losses of or changes in consciousness (awareness/orientation) that are usually caused by a blow to the head. Varney and Varney (1995) persuasively argue that mild brain injury can also occur in the absence of overt head injury, secondary to the physics of acceleration, deceleration, and rotation. Such injuries rarely result in identifiable cerebral lesions, yet like moderate and severe head trauma can be associated with contusions (bruises), most commonly occurring on the frontal and temporal lobes. Underlying white matter may be affected by edema, along with shearing and cytoskeletal injury of neuronal axons (Duckett & Duckett, 1993). Research (Dixon, Taft, & Hayes, 1993) has also suggested myriad acute and chronic changes in the brain's neurochemical functions following injury (e.g., neurotransmitter release/deficits, changes in receptor binding, alterations in cholinergic functioning, etc). Animal models of mild brain injury echo the possibility that concussion can occur without loss of consciousness, and that axonal swelling is present acutely postinjury (Ommaya & Gennarelli, 1974; Povlishock & Lontos, 1985). Although CT and MRI scans are useful in detecting bleeding and swelling in more severe traumatic injuries, they are less able to detect the more subtle, microscopic lesions that are typical of mild head injury. However, positive results in detecting brain abnormalities with functional neuroimaging (e.g., PET, SPECT, fMRI) have been reported by Ruff et al. (1994).

The most common classification method for severity of head injury is the Glasgow Coma Scale (GCS), which assesses motor and verbal responses, orientation, and eye opening to command to evaluate gross levels of consciousness after head injury. A score of 13 or above (out of 15 possible) places patients in the "mild" category for head trauma. Length of unconsciousness (less than 30 minutes), less than a 48-hour stay in the hospital (Rimel et al., 1981), and lack of neuroimaging evidence (Levin, Eisenberg, & Benton, 1989) have also been used to categorize mild head injury. Unfortunately, for some time there was no consensus on diagnostic criteria (Jordan, 1989), and varying definitions of mild head injury or mild TBI were found in research and clinical practice (Harrington, Malec, Cicerone, & Katz, 1993). To remedy this situation, the Mild Traumatic Brain Injury Committee of the Head Injury Interdisciplinary Special Interest Group of the American Congress of Rehabilitation Medicine (1993) published a consensus definition of mild TBI which included the following:

1. a GCS score of 13 to 15 (after 30 minutes)
2. less than 30 minutes loss of consciousness

3. 24 hours or less of posttraumatic amnesia (PTA)
4. at least one of the following symptoms: loss of consciousness, altered mental state at the time of trauma, retrograde amnesia or PTA, and transient or permanent focal neurological deficits

Prior to 1981, conventional wisdom held that mild head injury was rather benign, and natural recovery from such trauma occurs quite rapidly. However, Rimel et al. (1981) and Barth et al. (1983) found that some cognitive symptoms, as measured by neuropsychological tests, persisted for weeks or months postinjury. A significant proportion of patients with mild head injury (34%) had not returned to work 3 months postinjury due to their symptoms. Although subsequent studies (Dikmen, Machamer, Winn, & Temkin, 1995; Dikmen, McLean, & Temkin, 1986; Levin et al., 1987; McLean, Temkin, Dikmen, & Wyler, 1983) have reported a lower rate of cognitive dysfunction and little long-term disability, there is a possibility of lasting effects from relatively mild head injury. Based on this research, the symptoms of problematic or complicated mild head injury, known as postconcussive syndrome (PCS), are now well recognized: headaches, dizziness, memory loss, nausea, diplopia (double vision), tinnitus (ringing in the ears), personality change (mainly irritability), attentional deficits, and information processing impairment (Barth et al., 1989).

Research on repeated concussions (Gronwall & Wrightson, 1975) has also suggested a cumulative effect, for example, a decrease in an individual's ability to process information if he or she had a prior mild head injury. Some case studies (e.g., Shell, Carico, & Patton, 1993) have even documented life-threatening complications after two mild head injuries were incurred in 1 week. These cases of the "second-impact syndrome," where the athlete is believed to be still at risk while symptomatic from a previous head injury, are helping to shape decisions about when a player should return to play. In years past, athletic team physicians often applied "Quigley's rule" when evaluating effects of multiple concussions. Essentially, the rule recommends that the athlete discontinue play after receiving three concussions (Schneider, 1973). Some of the above research suggests that this practice may not be conservative enough to protect athletes from incurring lasting cognitive deficits; more specific decision rules have been proposed (Cantu, 1986; Saal & Sontag, 1987).

Building on previous research, the American Academy of Neurology Quality Standards Committee (1997) issued practice parameters for the management of concussion in sports, which include guidelines for assessment, treatment, and return-to-play decisions. Depending on the severity of injury, the athlete can return to play after evaluation anywhere from 15 minutes to 1 month postinjury. A relatively new sideline screening measure for the presence and severity of concussion is the *Standardized Assessment of Concussion* (SAC) (McCrea, Kelly, Kluge, Ackley, & Randolph, 1997). The athlete is given a brief neurological screening and physical exertion tests, then assessed on four domains: orientation, immediate memory, concentration (e.g., digits and months of the year backwards), and delayed memory. As concentration and speed of information processing appear to be particularly affected acutely post-concussion (Hinton-Bayre, Geffen, & McFarland, 1997), there has been further study on the sensitivity of these aspects of the SAC to mild TBI (Young, Jacobs, Clavette, Mark, & Guse, 1997).

Severe Brain Injury in Boxing

Boxing is one of the few sports where the primary goal is to render the opponent unconscious, cause a concussion, or inflict brain damage (Jordan, 1987). Due to the brutal nature of the sport, there have been many calls to abolish boxing. For example, both the American Academy of Neurology (1983) and American Academy of Pediatrics (1997) oppose the sport of boxing.

Although the chances of a boxer dying in the ring (0.13 per 1,000 participants, according to McCunney & Russo, 1984) are less than those for athletes in horse racing, parachuting, hang gliding, mountaineering, scuba diving, motorcycle racing, or football, the professional boxer is at risk for chronic brain injury (Haglund & Eriksson, 1993). Reportedly, 9% to 25% of professional boxers eventually become "punch drunk"; Ryan (1987) concluded that there is "clearly a significant relationship between the numbers of bouts fought and the presence of severity of chronic encephalopathy [brain damage]" (p. 38). Physicians have observed that "punch-drunkenness" occurs more often in professional boxers than in amateurs, and in boxers notorious for being able to "take a punch," who are sluggers rather than tacticians. Although the syndrome occurs across all weight classes, it appears to occur in smaller men who fight heavier opponents. Symptoms typically occur in three stages, where initial disturbances are noted in coordination and affect/emotionality. As the syndrome progresses, psychiatric symptoms increase along with dysarthria (speech difficulties) and a resting tremor. The third stage includes hearing problems, increased tremors, worsening incoordination, and decreased ability to think clearly and to remember. Changes in personality and decreased social skills have also been described. Symptoms similar to Parkinson's disease can be observed, and the course of this syndrome is generally progressive (Jordan, 1987).

Postmortem studies often find Alzheimer-like levels of apolipoprotein E (APOE) and amyloid plaques (Jordan et al., 1995). Research has documented an increased risk of Alzheimer's disease if patients have a positive history of head injury with loss of consciousness (Schofield et al., 1997) and/or the APOE e4 genotype (O'Meara et al., 1997). Reflecting the scientific trend, Jordan and colleagues' follow-up study (1997) suggested that possession of an APOE e4 allele was associated with increased severity of chronic neurological deficits in professional boxers. Undoubtedly, future research will help elucidate any possible connection between concussion, genetics, and cognitive decline.

Professional boxers without "dementia pugilistica" also display a higher rate of cortical atrophy than control subjects on neuroimaging studies (CT/MRI), and cognitive abnormalities on neuropsychological tests (Haglund & Eriksson, 1993). Ross, Casson, Siegel, and Cole (1987) found deficits in attention, memory, and visuospatial abilities that correlated with the number of professional bouts. The amount of sparring done by professionals also correlates with poorer performance on tests of attention, concentration, and memory (Jordan, Matser, Zimmerman, & Zazula, 1996). As abnormalities may not always be evident through neurological examinations or structural neuroimaging, neuropsychological tests are often considered the most sensitive diagnostic methods, and have been proposed as part of the routine screenings of boxers (Levin & Jordan, 1993).

Mild Concussion in Boxing

Although the mechanisms of injury (linear acceleration, rotational and deceleration forces, and carotid injuries due to blows) remain the same for professional and amateur boxers, stricter rules offer more protection for the amateur (Lampert & Hardman, 1984). These boxers have fought fewer and shorter fights than professionals, engaged in less sparring, and also wear headgear. Knockout rates are also low in amateur boxing: 1% to 4% of all fights end in a knockout (McKunney & Russo, 1984). In addition, a certain amount of self-selection may take place in the amateur ranks; poor boxers will lose early and often and leave the sport, whereas proficient boxers may choose to become professionals. Generally, the "punch drunk" syndrome of permanent and irreversible brain dysfunction seems rare for amateurs (Jordan, 1987), making them excellent candidates for the study of simple and repeated mild head injuries.

A large-scale retrospective study of amateur boxers in Sweden, where professional boxing is banned, found no differences between amateur boxers and control subjects in general mental status, physical and neurological examinations, neuroimaging, and personality functioning. After factoring in age, education, and vocabulary, neuropsychological deficits were minimal (decreased fine-motor speed). The number of abnormal EEGs (a measure of gross brain activity) for boxers was slightly higher than normal. In general, the researchers found no clinical evidence of deficits due to repeated blows to the head. There is, however, some question regarding the strictness of Swedish amateur boxing rules compared to their European or American counterparts, which may have limited some of the potential harmful effects of boxing in these studies (Haglund & Bergstrand, 1990; Haglund, Edman, Murelius, Oreland, & Sachs, 1990; Haglund & Eriksson, 1993; Haglund &

Persson, 1990). Another study (Holzgraefe, Lemme, Funke, Felix, & Felten, 1992) found that only a minority of amateur boxers demonstrated signs of structural damage to the brain.

At the other end of the spectrum, research with 20 active boxers revealed 7 amateurs with abnormal neurological examinations, 8 with EEG abnormalities, and 9 with deficiencies on neuropsychological testing, especially in the areas of attention and verbal and visual memory (McLatchie et al., 1987). Research has also examined performance on neuropsychological measures before and after fights. After an amateur bout, boxers' verbal and incidental memory skills were diminished, whereas their executive functions (higher order problem solving) and motor functions were enhanced. This study, however, lacked a matched control group to examine the impact of exercise on general mental and motor abilities or to account for practice effects (Heilbronner, Henry, & Carson-Brewer, 1991).

Two prospective studies have attempted to address the weaknesses of the previously noted research. Butler, Forsythe, Beverly, and Adams (1993) used neuropsychological assessment before the bout, immediately after the bout, and at a follow-up within 2 years. The authors found no evidence of neuropsychological dysfunction, although their subjects were relatively inexperienced (less than 20% with 30 or more contests). A much larger study (n = 393 at 2 year follow-up) found statistically significant relationships between the total number of bouts before baseline examination and changes in memory, visuoconstructive skills, and perceptual/motor ability (although the changes were not considered clinically significant). There were no significant findings at follow-up, suggesting that stricter safety rules enacted just prior to the study may be a confounding factor. The examiners will continue to follow this cohort to examine possible late effects of repeated blows to the head (Stewart et al., 1994).

Finally, a more recent study has attempted to integrate functional neuroimaging and neuropsychology (Kemp, Houston, Macleod, & Pethybridge, 1995). This research found abnormalities in both neuropsychological measures and cerebral SPECT perfusion scans in amateur boxers when compared to control subjects. Individuals with more bouts tended to have poorer neuropsychological test scores, although groups divided by abnormal versus normal SPECT imaging did not differ on psychometric testing. Unfortunately, correlation of abnormal SPECT scans with number of bouts was not addressed.

Mild Concussion in Football

Numerous studies have reported the incidence of concussion in football at 2% to 5% of all injuries incurred (DeLee & Farney, 1992; Karpakka, 1993; Zemper, 1989). This may be an underestimation of the actual occurrence of head trauma, however, because "injuries" were often defined as those reported to the trainer or those which kept a player out of a game or practice for a day or more. One team physician titled his article "When a Knee Injury Becomes a Head Injury" to underscore that the "grogginess," temporary amnesia, and confusion that accompany a mild (grade 1) concussion or "ding" are often missed, not reported, or dismissed (Magnes, 1990). It has been estimated that 85% to 90% of all sports related concussions are "grade 1," defined by Cantu (1986) as no loss of consciousness and PTA of less than 30 minutes. For other severity rating systems see Torg (1982), Jordan (1994), and the American Academy of Neurology Quality Standards Committee (1997) practice parameters.

A study of Minnesota high-school varsity football players revealed that approximately 5% of injuries were diagnosed as "concussions" that required temporary removal from play (Gerberich et al., 1983). However, 20% of the players indicated that they had previously suffered a loss of consciousness or change in awareness consistent with undiagnosed mild concussions. This percentage would predict approximately 250,000 concussions in high-school football each year. The study also found that individuals who had previously lost consciousness were 4 times more likely to sustain another head injury. At follow-up, approximately 3% of the players stated some lingering cognitive symptoms 6 to 9 months postinjury. Still, most of the athletes asked to return to play the same day of their injury.

In an attempt to characterize the nature, incidence, and consequences of mild head injury, the University of Virginia prospective study evaluated 2,350 football players from eight Ivy League schools, the University of Pittsburgh, and the University of Virginia (Alves, Rimel, & Nelson, 1987; Barth et al., 1989; Macciocchi, Barth, Alves, Rimel, & Jane, 1996). The 195 (8% of total sample) players who sustained a mild head injury, defined as a change in or loss of consciousness for less than 2 minutes and immediate demonstration of attention/memory problems, were evaluated with neuropsychological testing and self-report questionnaires up to four times postinjury. The injured players were compared against 59 red-shirted (non-playing) football players suffering orthopedic injuries and 48 non–football-playing students to control the effects of repeated testing. Forty-two percent of the football players with head injuries indicated a history of at least one prior minor head trauma, and 12% had sustained three or more such injuries. Results of the study indicate that a single mild head injury can cause deficits in global cognitive functioning and information processing within 24 hours. Rapid recovery generally takes place over the next 5 to 10 days. Symptoms unique to PCS, such as headache, nausea, dizziness, weakness, and memory problems, also appeared to be resolved by 5 to 10 days postinjury. Consistent with other studies, over 90% of the head trauma was mild (grade 1); hence, football players have significantly greater chances of injuring a knee, arm, or other body part than experiencing cerebral trauma. With mild concussion, rapid recovery will probably ensue, although some data suggest that recovery can take longer. The effects of repeated mild insults were unresolved by this study, as the number of players sustaining multiple concussions in the same season was not large enough to be statistically meaningful.

Concussion in Soccer

The frequency of soccer players "heading" a hard and fast-moving ball and of head-to-head or head-to-foot impact has caused some concern about possible lasting effects of repeated mild head trauma. Head injuries are believed to account for 4% to 22% of soccer injuries. As with other sports, concussion data are limited but growing, and the results are mixed. For example, in one study of active and former professional soccer players, no abnormalities were found on neuroimaging (CT/MRI scans) or on a brief neuropsychological battery (Haglund & Eriksson, 1993). Mild EEG disturbances have been found in soccer players, along with complaints of chronic PCS (Tysvaer, Storli, & Bachen, 1989). In one of the studies that found more cognitive deficits, 69 active players and 37 former players were examined; 30% of the retired players complained of chronic postconcussive symptoms (Tysvaer, 1992). One third of the former players displayed unexpected cerebral atrophy on CT scan. Eighty-one percent of the former players had mild to moderate deficits on neuropsychological tests, especially in the areas of memory, attention, concentration, and judgment, as opposed to a 40% impairment rate in age-matched control subjects. As with other studies, this study revealed the inadequacies of a standard neurological examination for detecting subtle cognitive changes, and screening through neuropsychological assessment was recommended. Witol & Webbe (1994) also suggested subtle cognitive dysfunction in soccer players, associated with repeated heading of a soccer ball and age/experience levels. Another study found an increase in reported postconcussive symptoms that correlated more with prior history of head trauma than with the number of times the soccer player had headed the ball in his career (Jordan, Green, Galanty, Mandelbaum, & Jabour, 1996). Further longitudinal research and control for variables such as body contact and body–ground contact are necessary before the question of soccer-related cognitive deficits can be answered.

Head Injuries in Other Sports

Surprisingly, the sport with the highest reported rate of head injuries is horseback riding. One of the earliest examinations of equestrian head injuries found five National Hunt Jockeys to have significant neurological impairment (Foster, Leiguarda, & Tilley, 1976). A review of medical records of three Alberta, Canada hospitals indicated that 91% of all horseback riding accidents involved a head injury. Although mild head injuries dominated the clinical picture (83% of head injuries), 3% of head injuries were moderate, and 14% were severe. The majority of accidents were associated with falling or being thrown from a horse (Hamilton & Tranmer, 1993). A study of pediatric equestrian head injuries found a significantly lower rate of injury (3% to 11%), perhaps because children wore headgear more frequently than adults (Bixby-Hammett, 1992).

The use of protective helmets is recommended for all sports in which there is a possibility of head injury. Ice hockey currently reports that 3% to 7.5% of all reported injuries are concussions; these figures have apparently declined over the years due to helmet use (Pelletier, Montelpare, & Stark, 1993; Tegner & Lorentzon, 1991). Sports where helmets have not been adopted (e.g., rugby, Australian football, and taekwondo) report a 2% to 11% concussion rate, although the incidence of minor concussions could be as high as 25% (Gibbs, 1993; O'Brien, 1992; Seward, Orchard, Hazard, & Collinson, 1993; Zemper & Pieter, 1989). Increased attention to safety features has reduced the rate of head injuries in automobile racing, yet 10.5% of all hospitalizations still involve head trauma. Competitive and recreational cycling also have head injury rates up to 13.8% (Fullerton & Becker, 1991; Jordan, 1989).

Conclusions

This review of the research suggests that for the majority of participants, mild head injury in sports is rare and is characterized by a brief loss or alteration of consciousness. Postconcussive symptoms can result from mild concussion, although in most cases, there is rapid recovery from these deficits. There is considerable variability among group data, and some individuals with complicated mild head injuries experience symptoms for more than 1 year. In addition, the cumulative effects of numerous mild head injuries are presently not well understood. The amateur boxing literature suggests some ability of the brain to withstand intermittent blows and manifest only minimal neurological or neuropsychological deficits. When there is less protection and increased force and number of blows, as in professional boxing or sparring with a professional, the risks for brain dysfunction increase. Given the recent rise in soccer participation and a late century trend for "white collar" men and women to engage in amateur boxing, it is hoped that ongoing prospective research, such as Stewart et al.'s (1994) study, will clarify both the short- and long-term effects of repeated mild head injuries (e.g., exactly who and when is a participant at greater risk for developing a degenerative neurological disorder). Continued integration of functional neuroimaging methods and neuropsychology will also contribute to better understanding of mild head trauma outcome.

Although the effects of a single concussion are often fairly innocuous, there is little consensus regarding deficits, symptoms, recovery, and outcome of repeated, sports-related, mild TBI. This lack of agreement is based upon the multifactorial nature of concussion (i.e., the magnitude and direction of impact, the physical reaction and structural features of the skull, and the position of the head at the moment of impact). Hence, each impact can cause unique injuries (Jordan, 1989). The variability in outcome and recovery from mild head injury also depends upon many individual (vulnerability) factors such as age, health, previous head injuries and neurological disorders, intellectual reserve, emotional status, pain, and so on. Many studies have methodological problems, for example, failure to account for base rates of postconcussive symptoms (e.g., Lees-Haley & Brown, 1993) and poor control groups. The extent to which neuropsychological assessment will contribute to successful future research depends on the resolution of some crucial issues, such as the sensitivity of particular test instruments to cognitive dysfunction, the question of estimating preinjury cognitive status, predictive and ecological validity, constructing a brief yet thorough test battery, and so on. Macciocchi (1990) also suggested that we must be cautious when considering the difficulty of repeated cognitive assessments of athletes, when practice effects are inevitable.

Although many of the mentioned studies of sports-related head injuries have been inconclusive, the use of professional and amateur sports as a laboratory to study mild head injury should continue. Professional and amateur sports are arenas in which phenomena such as the acceleration/deceleration forces commonly seen in automobile accidents can be prospectively and innocuously examined. In addition, although mild head trauma is less frequent than many other injuries and is downplayed by athletes, the possible serious effects of sports-related concussion have spurred the development of protective equipment that has filtered into everyday life (e.g., bicycle helmets, automobile design, etc.). Accordingly, it is hoped that the number of head injuries in the general public will decline. Ongoing study of this sample of the population should reap continued benefits for society as a whole.

References

Alves, W. M., Rimel, R. W., & Nelson, W. E. (1987). University of Virginia prospective study of football-induced minor head injury: Status report. *Clinics in Sports Medicine: Head and Neck Injuries, 6*(1), 211–218.

American Academy of Neurology. (1983). The American Board of Neurology opposes the practice of boxing [Policy statement]. Executive Board Meeting, American Academy of Neurology, May, 1983.

American Academy of Neurology Quality Standards Committee. (1997). Practice parameter: The management of concussion in sports [summary statement]. *Neurology, 48,* 581–585.

American Academy of Pediatrics Committee on Sports Medicine and Fitness. (1997). Participation in boxing by children, adolescents, and young adults. *Pediatrics, 99*(1), 134–135.

Barth, J. T., Alves, W. M., Ryan, T. V., Macciocchi, S. N., Rimel, R. E., Jane, J. A., & Nelson, W. E. (1989). Mild head injury in sports: Neuropsychological sequelae and recovery of function. In H. S. Levin, H. M. Eisenberg, & A. L. Benton (Eds.), *Mild head injury* (pp. 257–275). New York: Oxford University Press.

Barth, J. T., Macciocchi, S. N., Giordani, B., Rimel, R., Jane, J. A., & Boll, J. T. (1983). Neuropsychological sequelae of mild head injury. *Neurosurgery, 13,* 529–533.

Bixby-Hammett, D. M. (1992). Pediatric equestrian injuries. *Pediatrics, 89,* 1173–1176.

Butler, R., Forsythe, W., Beverly, D., & Adams, L. (1993). A prospective controlled investigation of the cognitive effects of amateur boxing. *Journal of Neurology, Neurosurgery, and Psychiatry, 56,* 1055–1061.

Cantu, R. C. (1986). Guidelines for return to contact sports after a cerebral concussion. *Physician and Sportsmedicine, 14,* 75–83.

DeLee, J. C., & Farney, W. C. (1992). Incidence of injury in Texas high school football. *American Journal of Sports Medicine, 20,* 575–580.

Dikmen, S., Machamer, J., Winn, R., & Temkin, N. (1995). Neuropsychological outcome at 1-year post head injury. *Neuropsychology, 9*(1), 80–90.

Dikmen, S., McLean, A., & Temkin, N. (1986). Neuropsychological and psychological consequences of minor head injury. *Neurosurgery, 48,* 1227–1232.

Dixon, C., Taft, W., & Hayes, R. (1993). Mechanisms of mild traumatic brain injury. *Journal of Head Trauma Rehabilitation, 8,* 1–12.

Duckett, S., & Duckett, S. (1993). The neuropathology of the minor head injury syndrome. In S. Mandel, R. T. Sataloff, & S. R. Shapiro (Eds.), *Minor head trauma: Assessment, management, and rehabilitation* (pp. 5–13). New York: Springer-Verlag.

Foster, J. B., Leiguarda, R., & Tilley, P. (1976). Brain damage in national hunt jockeys. *Lancet, i,* 981–983.

Fullerton, L., & Becker, T. (1991). Moving targets: Bicycle-related injuries and helmet use among university students. *Journal of American College Health, 39,* 213–217.

Gerberich, S. G., Priest, J. D., Boen, J. R., Staub, C. P., & Maxwell, R. E. (1983). Concussion incidences and severity in secondary school varsity football players. *American Journal of Public Health, 73,* 1370–1375.

Gibbs, N. (1993). Injuries in professional rugby league: A three year prospective study of the South Sydney Professional Rugby Football Club. *American Journal of Sports Medicine, 21,* 696–700.

Gronwall, D., & Wrightson, P. (1975). Cumulative effect of concussion. *Lancet, ii,* 995–997.

Haglund, Y., & Bergstrand, G. (1990). Does Swedish amateur boxing lead to chronic brain damage? 2. A retrospective study with CT and MRI. *Acta Neurologica Scandinavia, 82,* 297–302.

Haglund, Y., Edman, G., Murelius, O., Oreland, L., & Sachs, C. (1990). Does Swedish amateur boxing lead to chronic brain damage? 1. A retrospective medical, neurological, and personality trait study. *Acta Neurologica Scandinavia, 82,* 245–252.

Haglund, Y., & Eriksson, E. (1993). Does amateur boxing lead to chronic brain damage? A review of some recent investigations. *American Journal of Sports Medicine, 21,* 97–109.

Haglund, Y., & Persson, H. E. (1990). Does Swedish amateur boxing lead to chronic brain damage? 3. A retrospective clinical neurophysiological study. *Acta Neurologica Scandinavia, 82,* 353–360.

Hamilton, M. G., & Tranmer, B. I. (1993). Nervous system injuries in horseback-riding accidents. *The Journal of Trauma, 34,* 227–232.

Harrington, D. E., Malec, J., Cicerone, K., & Katz, H. (1993). Current perceptions of rehabilitation professionals towards mild traumatic brain injury. *Archives of Physical Medicine and Rehabilitation, 74,* 579–586.

Heilbronner, R. L., Henry, G. K., & Carson-Brewer, M. (1991). Neuropsychologic test performance in amateur boxers. *American Journal of Sports Medicine, 19,* 376–380.

Hinton-Bayre, A. D., Geffen, G., & McFarland, K. (1997). Mild head injury and speed of information processing: A prospective study of professional rugby league players. *Journal of Clinical & Experimental Neuropsychology, 19*(2), 275–289.

Holzgraefe, M., Lemme, W., Funke, W., Felix, R., & Felten, R. (1992). The significance of diagnostic imaging in acute and chronic brain damage in boxing. *International Journal of Sports Medicine, 13,* 616–620.

Jordan, B. D. (1987). Neurologic aspects of boxing. *Archives of Neurology, 44,* 453–459.

Jordan, B. D. (1989). Head injury in sports. In B. D. Jordan, P. Tsairis, & R. F. Warren (Eds.), *Sports neurology* (pp. 75–83). Rockville, MD: Aspen.

Jordan, B. D. (1994, April). Sports injuries. In *Proceedings of the Mild Brain Injury in Sports Summit of the National Athletic Trainers' Association Research and Education Foundation, Washington, DC,* 43–46.

Jordan, B., Kanik, A., Horwich, M., Sweeney, D., Relkin, N., Petito, C., & Gandy, S. (1995). Apolipoprotein E e4 and fatal cerebral amyloid angiopathy associated with dementia pugilistica. *Annals of Neurology, 38*(4), 698–699.

Jordan, B., Matser, E., Zimmerman, R., & Zazula, T. (1996). Sparring and cognitive function in professional boxers. *The Physician and Sportsmedicine, 24*(5), 87–98.

Jordan, B. D., Relkin, N. R., Ravdin, L. D., Jadcobs, A. R., Bennett, A., & Galndy, S. (1997). Apolipoprotein E e4 associated with chronic traumatic brain injury in boxing. *Journal of the American Medical Association, 278*(2), 134–140.

Jordan, S. E., Green, G. A., Galanty, H. L., Mandelbaum, B. E., & Jabour, B. A. (1996). Acute and chronic brain injury in United States national team soccer players. *The American Journal of Sports Medicine, 24*(2), 205–210.

Karpakka, J. (1993). American football injuries in Finland. *British Journal of Sports Medicine, 27,* 135–137.

Kemp, P., Houston, A., Macleod, M., & Pethybridge, R. (1995). Cerebral perfusion and psychometric testing in military amateur boxers and controls. *Journal of Neurology, Neurosurgery, and Psychiatry, 59,* 368–374.

Lampert, P. W., & Hardman, J. M. (1984). Morphological changes in brains of boxers. *Journal of the American Medical Association, 251,* 2676–2679.

Lees-Haley, P., & Brown, R. (1993). Neuropsychological complaint base rates of 170 personal injury claimants. *Archives of Clinical Neuropsychology, 8*(3), 203–209.

Levin, H. S., Eisenberg, H. M., & Benton, A. L. (Eds.). (1989). *Mild head injury.* New York: Oxford University Press.

Levin, H. S., & Jordan, B. J. (1993). Neuropsychological assessment of brain injury in boxing. In B. J. Jordan (Ed.), *Medical aspects of boxing* (pp. 197–206). Boca Raton, FL: CRC Press.

Levin, H. S., Mattis, S., Ruff, R. M., Eisenberg, H. M., Marshall, L. F., Tabaddor, K., High, W. M., & Frankowski, R. F. (1987). Neurobehavioral outcome following minor head injury: A three center study. *Journal of Neurosurgery, 66,* 234–243.

Macciocchi, S. N. (1990). Practice makes perfect: Retest effects in college athletes. *Journal of Clinical Psychology, 5,* 628–631.

Macciocchi, S. N., Barth, J. T., Alves, W., Rimel, R. W., & Jane, J. J. (1996). Neuropsychological functioning and recovery after mild head injury in collegiate athletes. *Neurosurgery, 39,* 510–514.

Magnes, S. A. (1990). When a knee injury becomes a head injury. *Physician and Sportsmedicine, 18,* 109–112.

McCrea, M., Kelly, J. P., Kluge, J., Ackley, A., & Randolph, C. (1997). Standardized assessment of concussion in football players. *Neurology, 48,* 586–588.

McCunney, R. J., & Russo, P. K. (1984). Brain injuries in boxers. *Physician and Sportsmedicine, 12,* 53–67.

McLatchie, G., Brooks, N., Galbraith, S., Hutchison, J., Wilson, L., Melville, I., & Teasdale, E. (1987). Clinical neurological examination, neuropsychology, electroencephalography and computed tomographic head scanning in active amateur boxers. *Journal of Neurology, Neurosurgery, and Psychiatry, 50,* 96–99.

McLean, A., Temkin, N. R., Dikmen, S., & Wyler, A. R. (1983). The behavioral sequelae of head injury. *Journal of Clinical Neuropsychology, 5,* 361–376.

Mild Traumatic Brain Injury Committee of the Head Injury Interdisciplinary Special Interest Group of the American Congress of Rehabilitation Medicine. (1993). Definition of mild traumatic brain injury. *Journal of Head Trauma Rehabilitation, 8,* 86–87.

O'Brien, C. (1992). Retrospective survey of rugby injuries in the Leinster province of Ireland 1987–1989. *British Journal of Sports Medicine, 26,* 243–244.

O'Meara, E. S., Kukull, W. A., Sheppard, L., Bowen, J. D., McCormick, W. C., Teri, L., Pfanschmidt, M., Thompson, J. D., Schellenberg, G. D., & Larson, E. B. (1997). Head injury and risk of Alzheimer's disease by apolipoprotein E genotype. *American Journal of Epidemiology, 146*(5), 373–384.

Ommaya, A. K., & Gennarelli, T. A. (1974). Cerebral concussion and traumatic unconsciousness. Correlation of experimental and clinical observations on blunt head injuries. *Brain, 97,* 633–654.

Pelletier, R. L., Montelpare, W. J., & Stark, R. M. (1993). Intercollegiate ice hockey injuries: A case for uniform definitions and reports. *American Journal of Sports Medicine, 21,* 78–81.

Povlishock, J. T., & Lontos, H. A. (1985). Continuing axonal and vascular change following experimental brain trauma. *Journal of Central Nervous System Trauma, 2,* 285–298.

Rimel, R. W., Giordani, B., Barth, J. T., Boll, T. J., & Jane, J. (1981). Disability caused by minor head injury. *Neurosurgery, 9,* 221–228.

Ross, R. J., Casson, I. R., Siegel, O., & Cole, M. (1987). Boxing injuries: Neurologic, radiologic, and neuropsychologic evaluation. In J. S. Torg (Ed.), *Clinics in sports medicine: Head and neck injuries* (pp. 41–52). Philadelphia: W. B. Saunders.

Ruff, R. M., Crouch, J. A., Troster, A. I., Marshall, L. F., Buchsbaum, M. S., Lottenberg, S., & Somers, L. M. (1994). Selected cases of poor outcome following a minor brain trauma: Comparing neuropsychological and positron emission tomography assessment. *Brain Injury, 8,* 297–308.

Ryan, A. J. (1987). Intracranial injuries resulting from boxing: A review (1918–1985). In J. S. Torg (Ed.), *Clinics in sports medicine: Head and neck injuries* (pp. 31–40). Philadelphia: W. B. Saunders.

Saal, J., & Sontag, M. (1987). Head injuries in contact sports: Sideline decision making. *Physical Medicine and Rehabilitation: State of the Art Reviews, 1*(4), 649–658.

Schneider, R. C. (1973). *Head and neck injuries in football: Mechanisms, treatment, and prevention.* Baltimore: Williams and Wilkins.

Schofield, P. W., Tang, M., Marder, K., Bell, K., Dooneief, G., Chun, M., Sano, M., Stern, Y., & Mayeux, R. (1997). Alzheimer's disease after remote head injury: An incidence study. *Journal of Neurology, Neurosurgery, & Psychiatry, 62*(2), 119–124.

Seward, H., Orchard, J., Hazard, H., & Collinson, D. (1993). Football injuries in Australia at the elite level. *Medical Journal of Australia, 159,* 298–306.

Shell, D., Carico, G. A., & Patton, R. M. (1993). Can subdural hematoma result from repeated minor head injury? *Physician and Sportsmedicine, 21,* 74–84.

Stewart, W., Gordon, B., Selnes, O., Bandeen-Roche, K., Seger, S., Tusa, R., Celentano, D., Shechter, A., Liberman, J., Hall, C., Simon, D., Lesser, R., & Randall, R. (1994). Prospective study of central nervous system function in amateur boxers in the United States. *American Journal of Epidemiology, 139,* 573–588.

Tegner, Y., & Lorentzon, R. (1991). Ice hockey injuries: incidence, nature, and causes. *British Journal of Sports Medicine, 25,* 87–89.

Torg, J. S. (1982). *Athletic injuries to the head, neck and face.* Philadelphia: Lea & Febiger.

Tysvaer, A. T. (1992). Head and neck injuries in soccer: Impact of minor trauma. *Sports Medicine, 14,* 200–213.

Tysvaer, A. T., Storli, O. V., & Bachen, N. I. (1989). Soccer injuries to the brain. A neurologic and electroencephalographic study of former players. *Acta Neurologica Scandinavia, 80,* 151–156.

Varney, N. R., & Varney, R. N. (1995). Brain injury without head injury. Some physics of automobile collisions with particular reference to brain injuries occurring without physical head trauma. *Applied Neuropsychology, 2,* 47–62.

Witol, A., & Webbe, F. (1994). Neuropsychological deficits associated with soccer play [Abstract]. *Archives of Clinical Neuropsychology, 9*(2), 204–205.

Young, C. C., Jacobs, B. A., Clavette, K., Mark, D. H., & Guse, C. E. (1997). Serial sevens: Not the most effective test of mental status in high school athletes. *Clinical Journal of Sports Medicine, 7*(3), 196–198.

Zemper, E. D. (1989). Injury rates in a national sample of college football teams: A two year prospective study. *Physician and Sportsmedicine, 17,* 100–113.

Zemper, E. D., & Pieter, W. (1989). Injury rates during the 1988 U.S. Olympic team trials for taekwondo. *British Journal of Sports Medicine, 23,* 161–164.

Medicolegal Issues II

Forensic Aspects of Mild Traumatic Brain Injury

7

Lawrence C. Hartlage

Whether serious brain injury has occurred is typically not an issue because there may be comprehensive data documenting the injury, including data from emergency medical technicians (EMTs); emergency room neurological or neurosurgical specialists; and complementary CT, MRI, or other neuroimaging or electrophysiological records. Thus, the forensic focus on such cases typically addresses the extent to which the injury may reasonably be expected to affect the lives of the individuals involved. In cases of mild TBI, however, two additional problems are likely to be encountered. These involve the related issues of recognition and documentation.

Recognition

It is probably safe to assume that the majority of mild brain injuries are neither detected nor even suspected (DeFilippis & Hartlage, 1997; Zasler, 1993). Statistics from sources like the National Head Injury Foundation (generally dealing with moderate to severe brain injury) estimate brain injury incidence in the range of 500,000 per year, largely based on documented hospital admissions with primary diagnosis of head injury (Frankowski, 1986). However, epidemiological studies have estimated an annual incidence in the United States ranging from 7 million to more than 10 million injuries (Annegers, Grabow, Kurland, & Laws, 1980; Caveness, 1977, 1979; Hartlage, 1984, 1990a; Sorenson & Krauss, 1991); the difference between estimated head injury and hospitalization for treatment of head injury may be used as

Reprinted, with changes, from "Forensic Aspects of Mild Brain Injury," by Lawrence C. Hartlage, 1997, *Applied Neuropsychology, 4*(1), pp. 69–74. Copyright 1997 by Lawrence Erlbaum Associates, Inc.

an approximation of the incidence of mild head injury. Indeed, a survey of hospital records indicates the likelihood of dramatic underreporting of mild head injury (Segalowitz & Brown, 1991), and for more than a decade the lay press has seen head injury as a largely unrecognized epidemic (Klein, 1982). Review of several hundred case reports offers a number of likely explanations for this failure to recognize mild head injury. At the accident site, a brief loss of consciousness may be resolved by the time EMTs or police arrive, so that the injured individual is described as suffering no loss of consciousness. Similarly, a superficial interview at the site may not reveal loss of consciousness because, typically, an individual who has been unconscious does not recall it. Even later questioning may fail to identify a loss of consciousness because the injured individual may fill in gaps in his or her recollection with what others have said and thus appear to have fairly complete recollection for the events surrounding the injury. Accordingly, official records may document no loss of consciousness, even when it has occurred.

Another factor that tends to mask mild head injury is the little-recognized fact that the head does not need to strike an external object for brain injury to occur (Hartlage & Rattan, 1992; Varney & Varney, 1995); the striking of the head against an external object is but one of four factors related to degree of brain injury and axonal shearing (Brenner & Enz, 1986; Gennarelli et al., 1987). As a result, individuals who complain of postconcussive symptoms when there has been no apparent trauma to the head, are at risk for having their complaints dismissed, even though research has documented both theoretical rationale and empirical evidence for brain injury without any injury to the head (Varney & Varney).

Even more problematic in the detection of mild head injury is the fact that brain injury may have occurred without loss of consciousness (Zasler, 1993); that is, loss of consciousness is not a sufficient indicator of residual brain injury (Cullum & Thompson, 1997). Indeed, there is considerable evidence supportive of the concept that initial subtle axonal changes resultant from mild brain injury become progressively severe, with axonal injury in humans representing an evolutionary process (Christman, Grady, & Povlishock, 1992; Kontos, Wei, & Povlishock, 1980; Povlishock, Becker, Cheng, & Vaughn, 1983). This could pose a substantial problem when symptoms of concussive head injury are dismissed due to no loss of consciousness, because once the case is settled, remaining problems may be considered psychopathological in origin rather than reasonably resultant from the head injury. When legal representatives of either side are skeptical of head injury because there is no confirmed loss of consciousness, the patient may be subject to ridicule of real neuropsychological problems resultant from the injury, and in frustration agree to settle without consideration of losses from head injury. In recent years, attorneys have begun taking a more aggressive stand on such issues, to the point of filing actions against plaintiffs' attorneys who did not fully recognize head injury and its sequelae when settling such cases (Chapman, 1991).

Clinically, failure to recognize the involvement of mild head injury—often unsuspected by the patient or family—in postinjury problems can result in considerable subjective distress for the patient, and anger toward and rejection of the patient by family members. Such common sequelae of mild head injury as forgetfulness, irritability and quickness to anger, fatigue, lethargy and diminished stamina, and impaired attention and concentration, when not recognized as realistically related to the injury, frequently make patients fear that they are losing their mind. These sequelae may also result in perceptions that the patient no longer loves his or her family or is no longer a conscientious employee or student. In my experience, one of the more important steps toward recovery is the patient's recognition that there is indeed a cause for his or her changed mental status; this recognition can provide a basis for addressing what sort of improvement may be hoped for, what future problems may be anticipated, and what steps can be taken to enhance recovery and minimize future problems.

Documentation

Documentation of mild head injury represents a reasonable forensic issue for attorneys who represent the patient and possibly family (plaintiff) and those who represent the liable party and his or her insurance carrier. From the patient's perspective, the very fact that he or she has experienced suffering, distress, or perceived loss of function is viewed as prima facie evidence that he or she is due compensation, and the patient may view demands for examination by the defendant's doctor as harassment. Defendants, logically and reasonably, are reluctant to consider compensation for injury until there is some convincing evidence that injury has in fact been sustained.

One historical problem hindering acceptance of long-term effects of mild brain injury involves the traditionally accepted maxim that severity of brain injury is related to (and can be inferred from) duration of coma. Thus it may be reasoned that if no loss of consciousness is documented, there is no reason to assume there will be any long-term consequence. When we look at the context in which the maxim was offered, it is clear that in an earlier era, when there was lower survival rate from very severe head injury, cases of moderately severe to severe brain injury showed a tendency of recovery grossly compatible with that predicted by the maxim (Hartlage, 1990b). A related and somewhat similar maxim predicted outcome based on duration of amnesia, with fairly similar accuracy (Russell, 1971). Formulated before an era in which the majority of head injuries resulted from high-speed motor vehicle accidents, this maxim was not intended to apply to the sorts of shear–strain problems encountered in such injury (Hartlage & Rattan, 1992), but it has nonetheless been cited in attempts to discredit long-term effects of mild head injury. The Glasgow Coma Scale (GCS) has also been used for outcome prediction. The GCS is an attempt to classify head injury severity on the basis of several relatively crude clinical indices. Rating and measurement error can seriously limit its potential for predicting outcome in mild head injury (Rimel, Giordani, Barth, Boll, & Jane, 1981), and may account for the wide range in recovery outcomes typically found in those with mild head injury (Dikmen & Levin, 1993). Further complicating this issue is the literature emphasizing that 80% to 85% of patients with mild TBI will make complete recovery, and briefly suffer only mild symptoms (Barth et al., 1983; Dikmen, McLean, & Temkin, 1986; Levin, Mattis, & Ruff, 1976). More recent literature demonstrates persistent symptoms, frequently of severity to produce disability in the remaining 15% to 20% of patients (Alexander, 1995; Hartlage, 1997; Kurtzke & Kurland, 1993).

Attorneys and psychologists may attribute different meaning to test results. Attorneys are likely to describe as subjective any test whose outcome may be influenced by the patient, and reserve the term "objective" for passive measures like X-rays. Psychologists typically describe as subjective tests with results dependent on subjective interpretation (e.g., inkblot personality tests), and consider objective those tests with numerical values for which interpretation would be equivalent by a trained psychologist (such as an IQ test). This differentiation can be quite important from a forensic perspective because demand for "objective" evidence of brain injury by plaintiff attorneys may result in failure to recognize mild brain injury, and such demand by defense attorneys may prolong settlement and require court action to resolve the case. The issue of validity of objective versus subjective test data is extremely important in mild head injury because the majority of mild head injury is best diagnosed by the sorts of neuropsychological measures that attorneys may consider to be subjective (Hartlage, 1990a; Tsushima & Popper, 1980; Tsushima & Wedding, 1979; Wells & Duncan, 1977). Support for the objective nature of neuropsychological test data is provided by the American Academy of Neurology, which states, "Neuropsychological evaluations have the advantage of being objective, safe, portable, and relevant to the functional integrity of the brain" (Therapeutics and Technology Assessment Subcommittee, 1996, p. 592). Furthermore, in mild TBI, the objective neurological and neurosurgical examination may produce a benign clinical picture, and added to other objective measures such as CT and EEG, commonly will not show any definitive abnormalities consistent with organic brain dysfunction (Zasler, 1993). Other researchers have shown similar lack of any clinical correlation between postconcussive disorder and standard EEG findings (Evans, 1992; Schoenhuber & Gentilini, 1989). Even more sophisticated EEG procedures, such as auditory-evoked potentials, do not seem to relate to postconcussive symptoms (Green, Leon-Barth, Dieter, Benfante, & Walker, 1992; Zasler, 1992). There is little doubt that examination with inappropriate or insensitive instruments, or by an unsophisticated examiner may result in conclusions of no evident brain injury, whereas competent examination including neuropsychological assessment may document clear evidence of such injury (Horn & Zasler, 1992).

For purposes of assessing effects of mild brain injury or an individual's functional status, a comprehensive neuropsychological examination is the best procedure currently available (Barth et al., 1983; Barth, Ryan, & Hawk, 1991; Gentilini, Nichell, & Schoenhuber, 1985; Hartlage, 1989b, 1991; Levin, Benton, & Grossman, 1982; Reitan & Wolfson, 1993; Stuss et al., 1985; Wells & Duncan, 1977; Williams, Levin, & Eisenberg, 1990). Although it may be more appealing to demonstrate X-ray, CT, or EEG evidence of brain abnormality as clear and irrefutable evidence of brain injury, such procedures contribute very little to understanding an individual's functional status subsequent to (or as a result of) minor brain injury. It is common for individuals with documented minor head injury and well documented residual sequelae to show absolutely no evidence of abnormality on CT, X-ray, or standardized EEG measures. Given a client with residual complaints of plausible sequelae of mild brain injury, in the absence of positive CT, X-ray, or EEG evidence, the attorney does a considerable disservice by not pursuing at least a neuropsychological examination, although defense attorneys' skepticism in absence of such evidence is appropriate and in keeping with their role. What are complaints that may be plausible indicators of minor (or more severe) brain injury? Although a wide variety of symptoms have been reported following mild brain injury (Boll, 1982; Fordyce, Roueche, & Prigatano, 1983; Goethe & Levin, 1984; Grigsby, 1986; Hartlage, 1989a, 1991; Klonoff, Crockett, & Clark, 1984; McLean, Temkin, Dikmen, & Wyler, 1983; Mendelson, 1987; Rutter, 1981; Sisler, 1978), the most common problems involve attention and concentration, decreased short-term memory, increased irritability and becoming easily upset, lethargy and diminished stamina, and increased anxiety and depression (Hartlage, 1989a; Hartlage & Williams, 1991; Kixmiller, Briggs, Hartlage, & Dean, 1993). Although mental ability may show signs of decline, the actual IQ may not be significantly lowered in cases of mild brain injury.

Neuropsychologist's Role in Documentation

Neuropsychological examination by a qualified neuropsychologist experienced with mild head injury can reasonably be expected to answer questions such as (a) has brain injury occurred and (b) if there is evidence of injury, how severe is it, how may it be expected to affect the individual, and can it reasonably be attributed to a given event? There may be evidence of a prior injury or drug or alcohol abuse problem, and the neuropsychologist may be able to distinguish problems unique to preexisting conditions from those unique to a specific event. A structural test such as CT or X-ray can document a severe brain injury, but cannot address such issues as how the injury may affect the individual to nearly the extent as can a measure of the individual's functional ability. Because structural measures such as X-ray or CT are relatively insensitive to mild brain injury, when compared with neuropsychological examination, any attempt by the plaintiff's attorney to focus on such measures and exclude neuropsychological procedures would be questionable, although such actions by defense attorneys would make considerable sense. One caveat worth keeping in mind when structural tests show negative findings, while mild head injury symptoms persist, is that absence of evidence does not prove evidence of absence. It is probably safe to say that it would be an extremely rare patient, well versed in correlative neuroanatomy, neuropsychological examination instruments, and head injury, who could successfully mislead an experienced and qualified neuropsychologist into egregious misdiagnosis of problems related to mild head injury.

Increasingly, documentation of mild head injury and the effects of its sequelae have recognized the associated behavioral problems, and this has altered to some extent the expectations of temporal relation between head injury and recognition of certain behavioral symptoms. Although attention, concentration, and memory problems may reasonably be expected to appear shortly after mild head injury, some of the behavioral problems appear to occur more gradually and, in fact, to become more severe over time (Williams & Hartlage, 1993). Depression, irritability, and lethargy, for example, are less likely to be reported immediately than they are several months or even longer afterward. Although the mechanisms underlying this phenomenon are not clear, frustration over inability to do things as before the injury may be one contributory factor. Whatever the cause, a number of behavioral changes relatively unique to TBI have been documented (Hartlage, 1989a, 1990b; Hartlage, Kixmiller, Brockett, Krug, & Dean, 1990; Hartlage & Williams, 1991; Kixmiller et al., 1993).

From a forensic perspective, mild head injury poses a special challenge to attorneys and neuropsychologists because it has high potential for being overlooked (especially if it occurs in conjunction with obvious physical injuries), and the sort of evidence commonly available is not so obvious to the untrained observer as open wounds or X-rays of broken bones. Yet, the problems resultant from mild head injury are very real and represent a significant health problem (Bennett, 1992). Although not reflected on common neurological, neurosurgical, or even neuropsychological examination, the very real nature of brain metabolism alteration is reflected in a number of studies involving receptor–agonist mechanisms in mild brain injury (Hayes, Jenkins, & Lyeth, 1992; Hayes, Lyeth, & Jenkins, 1989), neurotransmitter release (Nilsson, Hillerud, Ponten, & Ungerstalt, 1990; Swedlow, Botscheller, Marion, Sciabassi, & Palmer, 1992), and receptor binding (Miller, Lyeth, & Jenkins, 1990). Research demonstrating morphological injury of axonal (Kontos et al., 1980; Oppenheimer, 1968) and cytoskeletal structures (Taft,

Yang, Dixon, & Hayes, 1992), and relating cholinergic mechanisms of memory impairment resultant from brain injury (Hamm, Dixon, & Gbadebo, 1992; Smith, Okiyama, Thomas, Claussen, & McIntosh, 1991; Squire & Davis, 1981), has further helped document the scientific bases of neuropsychological dysfunctions following mild brain injury (Barth et al., 1983; Levin, Amparo, & Eisenberg, 1987; Levin, High, & Goethe, 1987). This can be an important issue in consideration of damages because minor brain injury can affect not only obvious matters such as future employability and earnings potential (Fraser, Dikmen, McLean, Miller, & Temkin, 1988; Rimel et al., 1981; Williams & Hartlage, 1993), but if occurring at an early age, may well be a source of developmental disabilities (Segalowitz & Brown, 1991). Additionally, mild head injury puts the individual at risk for potential catastrophic sequelae of a second impact (Saunders & Harbaugh, 1984), and has even been implicated as a risk factor for Alzheimer's disease (Mortimer, French, Hutton, & Schuman, 1985).

It is perhaps unfortunate that the descriptor *mild* for mild brain injury may encourage attorneys to assume that Webster's definitions of "clement," "gentle in nature," or "moderate in effect" can automatically be applied to the effects of brain injury that is mild in severity. To the extent that the scientific community has developed such an adjective to define a condition with such potential for disruption of lives, it must accept some of the responsibility for the confusion and misunderstanding too often attached to mild brain injury. It is hoped that promulgation of parameters of mild brain injury will help alleviate some of this misunderstanding and help ensure that neuropsychologists take appropriate actions to mitigate such confusion.

References

Alexander, M. P. (1995). Mild traumatic brain injury: Pathophysiology, natural history, and clinical management. *Neurology, 45,* 1253–1260.

American Academy of Neurology. (1996). Assesment: Neuropsychological testing of adults. *Neurology, 47,* 592–599.

Annegers, J. E., Grabow, J. D., Kurland, L. T., & Laws, E. R. (1980). The incidence, causes, and secular trends of head trauma in Olmstead County, Minnesota. *Neurology, 30,* 912–919.

Barth, J. T., Macciocchi, S. N., Giordani, B., Rimel, B., Jane, R. A., & Boll, T. J. (1983). Neuropsychological sequelae of minor head injury. *Neurosurgery, 13,* 529–533.

Barth, J. T., Ryan, T. V., & Hawk, G. L. (1991). Forensic neuropsychology: A reply to the method skeptics. *Neuropsychology Review, 2,* 251–256.

Bennett, T. L. (1992). Conceptualizing traumatic brain injuries. *The Journal of Head Injury, 3*(2), 21–28.

Boll, T. J. (1982). Behavioral sequelae of head injury. In D. Cooper (Ed.), *Head injury* (pp. 363–375). Baltimore: Williams & Wilkins.

Brenner, R., & Enz, B. E. (1986). Classification of information generated in a motor vehicle crash sequence. In A. Sances, D. Thomas, C. Ewing, S. Larson, & F. Unterharnscheidt (Eds.), *Mechanisms of head and spine trauma* (pp. 114–129). Goshen, NY: Alvray.

Caveness, W. F. (1977). Incidence of cranio-cerebral trauma in the United States. *Transitions of the American Neurological Association, 102,* 136–138.

Caveness, W. F. (1979). Incidence of craniocerebral trauma in the United States 1976, and trend from 1970–1975. In R. Thompson & J. Green (Eds.), *Advances in neurology* (pp. 1–3). New York: Raven.

Chapman, R. W. (1991, April). *The pending settlement: Issues to consider.* Paper presented at the JMA Foundation/National Brain Injury Research Foundation Annual Meeting, Washington, DC.

Christman, C. W., Grady, M. S., & Povlishock, J. T. (1992). Electron microscopic immunocytochemical study of diffuse axonal injury in man. *Neuroscience Abstracts, 18*(1), 988.

Cullum, C. M., & Thompson, L. L. (1997). Neuropsychological diagnoses and outcome in mild traumatic brain injury. *Applied Neuropsychology, 4*(1), 6–15.

DeFilippis, N. A., & Hartlage, L. C. (1997). *Traumatic brain injury.* Eau Clair, WI: Lorman Educational Services.

Dikmen, S. S., & Levin, H. S. (1993). Methodological issues in the study of mild head injury. *Journal of Head Trauma Rehabilitation, 8*(3), 30–37.

Dikmen, S., McLean, A., & Temkin, A. (1986). Neuropsychological and psychosocial consequences of minor head injury. *Journal of Neurology, Neurosurgery and Psychiatry, 49,* 1227–1232.

Evans, R. W. (1992). The postconcussion syndrome and the sequelae of mild head injury. *Neurologic Clinics,* 815.

Fordyce, D. J., Roueche, J. R., & Prigatano, G. P. (1983). Enhanced emotional readiness in clinic head trauma patients. *Journal of Neurology, Neurosurgery and Psychiatry, 46,* 620–624.

Frankowski, R. F. (1986). Descriptive epidemiologic studies of head injury in the United States (1974–1984). *Advances in Psychosomatic Medicine, 16,* 153–172.

Fraser, R., Dikmen, S., McLean, A., Miller, B., & Temkin, N. (1988). Employability of head injury survivors: First year post-injury. *Rehabilitation Counseling Bulletin, 31,* 276–285.

Gennarelli, T. A., Thibault, G., Tomei, G., Wiser, R., Graham, D., & Adams, J. (1987). Directional dependence of axonal brain injury due to central and noncentroidal alteration (SAS Paper No. 872197). *Proceedings of 31st Stapp Car Crash Conference,* 49–53.

Gentilini, M., Nichell, P., & Schoenhuber, R. (1985). Neuropsychological evaluation of mild head injury. *Journal of Neurology, Neurosurgery and Psychiatry, 48,* 137–140.

Goethe, K. E., & Levin, H. S. (1984). Behavioral manifestations during the early and long stages of recovery following head injury. *Psychiatric Annals, 14,* 540–546.

Green, J., Leon-Barth, C., Dieter, J., Benfante, P., & Walker, D. (1992). Somatosensory evoked responses via electronic brain imaging (EBI). *Clinical Electroencephalograph, 23,* 79–88.

Grigsby, J. P. (1986). Depersonalization following minor closed head injury. *International Journal of Clinical Neuropsychology, 7,* 65–68.

Hamm, R. J., Dixon, C. E., & Gbadebo, D. M. (1992). Cognitive deficits following traumatic brain injury produced by controlled cortical impact. *Journal of Neurotrauma, 9,* 11–20.

Hartlage, L. C. (1984). Unsuspected consequences of apparently insignificant head injuries. *Auto Torts, 7,* 187–191.

Hartlage, L. C. (1989a). *Behavior change inventory (inventory of pre- versus post-behaviors with brain injury).* Brandon, VT: Clinical Psychology Publishing.

Hartlage, L. C. (1989b). The neuropsychological and traumatic brain injury. *The JMA Journal, 1*(3), 6–8.

Hartlage, L. C. (1990a). Behavior and emotional changes after head injury. *Journal of Head Injury, 2*(1), 17–19.

Hartlage, L. C. (1990b). *Neuropsychological evaluation of head injury.* Sarasota, FL: Professional Resource Exchange.

Hartlage, L. C. (1991). Major legal consequences of minor head injuries. *The Journal of Head Injury, 2*(3), 8–11.

Hartlage, L. C. (1997). Is mild brain injury an epidemic, a fad, or a scam? *ATLA Brain Injury Newsletter, 4*(2), 5–10.

Hartlage, L. C., Kixmiller, J. S., Brockett, D. R., Krug, D. K., & Dean, R. S. (1990). Examination of factor structure of common symptoms following head injury [Abstract]. *Archives of Clinical Neuropsychology, 5*(2), 176.

Hartlage, L. C., & Rattan, G. (1992). Brain injury from motor vehicle accidents. In D. Templer, L. Hartlage, & W. Cannon (Eds.), *Preventing brain damage: Brain vulnerability and brain health* (pp. 3–14). New York: Springer-Chyler.

Hartlage, L. C., & Williams, B. L. (1991). Assessment of behavioral sequelae of traumatic and chemical CNS insult. *Archives of Clinical Neuropsychology, 6,* 279–286.

Hayes, R. L., Jenkins, L. W., & Lyeth, B. G. (1992). Neurotransmitter mediated mechanisms of traumatic brain injury: Acetylcholine and excitatory amino acids. *Journal of Neurotrauma, 9,* 173–187.

Hayes, R. L., Lyeth, B. G., & Jenkins, L. W. (1989). Neurochemical mechanisms of mild and moderate head injury: Implications for treatment. In H. Levin, H. Eisenberg, & A. Benton (Eds.), *Mild head injury* (pp. 54–79). New York: Oxford University Press.

Horn, L. J., & Zasler, N. D. (1992). *Rehabilitative management of post-concussive disorders.* Philadelphia: Hanley & Belfus.

Kixmiller, J. S., Briggs, J. R., Hartlage, L. C., & Dean, R. S. (1993). Factor structure of emotional and cognitive behaviors for normals and neurologically impaired patients. *Journal of Clinical Psychology, 3*(2), 233–241.

Klein, F. C. (1982, November 24). Silent epidemic: Head injuries difficult to diagnose, set rising attention. *The Wall Street Journal,* p. 1.

Klonoff, H., Crockett, D. D., & Clark, K. (1984). Head injuries in children: A model for predicting course of recovery and prognosis. In R. Tarter & G. Golstein (Eds.), *Advances in clinical neuropsychology* (Vol. 2, pp. 139–157). New York: Plenum.

Kontos, H. A., Wei, E. P., & Povlishock, J. T. (1980). Pathophysiology of vascular consequences of experimental concussive brain injury. *Clinical Association Transactions, 92,* 111.

Kurtzke, J. F., & Kurland, L. T. (1993). The epidemiology of neurologic disease. In R. J. Joint (Ed.), *Clinical neurology* (pp. 66). Philadelphia: J. B. Lippincott.

Levin, H. S., Amparo, E., & Eisenberg, H. M. (1987). Magnetic resonance imaging and computerized tomography in relation to the neurobehavioral sequelae of mild and moderate head injuries. *Journal of Neurosurgery, 66,* 706–713.

Levin, H. S., Benton, A. C., & Grossman, R. G. (1982). *Neurobehavioral consequences of closed head injury.* New York: Oxford University Press.

Levin, H. S., High, W. M., & Goethe, K. E. (1987). The Neurobehavioral Rating Scale: Assessment of the behavioral sequelae of head injury by the clinician. *Journal of Neurology, Neurosurgery and Psychiatry, 50,* 183–193.

Levin, H. S., Mattis, S., & Ruff, R. M. (1976). Neurobehavioral outcome following minor head injury: A three center study. *Journal of Neurosurgery, 66,* 234–243.

McLean, A., Temkin, N. P., Dikmen, S., & Wyler, A. R. (1983). The behavior sequelae of head injury. *Journal of Clinical Neuropsychology, 54,* 361–376.

Mendelson, G. (1987). The concept of post-traumatic stress disorder: A review. *International Journal of Law and Psychiatry, 10,* 46–62.

Miller, L. P., Lyeth, B. G., & Jenkins, L. W. (1990). Excitatory amino acid receptor subtype binding following traumatic brain injury. *Brain Research, 526,* 103–107.

Mortimer, J. A., French, L. R., Hutton, J. T., & Schuman, L. M. (1985). Head injury as a risk factor for Alzheimer's disease. *Neurology, 35,* 264–267.

Nilsson, P., Hillerud, L., Ponten, U., & Ungerstalt, U. (1990). Changes in cortical extracellular levels of energy-related metabolites and amino acids following concussive brain injury in rats. *Journal of Cerebral Blood Flow Metabolism, 10,* 631–637.

Oppenheimer, D. R. (1968). Microscopic lesions in the brain following head injury. *Journal of Neurology, Neurosurgery and Psychiary, 31,* 299–306.

Povlishock, J. T., Becker, D. P., Cheng, C. L., & Vaughn, G. W. (1983). Axonal change in minor head injury. *Journal of Neuropathology and Experimental Neurology, 42,* 225.

Reitan, R. M., & Wolfson, D. (1993). *The Halstead-Reitan Neuropsychological Test Battery.* Tucson, AZ: Neuropsychology Press.

Rimel, R. W., Giordani, B., Barth, J. T., Boll, T. J., & Jane, J. A. (1981). Disability caused by minor head injury. *Neurosurgery, 9,* 225–228.

Russell, N. R. (1971). *The traumatic amnesias.* New York: Oxford University Press.

Rutter, M. (1981). Psychological sequelae of brain damage in children. *The American Journal of Psychiatry, 138,* 1433–1544.

Saunders, R. L., & Harbaugh, R. E. (1984). The second impact in catastrophic contact-sports head trauma. *Journal of the American Medical Association, 252,* 536–539.

Schoenhuber, R., & Gentilini, M. (1989). Neuropsychological assessment of mild head injury. In H. Levin, H. Eisenberg, & A. Benton (Eds.), *Mild head injury* (pp. 142–150). New York: Oxford University Press.

Segalowitz, S. J., & Brown, D. (1991). Mild head injury as a source of developmental disabilities. *Journal of Learning Disabilities, 24,* 551–558.

Sisler, G. E. (1978). Psychiatric disorder associated with head injury. *Psychiatric Clinics of North America, 1,* 137–152.

Smith, D. H., Okiyama, K., Thomas, M. J., Claussen, B., & McIntosh, T. K. (1991). Evaluation of memory dysfunction following experimental brain injury using the Morris Water Maze. *Journal of Neurotrauma, 8,* 259–269.

Sorenson, S., & Krauss, J. (1991). Occurrence, severity, and outcomes of brain injury. *The Journal of Head Trauma Rehabilitation, 6,* 1–10.

Squire, L. R., & Davis, H. P. (1981). The pharmacology of memory: A neurobiological perspective. *Annual Review of Pharmacology and Technology, 21,* 325–356.

Stuss, D. T., Ely, P., Hugenholz, H., Richard, M., La Rochelle, S., Pirier, C., & Bell, I. (1985). Subtle neuropsychological deficits in patients with good recovery after closed head injury. *Neurosurgery, 17,* 41–45.

Swedlow, P. E., Botscheller, M. L., Marion, D. W., Sciabassi, R. J., & Palmer, A. M. (1992). Controlled cortical impact induces sustained evaluations in the extracellular concentration of excitatory amino acids. *Society for Neuroscience Abstracts, 18,* 172.

Taft, W. C., Yang, F., Dixon, C. E., & Hayes, R. L. (1992). Microtubule associated protein 2 levels decreased in hippocampus following traumatic brain injury. *Journal of Neurotrauma, 9,* 281–290.

Tsushima, W. T., & Popper, J. S. (1980). Computerized tomography: A report of false negative errors. *Clinical Neuropsychology, 2,* 130–133.

Tsushima, W. T., & Wedding, D. (1979). A comparison of the Halstead-Reitan battery and computerized tomography in the identification of brain damage. *Journal of Nervous and Mental Disease, 167,* 704–707.

Varney, N. R., & Varney, R. N. (1995). Brain injury without head injury: Some physics of automobile collisions with particular reference to brain injuries occurring without physical head trauma. *Applied Neuropsychology, 2,* 47–62.

Wells, C. E., & Duncan, G. W. (1977). Danger of over reliance on computed cranial tomography. *American Journal of Psychiatry, 134,* 811–813.

Williams, B. L., & Hartlage, L. C. (1993). Factors influencing return to work following head injury. *The Journal of Head Injury, 3*(2), 48–52.

Williams, D. H., Levin, H. S., & Eisenberg, H. M. (1990). Mild head injury classification. *Neurosurgery, 27,* 442–448.

Zasler, N. D. (1992). Neuromedical diagnosis and treatment of postconcussive disorder. In L. Horn & N. Zasler (Eds.), *Rehabilitation of post-concussive disorders* (pp. 33–68). Philadelphia: Hanley & Belfus.

Zasler, N. D. (1993). Post-concussive disorders: Facts, fallacies and foibles. *The Journal of Head Injury, 3*(2), 8–13.

Litigation Perspectives for the Health Professional

8

Rex D. Smith and
Ian R. Rapaport

Whereas many lawyers and laymen complain that the world of medicine and psychology is complex and difficult to understand, many health professionals have the same complaint when first exposed to the American civil justice system. This chapter addresses the civil process and the health professional's role within it. Honesty, integrity, and the ability to clearly communicate one's thoughts are any witness's touchstones. This is especially true for the health professional expert in the evolving and often esoteric science of mild TBI.

Of the millions of cases of TBI annually in the United States (Davis, 1990), many lead to litigation over the cause and the extent of the injury. The claims and lawsuits that arise from TBI primarily are based on negligence or product liability. The injury can be from an automobile accident, fall, faulty product, and so on. As the medical and neuropsychological aspects of these injuries are becoming more generally understood by attorneys, health professionals such as neurologists, neurosurgeons, neuropsychologists, clinical psychologists, psychiatrists, audiologists, and others are being called upon to testify in increasing numbers.

The Claims Process

The first step in the litigation process often has nothing to do with litigation per se, but is simply the making of a claim by the injured party. The injured party makes a claim against the individual or company alleged to have caused the injury; this can be done with or without an attorney. Many times, the health care professional is first involved when the patient or patient's attorney requests a report to be used in this claims process.

Once the health professional is aware that litigation is a possibility for his or her patient, several matters become important. First, it is both proper and prudent for the health professional to inquire into the status of the patient's claim and the health professional's role. If it appears that the health professional will be called upon to participate in the claims process, either through a report or testimony, he or she should take the steps necessary to insure that there is sufficient and appropriate support for his or her opinions. Many times a treating physician will make treatment recommendations based on only an interview and screening test. Although this may be an acceptable, standard medical practice, a higher standard is recommended for the scrutiny of cross-examination and judicial review.

When the health professional is first notified that he or she may be called upon to testify, he or she should do the following:

1. Review the patient's records to insure that all pertinent records or testimony have been obtained. Prior school records, work records, and patient interviews, although not necessarily essential for treatment, will take on new significance in the litigation process. The health professional should also obtain and review all of the records necessary to support his or her professional opinions.
2. Understand the mechanism of the injury. Whereas the patient's self-report may be sufficient for treatment and analysis, a full review of accident reports and emergency records helps support any opinions offered in litigation. Many times I have seen a health professional render an opinion, based on a patient's self-report, that is clearly contradicted by earlier reports or other statements by the patient. Having a complete understanding of the entire record and history of the patient will give the health professional credibility in a judicial inquiry and assist him or her in helping the patient.
3. If the patient is represented, discuss the case with the patient's attorney. An understanding of the claims process and the health professional's role can better prepare this professional to assist the patient, the court, and himself or herself. A well prepared attorney or neurolawyer will be able to give a specific roadmap to the patient's claim and the health professional's role in it. Learning early on when and where he or she will be needed helps the health professional avoid the crisis that often occurs in litigation.
4. Perform any additional testing that may be necessary. If the passage of time from the initial treatment to the time of report or testimony calls for additional testing, the health professional should go ahead and perform it. If the initial treatment and opinions were made with only partial or screening testing, the professional should complete the testing with generally accepted instruments. Basing opinions on test batteries or instruments that are not generally accepted can lead to a damaging cross-examination by defense counsel.

5. Update the curriculum vitae to include all new professional achievements. The health professional's curriculum vitae will be critically reviewed by defense counsel and the court. It must be ready for cross-examination.

During the claims process the health professional will often receive requests for his or her records. Most states provide a privilege for medical, psychiatric, and neuropsychological records (e.g., see Official Code of Georgia Annotated, 1987, § 24-9-21 & § 24-9-40). In general, these records should be released only with an appropriate authorization or subpoena. Many neuropsychologists take the position that their records may be released only to another psychologist as per the Ethical Principles for Psychologists from the American Psychological Association. Frankly, this is viewed rather skeptically by the defense bar and often by juries as well. If the patient has provided an appropriate release of records, and the health professional is not constrained by other ethical considerations, it is recommended that the records be released without delay. A refusal often leads to cross-examination questions that could be harmful to the patient's claim. If there are any questions about disclosure, the health professional should consult with either his or her personal counsel or the patient's counsel.

During the informal claims process, the health professional may be asked to prepare a new report specifically for that process. At this point the standard of scrutiny has been raised. The health professional should carefully document the basis for his or her opinions, what has been done, what records have been reviewed, and what assumptions are being made. Calculations should be reviewed for errors.

A common point of attack by a defense attorney is the neuropsychologist or other treating health professional's preinjury estimate of functioning. Often, I have seen a neuropsychologist state that a patient has seen a significant decline in functioning, based on the patient's self-report of good or superior academic achievement. However, upon receipt of additional school records, the patient's history is not supported and often in severe disagreement.

The Complaint and Answer

In a significant number of cases, the informal claims process is not successful, and formal litigation is instituted. The litigation process is most often begun by the filing of a complaint in either state or federal court. The civil action is begun when the patient, who is referred to as the plaintiff, files a document that contains "a short sworn statement of the claim showing that the pleader is entitled to relief" (Federal Rules of Civil Procedure [F.R.C.P.] 7) against the defendant, who is the party claimed to have caused the injury.

The defendant is given time to file a response in a document known as an answer, which "shall state in short and plain terms the party's defenses to each claim asserted" (F.R.C.P. 8).

Discovery—Subpoenas and Request To Produce

After the plaintiff and defendant have filed their complaint and answer, the parties enter into a period known as discovery. During this phase of litigation, the parties have the power to subpoena records, take depositions, and conduct other formal discovery through the power of the courts. In general, the parties may discover "any evidence that may lead to admissible evidence" (F.R.C.P. 26; see also Official Code of Georgia Annotated, 1987, § 9-11-26). This rule is often applied very broadly and can lead into inquiries about the health professional's qualifications, treatment, and other areas that might show bias to one side or the other. In many cases, a health professional's prior testimony will be obtained by the defendant and studied for contradictory testimony or opinions.

The first step in the discovery process for the health care professional is usually the service of a subpoena or other court process compelling production of the patient's records. Often these requests will be quite extensive—they may request a curriculum vitae, patient records, and even raw data. Although questions about complying with a subpoena should be referred to counsel, a few observations may be helpful here.

The subpoena should be carefully reviewed and fully complied with if there are no constraining ethical considerations. A partial response will be questioned closely and may be cast in a poor light before the jury. Consultation with counsel is appropriate if any questions arise as to the scope or sufficiency of the subpoena, but the scope of discovery is usually very broad, including "any matter, not privileged, which is relevant to the subject matter involved in the pending action" (F.R.C.P. 26(b)(1)). Records should be produced to both sides in the litigation process.

When a subpoena is received it should be forwarded to the opposing party with an inquiry of any objection to compliance. The requesting party should receive a copy of transmittal correspondence so that all parties will be fully apprised. If there is no objection, the health professional should file his or her response in a timely manner. When filing a response, the health professional should fully and carefully catalog what is being produced. If any records are being withheld, a specific objection or explanation should be provided along with a description of the records being withheld. The health professional should avoid appearing to have withheld records without a proper disclosure. The professional must not let the shadow of doubt be cast upon his or her integrity—it can hurt the patient in litigation.

If an objection is received by the opposing party, the health professional should consult with that party and honor the objection. However, the professional is still under an obligation to file a timely response, usually 30 days from the date of service (F.R.C.P. 34; see also Official Code of Georgia Annotated, 1987, § 9-11-34). The objection should be disclosed in the response.

After receiving the response, the litigating parties are then under a duty to confer with each other and attempt to resolve any discovery dispute (see Georgia Uniform Court Rules, Local Rule 6.4). In the vast majority of cases, the parties resolve the discovery dispute and notify the health professional of their agreement. If not otherwise constrained by a professional code of ethics, the health professional should then comply pursuant to the agreement. In the rare case where an amicable resolution is not reached by the parties, the moving party has the option to bring the dispute before the judge in a motion to compel (F.R.C.P. 37; see also Official Code of Georgia Annotated, 1987, § 9-11-37). This motion may very well be directed to the health professional as the records custodian and require an appearance before the court. Prompt consultation with personal counsel or the patient's counsel is recommended. A written response to the court will often be required. In some states, the motion may be directed to the patient. It is necessary to thoroughly understand the motion and how to respond.

After all parties have had an opportunity to file their legal briefs stating their position to the court, the judge will issue an order deciding the issue. The order will usually be specific as to what documents must be produced, when and where. Failure to comply with the court's order can have significant consequences. Although there are procedures for appealing a discovery order, this must be done within time limits and in compliance with specific appeals procedures. It is extremely rare for an appeal of a discovery order to be heard and overruled by an appellate court, because the trial judge is given broad discretion in discovery matters.

Independent Medical Exam

Most of my previous comments have been made with the treating medical professional in mind. During the litigation process, a medical or psychological professional will often be called upon to render a "second" opinion. This second opinion is often referred to as an independent medical examination (IME). The basis for this exam under the Federal Rules of Civil Procedure is Rule 35, which states in pertinent part:

(a) Order for Examination. When the mental or physical condition . . . of a party . . . , is in controversy, the court . . . may order the party to submit to a physical or mental examination by a suitably licensed or certified examiner. . . .

(b) Report of Examiner.

The professional called on to render an examination and opinion under this rule is in a unique position. He or she is not a treating professional, but is being called on to do an examination and render a written report under the Rules of Civil Procedure. The IME process will begin by an inquiry, generally by the defense counsel, as to whether the professional is willing to fulfill this function. Several observations of this process will be helpful.

First, the health professional must have an understanding of the parties and studiously avoid any conflict of interest. A conflict may arise through the parties, their attorneys, the insurance carriers involved, or the judge who will hear the case. The professional should analyze potential conflicts of interest and reject any proposed assignment that would call into question his or her objectivity. All relevant potential conflicts should be reviewed early in the process with the retaining party.

Second, the health professional must thoroughly understand the case. He or she should request to review all pertinent documents including the original complaint, all pertinent discovery, the depositions of the parties, and the reports and depositions of any other expert who has testified in the case. After reviewing the preliminary materials from the retaining counsel, the health professional should submit a list of materials important for his or her review and opinions.

Third, it is essential that the health professional thoroughly understand his or her duties and the time constraints imposed by the court. A clear written directive from the referring counsel is essential, and all issues related to the professional's retention and service, including fees, should be agreed to before an examination takes place. It is possible that the professional who conducts the IME will be asked to testify as to his or her findings and opinions. Any limitations on availability must be expressed prior to acceptance of this court-sanctioned assignment.

Rule 35 allows for an examination of the patient. Most often, the examination is agreed to by the parties and there is no written order. Occasionally, the parties will not be able to agree, and the court will issue a written order to control the time and scope of the examination. When the examination is being done pursuant to a court order, the health professional needs to obtain a copy of the order and thoroughly review it to insure that he or she can comply with its restrictions. Any issues related to the terms of the order should be immediately brought to the attention of the retaining counsel and resolved prior to the exam.

The examination itself will vary among professions. The examination should be conducted pursuant to accepted standards within the health professional's specialty, as the tests and techniques used will need to be admissible into evidence. The standard of admissability of evidence will be governed either by the "generally accepted" standard used in many state courts (first enunciated in *Frye v. United States,* 1923) or the Daubert test used by the federal courts (*Daubert v. Merrell Dow Chemical Co.,* 1993). Under the Daubert test, the trial court should allow an expert to testify only if the expert is proposing to testify to "scientific knowledge that will assist the jury to understand or determine a fact in issue." To determine whether scientific evidence meets this standard, the court looks to four key issues:

1. whether the theory or technique can be and has been tested
2. whether the theory or technique has been subjected to peer review and publication
3. the known or potential rate of error and the existence and maintenance of standards controlling the technique's operation
4. whether the theory or technique has gained general acceptance in the relevant scientific community (the "general acceptance" test)

In conducting the examination the health professional should document thoroughly what the examination consisted of, the tests administered, and the results obtained. Neither the parties, the judge, nor jury should have any questions about the examination and results because of the professional's record keeping.

When conducting the examination of the plaintiff, the health professional should remember that the individual is not his or her patient. The examination is being conducted pursuant to the civil litigation process and appropriate rules of civil procedure. A thorough, well documented examination should be conducted with the highest standard of professionalism. The plaintiff may be hostile or suspicious, and although the health professional should use his or her professional training to set the plaintiff at ease so that a thorough examination can be conducted, any disagreement, hostility, or noncompliance should be properly documented.

The examination must be thorough and complete. It is unlikely there will be an opportunity for a follow-up examination, so the examination should be planned and conducted accordingly. Any questions concerning follow-up examinations should be discussed with the retaining counsel prior to the examination.

As a Rule 35 examiner, the health professional will be asked to prepare a written report. In general, that report should be prepared according to the standard practice of the health profession. Findings and opinions should be clearly communicated within the report. The report should document what the professional reviewed, the tests performed, and all factors that led to his or her opinion. Any limitation on the review or examination should be reported. The health professional's entire file, including correspondence between counsel, time sheets, and administrative records, are generally discoverable and most likely will be reviewed by the plaintiff's attorney.

Testimony

The health professional may be asked to testify by deposition or at trial. Both require careful preparation and consideration, but there are significant differences between the two methods.

A deposition is a procedure established by Rule 30 of the Federal Rules of Civil Procedure and comparable state laws. The deposition may be taken at any reasonable time and place. Commonly it is taken at the professional's (deponent's) office, but it could be taken at an attorney's office, a court reporter's office, a meeting room at the courthouse, or virtually anywhere.

The deposition consists of a question and answer session that will be recorded and transcribed verbatim by a certified court reporter. Although retained by the party taking the deposition, the court reporter is an officer of the court and holds no affiliation to any party. After the deposition is completed, the court reporter is responsible for transcribing the testimony into a booklet and providing certified copies to the parties and the deponent. The deponent then has an opportunity to review the deposition and make any changes that are necessary to insure its accuracy (Van Brunt & Strider, 1997). The changes or corrections are made on a document called an errata sheet. After the errata sheet is completed the deposition must be signed before either the court reporter or a notary public.

Depositions are taken in a format similar to that of live testimony at trial. The deponent takes an oath, swearing or affirming that the testimony given will be truthful. The party taking the deposition will often place preliminary stipulations and agreements on the record, then testimony of the deponent will begin in a question and answer format.

There are two types of depositions that are substantially different. The most common deposition is the discovery deposition, in which the party taking the deposition is simply gathering information to understand the deponent's qualifications, what he or she did in relation to the case, and his or her opinions. A skilled attorney will seldom be argumentative, but will be precise. The object is to uncover any weakness in the testimony that can be exploited at trial. Although a discovery deposition can be used at trial, that is not its primary purpose. Many times the attorney who plans to call the professional as a witness at trial will not even ask any questions, in order not to disclose his or her strategy at the deposition.

The second type of deposition is commonly known as a preservation deposition, which is used to preserve the deponent's testimony for use at trial. The courts often excuse medical professionals from attending trial, and will allow their testimony to be presented by way of the deposition. However, this technique is being used less and less often. The more common procedure is to take a preservation deposition on videotape, which is often played to the jury in lieu of live testimony.

Prior to the deposition, the health professional should understand the role of the parties. He or she should not hesitate to ask questions about the procedures. If the deposition is being taken by videotape, the professional should make sure he or she is comfortable and knows the location of the microphone and camera. The health professional should speak directly to the camera so that he or she will seem to make eye contact with the judge and jury when the video is played at trial. Consideration should be given to the backdrop and dress as if the professional were speaking live at trial. He or she should be comfortable with the location of the deposition taping and how he or she is being portrayed.

Whether the health professional is preparing to testify by deposition or at trial, he or she should understand the judge's charges regarding witnesses, experts, and credibility. The judge will charge the jury after the close of all the evidence by reading the law that will be applied to the case. The exact language of the judge's charge will vary from state to state, and often from judge to judge, but in matters regarding experts that language will be similar to the following:

> The rules of evidence provide that a scientific, technical or other specialized knowledge might assist the jury in understanding the evidence or in determining a fact in issue, a witness qualified as an expert by knowledge, skill, experience, training, or education, may testify and state his opinion concerning such matters. You should consider each expert opinion received in evidence in this case and give it such weight as you may think it deserves. If you should decide that the opinion of an expert witness is not based upon sufficient education and experience, or if you should conclude that the reasons given in support of the opinion are not sound, or that the opinion is outweighed by other evidence, then you may disregard the opinion entirely. (Fifth Circuit Pattern Jury Instructions, Civil Cases No. 6, "Expert Witnesses")

As you can see, the jury may consider many factors in deciding what weight to give an expert's testimony.

Another statement of law that may be read to the jury is that of impeachment:

> A witness may be discredited or "impeached" by contradictory evidence, by a showing that he testified falsely concerning a material matter, or by evidence that at some other time the witness has said or done something, or has failed to say or do something, which is inconsistent with the witness's present testimony. (Fifth Circuit Pattern Jury Instructions, Civil Cases No. 5A, "Impeachment [Contradictory Evidence—Inconsistent Statements]")

As you can see, a witness can be impeached in any number of ways. The health care professional should be aware that the opposing attorney will seek to impeach his or her testimony in some form. Often the impeachment is that the facts the professional relied on are incorrect. However, a medical professional could be placed under attack because of some bias he or she may have regarding the case. These issues should be carefully considered by the professional in preparing for testimony.

The health professional should not take preparation lightly. He or she will be placed under oath, and his or her testimony will be subject to cross-examination. Careful preparation is a necessity. The professional must review reports, notes, and all supporting documents carefully. A follow-up appointment with the patient should be considered if appropriate. A personal meeting between the health professional and the attorney who will call him or her as a witness is recommended. The professional's thorough understanding of the areas he or she will be called on to testify will be helpful to him or her in both the preparation and actual testimony.

Exhibits and visual aids are regularly used in today's litigation environment. The health professional should have all exhibits to be used during testimony prepared well ahead of time and properly marked, and he or she should have a careful understanding of how they will be used.

The actual act of testifying is a very important part of the litigation process. The jury will watch and listen closely to the professional's testimony and demeanor. It is important that the professional speak clearly and in lay terms. He or she should listen carefully to the question asked and respond directly to that question. The professional might think of the testimony as a lecture in which he or she is teaching people about the area of specialty for the first time. Any exhibits produced from the professional's work, such as MRIs, graphs, charts, and so on, should be explained succinctly as to what they are, how they are produced, and how they apply to the patient.

Ultimately, a calm and deliberate demeanor will be important in the jury's consideration of the testimony. Sincerity and objectivity will be strong assets for the health professional. It can at times be difficult to maintain a calm demeanor during cross-examination. The health professional must remember that he or she is not an advocate, but a witness sworn to tell the truth. In essence, the professional is not testifying for or against anyone, but simply testifying to his or her own personal knowledge and opinion. An objective witness is generally much more believable to a jury than one who appears to be an advocate for one side or the other.

Conclusions

Although many health professionals who treat patients with mild TBI find litigation and testifying difficult, it can be a positive experience if the professional is properly prepared. Once the professional is notified that he or she will be called upon to testify, he or she should reexamine every aspect of the evaluation and treatment to ensure there is sufficient and appropriate support for his or her opinions. To stand up to the strict scrutiny of cross-examination and judicial review, it is necessary to conduct a thorough review of a patient's background and the accident that caused the injury.

If the health professional has properly prepared himself or herself and documented the file to substantiate his or her opinions, the act of testifying will be much easier. When testifying, the professional should listen carefully to the question and answer clearly and in terms an average person can understand. Most importantly, the professional should be objective and remain calm, remembering that he or she is a witness, not an advocate for the patient.

In their article "Ten Commandments for Expert Witnesses," Van Brunt and Strider (1997) had two commandments for the testifying expert:

1. Thou shalt prepare for testimony with great care.
2. Thou shalt testify efficiently. (p. 7)

Although their style might be sacrilegious, their points are built on solid rock.

References

Davis, M. E. (1990). Mild to moderate brain injury, a silent epidemic. *Trial,* 109.

Daubert v. Merrell Dow Chemical Co., 509 U.S., 113 S.Ct. 2786, 125 Ed.2d 469 (1993).

Frye v. United States, 293 F. 1013 (D.C. Cir. 1923).

Van Brunt, R. T., & Strider, J. S. (1997, July 25). Ten Commandments for Expert Witnesses. *Fulton County Daily Report,* p. 7.

Forensic Misconceptions in Mild Traumatic Brain Injury

9

Anjali Palav, Kevin Duff, and Robert J. McCaffrey

Introduction

In light of the recent increase in popularity of neuropsychology and its recognition as a specialty by the APA Commission for the Recognition of Specialties and Proficiencies in Professional Psychology (CRSPPP) in 1996, there is an increasing presence of clinical neuropsychologists in courtrooms across the country. The role of clinical neuropsychologists in the context of mild brain injury litigation is that of the expert. As such, they provide valuable assistance to the trier of fact by helping him or her understand neuropsychological evidence. To fulfill this role, however, clinical neuropsychologists must keep several guidelines in mind. This chapter outlines these guidelines while dispelling myths that are prevalent in forensic neuropsychology. Where possible, actual courtroom testimony, with only identifying information altered, is provided to illustrate key topics. Topics discussed include the definition of a clinical neuropsychologist, the role of clinical neuropsychologists in legal proceedings, the selection and interpretation of neuropsychological tests, and the formation of opinions that are within a reasonable degree of neuropsychological certainty.

Role of the Clinical Neuropsychologist as an Expert

Although some have debated the validity and utility of forensic neuropsychology (Barth, Ryan, & Hawk, 1991; Faust & Ziskin, 1988; Wedding, 1991), the presence of the clinical neuropsychologist in the courtroom is well established. This is especially apparent in cases involving individuals who have allegedly suffered brain injuries. Neuropsychologists are often called as experts in such proceedings to assist the trier of fact. Clinical neuropsychological testimony may have dramatic effects on the outcome of a case. But who is an expert? What is expected of the expert? What types of testimony should and shouldn't experts provide? How can they best serve the trier of fact?

To answer the first question of "What is an expert?" it may be beneficial to present the view of the court. As stated in Rule 702 of the Federal Rules of Evidence (Moore, 1985),

> If scientific, technical, or other specialized knowledge will assist the trier of fact to understand the evidence or to determine a fact in issue, a witness qualified as an expert by knowledge, skill, experience, training, or education, may testify thereto in the form of an opinion or otherwise.

An expert is an individual who is engaged to assist the trier of fact in understanding the evidence in the case. Usually the trier of fact, the judge or jury, is not familiar with the evidence presented and needs the expert to clarify certain aspects it. Education, experience, and training qualify the expert to give an opinion. In the proceedings, the expert should act as an unbiased educator (Saks, 1990), that is, he or she should be impartial and objective and attempt to educate the trier of fact about his or her area of expertise. Saks (1992) referred to this role as the "Mere Conduit-Educator" in that the trier of fact wants to hear from "the field," in this case clinical neuropsychology, and not necessarily from "the individual." The testifying clinical neuropsychologist should only provide input; the trier of fact is responsible for determining the outcome in the case (Newman, 1991).

Consider the following testimony.

Q: What is your profession?

A: I'm a neuropsychologist.

Q: Would you explain to the jury what a neuropsychologist is?

A: A neuropsychologist is kind of a specialist in psychology. They try to understand if there's a relationship between the brain and the way people behave. They try to see if there is a relationship between problems you may have with your brain and how you behave, what you do, your ability to work, your ability to solve problems, your emotions.

Q: What kind of training did you have to become a neuropsychologist?

A: After getting my undergraduate degree, I was in a master's program in counseling for 2 years. After I completed that program, I worked for a number of years in different private and state human services agencies as a vocational rehabilitation counselor. I returned to school and worked towards a PhD in counseling psychology. While in school I did a summer practicum for a head trauma program in a medical center. When I completed my degree, the medical center hired me as a psychologist to work in the head trauma program. Eventually I became the coordinator for this program.

Q: And what were your duties as the coordinator of the head trauma program?

A: I was responsible for performing neuropsychological assessments of persons who suffered head injuries, determining what treatments they needed, and delivering treatment to those individuals. I supervised other psychologists who were working on staff to maintain quality control. And I also was involved with the training of interns for the program.

Q: And what did you do after you left there?

A: Then I went into practice for myself doing the same thing that I did at the head trauma program, assessment and treatment of persons with head injury.

Q: Are you aware of the fact that Division 40 of the American Psychological Association sets definitive training modules for neuropsychologists?

A: Yes. I am.

Q: Do your qualifications, in any fashion, fit that particular module as set by Division 40 for neuropsychology?

A: I really couldn't answer that question. I'm not sure at this point.

In this initial portion of testimony, the questions and answers are designed to qualify the clinical neuropsychologist as an expert. Defining what a clinical neuropsychologist is and does helps the trier of fact develop a foundation on which further, more relevant questions and answers will be built. One commonly used definition of a clinical neuropsychologist is spelled out by Division 40 of the American Psychological Association (APA). Professionals within this field should be familiar with this definition and its requirements. The definition states that the "Clinical Neuropsychologist is a professional psychologist who applies principles of assessment and intervention based upon the scientific study of human behavior as it relates to normal and abnormal functioning of the central nervous system" (Division 40 of the APA, 1995). Although the definition given in the testimony above conveys much of the same information, Division 40's definition is clear, succinct, and avoids unnecessary and confusing jargon.

Many models have been suggested for the education and training needed to become a clinical neuropsychologist. For example, Meier (1981) outlined four educational models to ensure competency in neuropsychology that were initially presented by the International Neuropsychological Society (INS) Task Force on Education, Accreditation, and Credentialing (INS Task Force,

1981). The models include (a) subspecialty in neuropsychology within a traditionally applied program (such as clinical or counseling), (b) interdepartmental program in neuropsychology and clinical neurosciences, (c) integrated scientist-practitioner program modified for neuropsychology, and (d) coordinated but separately credentialed PhD and PsyD program. Division 40 also requires competence in neuropsychology, as indicated by (a) successful completion of training in neuropsychology and neuroscience at an accredited university, (b) at least 2 years of supervised training by a clinical neuropsychologist applying neuropsychological services in a clinical setting, (c) achieving licensure or certification to provide psychological services, and (d) peer review of abilities and skills. If the clinical neuropsychologist is engaging in forensic activities, it is suggested that they also receive education in basic law issues and ethical general forensic psychology (Giuliano, Barth, Hawk, & Ryan, 1997). These models may be used as a yardstick with which clinical neuropsychologists can measure their educational preparedness and, perhaps, suitability to testify as an expert. If, as in the sample testimony, the qualifications of the clinical neuropsychologist are suspect, this expert may not be providing the trier of fact with the information needed to make an informed decision.

If the clinical neuropsychologist is qualified as an expert, what is expected of him or her in the proceedings? Clarifying issues, conveying accurate knowledge, and providing opinions are three expectations of the expert clinical neuropsychologist.

The following testimony addresses clarification of issues.

> Q: Can you tell the jury what is meant by mild head injury?
>
> A: Mild head injury really refers to someone who most probably was not in a coma, suffered a blow to the head, was dazed or suffered a brief loss of consciousness but otherwise appears to have not suffered any kind of damage. Mild refers to the degree of head injury; it can include bruising of the brain, axonal tearing, or shredding where the fibers are torn.

The clinical neuropsychologist is expected to assist in clarifying issues that fall outside the realm of a layperson's knowledge and experiences. The clarification, however, should not come at the expense of oversimplification. For example, in the preceding testimony, the clinical neuropsychologist's description of mild head injury seems vague and lacks the scientific precision that a trier of fact might expect from an expert witness.

There are several definitions of mild head injury that are both understandable and objective. Mild TBI, as defined by The Mild Traumatic Brain Injury Committee of the Head Injury Interdisciplinary Special Interest Group of the American Congress of Rehabilitation Medicine (1993), requires at least one of the following:

1. any loss of consciousness
2. any loss of memory for events immediately surrounding the accident
3. alteration in mental state at the time of the accident
4. focal neurological deficits, but where the severity of the injury is limited by 30 minutes or less of loss of consciousness, initial Glasgow Coma Scale (GCS) score of 13–15, and less than 24 hours of posttraumatic amnesia (PTA)

The *Diagnostic and Statistical Manual of Mental Disorders, Fourth Edition* (*DSM–IV;* American Psychiatric Association, 1994) requires two or more of the following criteria for mild neurocognitive disorder:

1. memory impairment
2. executive functioning disturbance
3. attention/speed of information processing difficulties
4. perceptual–motor impairments
5. language disturbances

Additional evidence, such as neuroimaging and neuropsychological performance, must also be present, along with impairment in social and occupational functioning. Alternatively, severity of head injury has been indexed by length of hospital stay or duration of recovery from the injury (Richardson, 1990). The choice of which criteria to use is up to the clinical neuropsychologist and his or her view of the supporting research. The clinical neuropsychologist needs to be aware that there are multiple definitions of mild head injury, and that they may be quite different. This becomes particularly important when reviewing research results on which opinions are based.

The following testimony addresses the level of knowledge expected of an expert.

Q: Doctor, what types of symptoms do you expect to see in an individual who has suffered a mild head injury?

A: In most cases, the person exhibits symptoms consistent with frontal lobe injury. Those might include difficulties paying attention, solving problems, and reasoning their way through different situations. Their emotional state may also be changed. But these changes are subtle, that is, they usually look fine to others.

Q: How do individuals with mild head injuries perform on neuropsychological tests?

A: One of the hallmarks would be inconsistency across time.

Whereas one of the expectations of the expert witness is to provide clarification, another, equally important one, is for the expert witness to be knowledgeable about the area on which he or she is testifying (Giuliano et al.,

1997). In this sample testimony, the clinical neuropsychologist is describing expected symptoms of a mild head injury. If the clinical neuropsychologist can clearly present accurate information, then the trier of fact will be in a better position to make an informed decision (McCaffrey, Williams, Fisher, & Laing, 1993). If, however, the clinical neuropsychologist presents erroneous information, the trier of fact has not gained anything from the testimony, and may actually have been misled. Such erroneous information might include base rates of symptoms attributed to head injury, inconsistency of neuropsychological performance, and myths of neuropsychology.

As stated in the sample testimony, an individual who suffered a head injury may present with memory problems, trouble with attention/concentration, irritability, and impatience, and it is often easy to attribute these symptoms to the head injury. Two findings, however, suggest that clinical neuropsychologists should be cautious about making this causal leap. First, the base rates of these and other symptoms attributed to head injury are high among individuals without head injury (Gouvier, Uddo-Crane, & Brown, 1988). For example, 27% of subjects with head injury reported being impatient, compared to 42% of subjects without head injury; and 38% of subjects with head injury reported memory problems, compared to 20% of subjects without head injury (neither difference was statistically significant). A second finding is that many classic symptoms of mild TBI are nonspecific (Williams, 1997). Nonspecific symptoms are those which are seen in many disorders and are thus unlikely to be related to one certain disorder. By presenting the base rate and nonspecific symptoms information, the clinical neuropsychologist will be painting a truer picture for the trier of fact to evaluate.

As noted in the sample testimony and by others (Smith, 1994), individuals with mild head injury may perform inconsistently on neuropsychological tests. Models of the path of recovery from head injuries tend to show a period of rapid recovery that gradually reaches a plateau (Long & Schmitter, 1992). Given the evidence for these recovery models, extreme variability from the recovery curve is atypical. Alternative explanations for inconsistent performance across time might include fatigue, effects of medication, psychiatric conditions, test anxiety, symptom exaggeration, litigation-related issues, or frank malingering.

As part of his or her educator role, the clinical neuropsychologist may assist the trier of fact by dispelling erroneous beliefs about the field of clinical neuropsychology. Dodrill (1997) presented six commonly held myths of clinical neuropsychology as a way of challenging the profession to challenge itself. The myths include (a) we know what our tests measure, (b) we have tests that are sensitive to the functioning of the frontal lobes, (c) patient self-report of cognitive functioning is reliable, (d) an above-average intelligence score should mean above-average neuropsychological performance on all tests, (e) clinical neuropsychologists lack the time to do research, and (f) relationships with other clinical neuropsychologists are not important. Awareness of these myths, and others like them, will aid the trier of fact in properly weighing the evidence.

The following testimony illustrates the need for clinical neuropsychologists to be familiar with current research.

Q: Doctor, you've been defending your choice of test batteries based on one particular monograph. What is the date of the monograph you've been relying on?

A: 1978.

Q: 1978, 19 years ago?

A: That's correct.

Q: Would you agree that the field of neuropsychology was in its infancy at that point and that there's been an explosion of literature both for and against various parts of neuropsychology since that time?

A: Yes, I would.

Proper education, training, and experience is not enough for one to be considered sufficiently knowledgeable. The clinical neuropsychologist must also stay current with his or her area of expertise (see Section VI. A. of the Specialty Guidelines for Forensic Psychologists; Committee on Ethical Guidelines for Forensic Psychologists, 1991, p. 661). Due to time limitations and the vast amount of research that is generated, it can be a daunting task to remain abreast of current research, but it is a vital part of the expert's role. Presenting out-of-date findings can lead the trier of fact astray in the search for justice.

The following testimony illustrates the role of the clinical neuropsychologist in providing opinions to the trier of fact.

Q: Doctor, what was the purpose of the referral?

A: The purpose of the referral was to establish if the patient had suffered any cognitive deficits as a result of the motor vehicle accident in question.

[More testimony follows, during which the results of the neuropsychological testing are presented.]

Q: Based upon your evaluation and testing and your review of the history, do you have an opinion, Doctor, to a reasonable degree of neuropsychological certainty as to the cause of that cognitive deficiency?

A: The cause is the motor vehicle accident in question.

When testifying as an expert witness, a clinical neuropsychologist may be asked to form an opinion, as in this sample testimony, as to the causation of impairments or deficits (Richardson & Adams, 1992). Given the complexity of the injury and the assessment and treatment procedures, it is not surprising that the trier of fact might need help sorting out the data. But "what is [also] useful is when the expert guides the trier of fact through the reasoning process which produced that opinion" (Newman, 1991, p. 247). By supplying the trier of fact with the data and the reasoning behind the opinion, the expert has provided only input, not outcome.

To best aid the trier of fact in the decision-making process, the expert clinical neuropsychologist is required to consider all possible alternative explanations for the data when forming his or her opinion (see Section VI. C. of the Specialty Guidelines for Forensic Psychologists; Committee on Ethical Guidelines for Forensic Psychologists, 1991, p. 661). Given the number of nonspecific symptoms of mild head injury, there are a number of differential diagnoses to consider. Williams (1997) suggested that poor neuropsychological performance and reported symptoms may also be due to depression, anxiety, PTSD, and the effects of certain medications. Additionally, alternative hypotheses could include previous exposure to toxins, genetic conditions, stress, cultural factors, personal habits (e.g., substance abuse, poor nutrition), and malingering (McCaffrey et al., 1993). If alternative explanations have been considered and ruled out, the expert can be more confident of his or her opinion.

The following testimony illustrates the value of behavioral observations in ruling out alternative explanations.

> Q: Now would you say that an individual who presented to you tapping her foot incessantly and showing clear nervous reaction with her hand or hands, would you say that those types of observations would be meaningful psychological observations?
>
> A: They may be meaningful psychological observations.
>
> Q: Can you show me anywhere in your records where those particular behaviors were recorded?
>
> A: I don't know if I necessarily recorded that information but I may have used it, along with other information, to say that this person had a nervous reaction to the testing situation.

Recording behavioral observations during the neuropsychological evaluation can aid the clinical neuropsychologist in ruling out alternative explanations. Support for or questioning of subjective complaints, and assessment of the individual's strengths and weaknesses can be gleaned from test-taking behaviors (Long & Collins, 1997). When making behavioral observations, some areas to include might be appearance, content/quality of speech, appropriateness of behavior, motivation, and response to failure. For example, an individual who performed poorly on an evaluation but had low motivation may indicate a different opinion than someone who performed poorly but was highly motivated. As noted in the sample testimony, behavioral observations are useful only if they are actually recorded, and in sufficient detail to re-create the scene for the trier of fact.

One final, noteworthy expectation of the expert witness is that he or she be aware of and stay within the limits of his or her expertise (Newman, 1991). As noted in Section 7.04(b) of the APA Code of Ethics (APA, 1992), "Whenever necessary to avoid misleading, psychologists [should] acknowledge the limits of their data or conclusions." Straying from the limitations of one's data and conclusions is not only an ethical violation but may also unduly influence the trier of fact in the decision-making process.

Selection and Interpretation of Neuropsychological Tests

A test is an instrument used to quantify behavior (Kaplan & Saccuzzo, 1993). All tests must possess adequate reliability and demonstrated validity (Anastasi & Urbina, 1997). The selection, use, and interpretation of test results in forensic neuropsychological evaluations needs to conform to the highest ethical and scientific standards (Committee on Ethical Guidelines for Forensic Psychologists, 1991; *Standards for Educational and Psychological Testing,* 1985).

Clinical neuropsychological assessments may be conducted through either a fixed battery or flexible battery. A fixed neuropsychological battery is a standardized group of tests administered to every patient, defendant, or litigant regardless of the presenting complaint or referral issue (Kane, 1991). A flexible neuropsychological battery is a collection of several neuropsychological tests that may or may not include subtests from a fixed battery. The selection of the tests in a flexible battery is based upon several factors including, but not limited to, the clinical neuropsychologist's perceptions of the examinee's presenting complaint and the referral question.

There are several important issues facing a clinical neuropsychologist who elects to use a flexible battery in forensic matters. The clinical neuropsychologist may be asked to defend the test selection strategy, the evaluation process, the interpretation of neuropsychological findings, and his or her opinions. As noted by Kane (1991, p. 297), "Once the clinical neuropsychologist chooses areas of neuropsychological function to assess, a number of test alternatives become available [cf. Lezak, 1983]. But little data are available to guide one's choice and personal preference, and bias often dictates test selection."

The following testimony illustrates questions a neuropsychologist might face if he or she used a flexible battery.

Q: Now you've told us that you use a set of tests, a flexible battery of tests. Doctor, can you point to any literature today that sustains and supports the use of the specific testing instruments you utilized, supports the use of those instruments in establishing the existence or nonexistence of traumatic brain injuries versus the normal population?

A: Absolutely.

Q: What literature can you point to that has tested the validity and reliability of the entire group of tests that you used?

A: There is a wealth of literature that talks about many of the tests within this battery as diagnostic in determining head injury.

Q: That's not what I'm asking. Is there literature to support the use of the entire battery of tests as a group, yes or no?

To assist clinical neuropsychologists in the selection of assessment instrunents and strategies for forensic use, Heilbrun (1992) proposed guidelines:

1. The test should be commercially available and have a test manual that describes the psychometric properties and administration procedures. In addition, the test should be reviewed in the *Mental Measurements Yearbook, Test Critiques,* or a related publication or peer-reviewed journal.
2. The reliability coefficients for the test should be greater than 0.80.
3. The test should be relevant to the legal proceeding.
4. The clinical neuropsychologist should follow the standardized administration procedures outlined in the test manual.
5. Tests should be neither selected nor used for purposes for which they were not developed.
6. Tests should be scored using objective procedures and interpreted with actuarial methods.
7. The examinee's response style must be specifically evaluated because neuropsychological test data can be influenced by a number of factors including the examinee's motivation, secondary gain issues, and so on.

The need to evaluate an examinee's response style is also in keeping with the *DSM–IV* guidelines regarding the need to strongly suspect malingering in any medicolegal evaluation (American Psychiatric Association, 1994, p. 683). For forensic neuropsychological evaluations Williams (1997) recommends the use of the *Halstead-Reitan Neuropsychological Test Battery* for adults (HRNB; Reitan & Wolfson, 1993), the *Memory Assessment Scales* (MAS; Williams, 1991), the *Western Aphasia Battery* (Kertesz, 1982), and the *Minnesota Multiphasic Personality Inventory* (MMPI; Hathaway & McKinley, 1951).

A number of tests used in neuropsychological evaluations contain data in the test manual on the differences necessary between subtests to achieve conventional statistical significance (i.e., $p < .05$). Perhaps the most commonly reported statistically significant differences are those for the Wechsler scales for VIQ and PIQ. On the WAIS–R, a difference of 10 points between VIQ and PIQ is statistically significant at the $p < .05$ level. Although this 10-point difference is statistically significant, the clinical neuropsychologist needs to consider the clinical significance, if any, of such a finding. The first question would be, "What is the base rate (frequency) of a difference of this magnitude in the population?" In their study of VIQ and PIQ differences in the WAIS–R normative sample, Matarazzo and Herman (1985) reported that a difference of at least 10 points was observed in 37.8% of the normative sample. Given that such a large percentage of the normative sample demonstrated a statistically significant difference, the clinical significance of such a finding is highly questionable. This example illustrates that statistically significant neuropsychological findings may not be clinically relevant or meaningful. The issue of clinical versus statistical significance, illustrated by the following testimony, is frequently encountered in mild brain injury litigation.

> Q: The performance score went up 13 points on the second testing session. Is that a good increase?
>
> A: Yes, it is impressive.
>
> Q: Is that something that's not usually seen in IQ testing and retesting?
>
> A: It depends on how you look at it. It's a question of statistical significance. I think it's impressive. Usually looking for a 15-point spread before we say we have a statistically significant score. This is a pretty big increase and in my opinion is quite significant.

Another example of the importance of considering base rate information is provided by Heaton, Grant, and Matthews (1991). Heaton et al. reported that on the WAIS and HRNB 15% of 455 neurologically normal subjects had two "abnormal" test scores out of a total of 40 test measures. Therefore it is important not to rely on a single impaired test score in arriving at an opinion within a reasonable degree of neuropsychological certainty.

The level of neuropsychological impairment is more readily determined when a fixed battery has been used because there are standardized administration procedures and scoring criteria. Deciding the level of impairment with a flexible battery is more difficult because each test is likely to have been normed on a different group of individuals. Tests included in flexible batteries may not have a test manual, may not have reported validity and reliability data, and may not have been used in combination with other tests to objectively detect the presence and severity of brain impairment. Thus, the flexible battery approach may fall short of Heilbrun's (1992) criteria, and may not meet the guidelines of the *Standards for Educational and Psychological Testing* (1985).

Clinical neuropsychologists frequently must evaluate an individual's neuropsychological performance over time. A key issue is whether improvement in objective test scores is due to spontaneous recovery of function or to specific treatment/rehabilitation interventions. Examining change in performance between two or more assessments involves consideration of not only the temporal variables, but also the role of practice effects (cf. McCaffrey & Westervelt, 1995). The following testimony provides an example of a clinical neuropsychologist's failure to consider the role of practice effects.

Q: The overall IQ score went up from 91 to 101. That's a 10-point increase. Does this indicate that your treatment program has to some extent worked?

A: I think it's a measure that something happened and there was some improvement, yes.

A key issue for clinical neuropsychologists is the proper interpretation of the data from the testing process. At the heart of this issue is knowledge of the normative sample and the standardized procedures for administering the tests. A standardized administration adheres to the procedures outlined in the test manual. If the clinical neuropsychologist does not follow the standardized administration procedures, then it is inappropriate to compare directly the examinee's performance to that of the normative sample.

It is fairly common practice among a subset of clinical neuropsychologists to administer only the immediate and delayed verbal memory and figural memory portions of the *Wechsler Memory Scale–Revised* (WMS–R; Wechsler, 1987). This does not constitute a standardized administration of the WMS–R, and in fact is contrary to the administration instructions that, "As much as possible, the prescribed subtest sequence should be maintained and additional interpolated activities avoided; otherwise, the norms for the delayed-recall trials may be misleading" (p. 9). This practice is illustrated by the following testimony.

Q: Because protocol is important, isn't it?

A: Yes, it is.

Q: And in order for these norms that we've been talking about to mean anything, folks who are administered tests should be administered those tests in exactly or as near as exactly as possible the same way?

A: That's correct.

Q: Because otherwise the norms may not mean anything.

A: The test should be administered as exactly as possible.

Q: Did you give her the entire *Wechsler Memory Scale–Revised*?

A: I gave her the logical memory section.

Q: Isn't it a fact that subtests like the logical memory should be administered to patients in the precise order in which they appear in the testing manual?

A: I believe that that's necessary only if you're administering the entire test.

Q: But you didn't administer the same tasks between the immediate and delayed portions of the logical memory subtest?

A: No.

Q: Then in a sense you were not following the protocol that had been followed by all the other people who took the test and set the standard for meaningful scores.

Forming Opinions Within a Reasonable Degree of Neuropsychological Certainty

Once the test battery is appropriately chosen, administered, and evaluated, the clinical neuropsychologist must synthesize the findings into opinions that will be requested during the deposition and/or trial. When a clinical neuropsychologist is asked for his or her opinion concerning interpretation of neuropsychological data, this opinion is required to be within a reasonable degree of neuropsychological certainty. Once an opinion is stated, it must be supported by both data collected during the assessment and prior information such as school records and medical histories (Heilbronner & Karavidas, 1997). To our knowledge, there are no published standards on this matter. Nevertheless, the clinician should not form an opinion that is not supported by the data. A good rule of thumb is to "leave no stone unturned." A thorough neuropsychological evaluation, including review of records, clinical interview, and neuropsychological testing, should be performed. If there are any limitations to the assessment, such as being unable to interview relatives or not having access to records, they should be clearly stated along with the opinion. In forming opinions, the clinical neuropsychologist should be aware of alternative explanations and be able to explain why his or her conclusion is more plausible. A well supported opinion is valuable in the context of mild brain injury litigation.

Opinion of Preinjury Functioning

In the context of mild brain injury litigation, a clinical neuropsychologist will first be asked to provide an opinion of whether any deficits in the patient's functioning can be attributed to the injury. When evaluating this possibility, it is important to obtain information concerning the patient's preinjury level of functioning. Without this standard against which to compare current cognitive, psychological, and physical functioning, the results of any neuropsychological evaluations performed after the injury are meaningless. Ideally, the results of the current evaluation would be compared to those of previous evaluations; however, comparable prior information is rarely available. Thus, the clinical neuropsychologist is often required to estimate the patient's preinjury functioning. Although the majority of studies indicate that IQ is not affected in mild brain injury (e.g., Binder, Rohling, & Larrabee, 1997; Dikmen, McLean, & Temkin, 1986), a few studies have found evidence to the contrary (e.g., Parker & Rosenblum, 1996). Nevertheless, preinjury IQ is frequently estimated in mild to moderate brain injury cases. There are a number of methods for accomplishing this task. Following is an overview of these methods; for a comprehensive review see Crawford (1989).

Present ability measures is one method for estimating preinjury IQ. Current performance on a task that is thought to be resistant to brain injury is used as the comparison standard. To be considered as a preinjury index, a test must meet two criteria in addition to being resistant to the effects of neurological and psychiatric disorders: (a) have adequate reliability and (b) correlate highly with measures of IQ. The Vocabulary subtest of the Wechsler intelligence scales and the *National Adult Reading Test* (NART; Nelson, 1982) are frequently used for this purpose. Of the two, the NART appears to be a better index of preinjury functioning. Both the Wechsler Vocabulary subtest and the NART meet the requirements of reliability and high loading on *g*, the general intelligence factor (Crawford, Parker, Stewart, Besson, & DeLacey, 1989; Matarazzo, 1972; Nelson, 1982; Wechsler, 1955). However, the Vocabulary subtest may be susceptible to cognitive decline resulting from mild brain injury (Crawford, Parker, & Besson, 1988; Russell, 1972; Vogt & Heaton, 1977), whereas the NART appears to be resistant to the effects of brain injury (Crawford et al., 1988). As a result, using the Vocabulary subtest as a measure of present ability may result in an underestimate of preinjury IQ, relative to using the NART. The NART, however, is not without its drawbacks. It is likely to produce inaccurate estimates for patients with language disturbances, patients in different age groups than the elderly population on which it was normed, and patients outside the United Kingdom (Lynch & McCaffrey, 1997; Stebbins, Gilley, Wilson, Bernard, & Fox, 1990). In the United States and Canada, the revised version of the NART (NART–R; Blair & Spreen, 1989) is a more appropriate choice. Recent studies have indicated that the *Wide Range Achievement Test–*

Revised (WRAT–R; Jastak & Wilkinson, 1984) Reading subtest may be another appropriate index of preinjury IQ (Johnstone, Callahan, Kapila, & Bouman, 1996; Johnstone & Wilhelm, 1996; Wiens, Bryan, & Crossen, 1993).

A more individual approach to estimating preinjury IQ is Lezak's (1995) best performance method. This method requires a thorough assessment of intellectual functioning including formal testing, clinical observation, and gathering of historical information. According to Lezak, any of the following can be considered as indicators of preinjury ability: "interview impressions, reports from family and friends, test scores, prior academic or employment level, school grades, army ratings, or an intellectual product such as a letter or an invention" (p. 107). The highest level of functioning indicated by this information is considered to be the estimate of preinjury IQ. Failure to gather a wide variety of information is likely to result in an inaccurate estimation of preinjury IQ. For example, the common practice of using the highest scale score of the Wechsler intelligence scales as an index of preinjury IQ is unjustified due to normal variation in performance on different subtests (intersubtest scatter) and the imperfect correlation of the individual subtests with FSIQ (Lynch & McCaffrey, 1997). When used responsibly, however, the best performance method appears to be an appropriate method for estimating preinjury intelligence.

Another approach to estimating preinjury IQ is the use of demographic variables that correlate highly with IQ (Matarazzo, 1972). This method, unlike the present ability measures, has the advantage of not being sensitive to brain impairment, and thus may be a more accurate measure of preinjury ability levels. Education and occupation levels are among the most frequently used demographic variables for this purpose. Clinical neuropsychologists can use tables, such as those found in Matarazzo and Herman (1984), Reynolds, Chastain, Kaufman, and McLean (1987), and Ryan and Sattler (1988), that provide WAIS–R IQ values that correspond to a variety of educational and occupational classifications. In this way, they can determine if the client's current IQ corresponds to the IQs of those with similar educational and occupational histories. For example, IQ can range from 63–141 for high school graduates, from 87–148 for college graduates, from 56–135 for semi-skilled workers, and from 81–148 for professional and technical workers (Kaufman, 1990, p. 170). Matarazzo and Herman (1984) caution, however, that this method provides at best a very rough estimate of preinjury functioning. They suggest that this method should be supplemented with other indices of preinjury ability, such as occupational history or SAT scores, and that clinical neuropsychologists should not rely solely on this method for estimating preinjury IQ.

Regression equations based on demographic variables provide another method for estimating preinjury IQ. Such equations have been developed for the WAIS (Wilson et al., 1978), WAIS–R (Barona & Chastain, 1986; Barona, Reynolds, & Chastain, 1984), and the WISC–R (Reynolds & Gutkin, 1979).

Although there is not much empirical support for the equations used to predict WISC–R IQs (Klesges, 1982; Klesges & Sanchez, 1981), those used to predict WAIS and WAIS–R IQs have been more successful (Eppinger, Craig, Adams, & Parsons, 1987; Goldstein, Gary, & Levin, 1986; Karzmark, Heaton, Grant, & Matthews, 1985; Klesges, Sanchez, & Stanton, 1981; Paolo & Ryan, 1992; Wilson, Rosenbaum, & Brown, 1979). However, these methods have been reported to overestimate preinjury IQ in a significant number of individuals. Silverstein (1987) examined the predictive accuracy of the equations for all three of the mentioned tests and found that the equation for the WAIS, which provides the best estimate of the three, still misclassified over half of the subjects. Both the Wilson Index for the WAIS and the Barona Index for the WAIS–R have poor predictive ability for persons with brain injury (Bolter, Gouvier, Veneklasen, & Long, 1982; Paolo, Ryan, Troster, & Hilmer, 1996). Given these reports, the regression equations should never be used as the only estimate of preinjury intelligence.

Regression equations that combine both demographic variables and present ability measures have also been developed, including those that combine demographic variables and NART errors (Berry et al., 1994; Crawford, Cochrane, Besson, Parker, & Stewart, 1990; Crawford, Stewart, Parker, Besson, & Cochrane, 1989; Wilshire, Kinsella, & Prior, 1991) and those that combine demographic variables and WAIS–R subtest scores (Krull, Scott, & Sherer, 1995). Overall, these equations have more predictive accuracy than either demographic variables or present ability measures alone, and load more highly on *g* than does either method alone (Lynch & McCaffrey, 1997). This illustrates the necessity of considering a variety of information sources when estimating preinjury IQ. Although further research is required on these equations, they appear promising as a method of estimating preinjury functioning.

Because each of the methods described above has its drawbacks, estimation of preinjury IQ should not be based on one method alone. No single method of estimating preinjury IQ produces an irrefutable measure of preinjury functioning. The quality of the estimate is strengthened if several estimates produce similar results. To provide the best estimate possible, the clinical neuropsychologist should employ a number of the above methods.

In the context of litigation, the clinical neuropsychologist's role is to assist the trier of fact in understanding the importance of the estimation of preinjury IQ as a comparison standard for current functioning, and the process by which the client's preinjury IQ was estimated. Consider the following testimony.

Q: And were you able to make a determination as to what her premorbid or preaccident intelligence level was?

A: The vocabulary test and the comprehension test gave us an indication of premorbid intelligence. They gave us a standard against which to

> measure other tests. Her vocabulary and comprehension were at the high school plus level. We also looked at her educational and occupational history to get an idea of her functioning before her accident.

Here the clinical neuropsychologist does support his opinion about the client's preinjury IQ with two methods of estimation. The neuropsychologist's role, however, is to explain the reasoning behind his or her opinion so that the trier of fact can follow it. To be of assistance to the trier of fact, the clinical neuropsychologist should explain his or her opinion in layman's terms.

Opinion of Future Outcome

A clinical neuropsychologist may next be asked to provide an opinion of the client's prospects for future independent living, environmental support, and, especially in the case of mild brain injury, employability (Heaton & Pendelton, 1981). To answer these questions, clinicians must assess not only deficits, but also residual strengths and the ways in which such strengths can compensate for any deficits (Chelune & Moehle, 1986). Unfortunately, many of the neuropsychological instruments in use today were designed only to detect and possibly localize the presence of brain damage; thus, they do not provide us all the necessary information for predicting outcome. As a result, any opinion stated under oath must be formulated with caution in order to avoid overstating the data.

Studies have indicated that performance on neuropsychological measures is correlated with vocational outcome (see Heaton & Pendleton, 1981 for a review). Neuropsychological measures are related to current occupational status and can be used to differentiate between employed and unemployed subjects. They are also related to future employment status and income (Chelune & Moehle, 1986). Multiple regression equations and discriminant functions using neuropsychological variables have been developed to predict outcome (Guilmette & Kastner, 1996); however, the predictive accuracy of these measures is not perfect (Heaton & Pendleton). This can be illustrated by the example of the surgeon who, despite a very low WAIS–R Block Design scaled score following head injury, continued to operate successfully until his retirement (Newcombe, 1987). In addition, it is not unlikely for two patients with similar test scores to have widely different amounts of success in reentering the work environment.

Why do some patients enjoy better outcomes than their neuropsychological performance may suggest? Conversely, why do other patients not return to work successfully following head injury, despite performing well on neuropsychological measures? In answering these questions, it is important to keep in mind the differences between the neuropsychological assessment setting and the work environment. Standard neuropsychological assessments are conducted in controlled settings; distractions are minimized, the patient is presented with one task at a time, and the patient is not criticized for mistakes (Long & Collins, 1997). This situation is markedly different from that of the average job, where there are often distractions, multiple tasks, and criticism for poor performance. Moreover, neuropsychological tests do not measure stamina, motivation, or insight, all of which play a role in how well a person performs on the job (Newcombe, 1987). As a result, specific predictions about vocational functioning are not reliable at the individual level; predictions from neuropsychological instruments are more accurate at the group level and for general predictions about vocational potential (Chelune & Moehle, 1986; Wilson, 1993).

Despite the limitations of neuropsychological tests for predicting vocational outcome, clinical neuropsychologists will be asked about their opinions on this matter. In this situation, it is best to acknowledge the limitations of these opinions. Obtaining as much supporting information as possible is also helpful. To this end, the following areas should be assessed in addition to the gathering of neuropsychological data: demographics, academic and occupational history, medical history, patient and relative reports of disability, behavior during the testing session, and personality test data (Chelune & Moehle, 1986). This information is critical because it provides a biopsychosocial background against which to interpret the test data (Long & Collins, 1997). In addition, ecologically valid measures, such as tasks performed in a work environment, should be used if possible (Guilmette & Kastner, 1996). All this information should be combined with the pattern of performance over the entire test battery to provide the most accurate prediction of possible vocational outcome (Long & Collins).

To assist the trier of fact, the neuropsychologist should make his or her testimony pertaining to future employment possibilities as thorough as possible, and clearly identify limitations. The following testimony illustrates this point.

Q: Now, did you perform what you defined for us yesterday as a vocational assessment?

A: No, we did not. A vocational assessment, I don't know that we would have gotten any more information. We know her scholastic skills, her academic skills. Although I wouldn't say that the neuroassessment that we did and the treatment that we did includes every particular piece that you might find in a vocational assessment, it really provided us with more than enough relevant information to give us an indication of how she might perform in a job situation. The testing indicated that she could in no way return to her former job as a social worker and that she could not work in a position that required quick responses, rapid thinking, and solving novel problems. She might be able to do jobs that are fairly rote in nature like filing, doing maybe library work, but even in that situation, this could only be success-

fully accomplished in a nonstressful environment within a limited period of time.

Because there are limitations on the ability of neuropsychological tests to predict vocational functioning, predictions based on these tests should be compared against reports of actual work performance, if possible. However, this was not done in the example case.

Q: Do you know if she was employed at any time following her injury?

A: She was employed as a waitress for 8 months at a resort restaurant.

Q: It seems that waitressing would require quick responses and rapid thinking. Did she encounter any problems while performing her duties as a waitress?

A: I don't know. Her performance at that position was irrelevant.

In this case, the clinical neuropsychologist has not provided the full picture to the trier of fact. As previously stated, the role of the clinical neuropsychologist is to provide the trier of fact with accurate information so that the trier of fact can understand it and reach a conclusion.

Opinion of Possible Malingering

Clinical neuropsychologists will also be asked if the patient's performance on the assessment represents his or her best ability. The clinician should consider the possibility of malingering when assessing neuropsychological functioning following mild brain injury. Malingering is defined by the *DSM–IV* as the "intentional production of false or grossly exaggerated physical or psychological symptoms, motivated by external incentives" (American Psychiatric Association, 1994, p. 683). Because external incentives, such as a large monetary award, may be linked with poor performance on neuropsychological measures in 20% to 60% of patients (Pankratz & Binder, 1997), clinical neuropsychologists should always evaluate the patient's attempt to put forth maximum effort during neuropsychological testing.

Malingering can be assessed with a number of methods. Because a thorough review of these methods is beyond the scope of this chapter, the interested reader is referred to Franzen, Iverson, and McCracken (1990) and Nies and Sweet (1994) for more detailed information. Neuropsychological tests themselves can be examined for evidence of malingering. Single tests, such as the MAS or the *California Verbal Learning Test* (CVLT; Delis, Kramer, Kaplan, & Ober, 1987), can be examined for the predicted superior performance on recognition memory over recall memory (Zielinski, 1994). Neuropsychological batteries, such as the HRNB, can be examined to determine if performance is consistent on tests that tap the same ability (Hart, 1995; Ruff, Wylie, & Tennant, 1993). Neuropsychological batteries can also be used in conjunction with patient report and behavioral observations to determine if the patient's complaints are consistent with his or her actions and test performance (Ruff et al., 1993). Consistency of performance across testing sessions can also be examined if a patient is assessed more than once; Reitan and Wolfson (1997) have developed the Retest Consistency Index, the Response Consistency Index, and the Dissimulation Index for the HRNB.

Specific tests for malingering can be administered as a supplement to the neuropsychological battery. The *Rey 15-Item Test* (Rey–15; Rey, 1964) is an example of a test that seems difficult to the patient but is in fact rather simple. Thus, those who are attempting to "fake bad" are likely to make mistakes to a greater degree than those who are trying their best. Because it is easy and quick to administer, the Rey–15 makes a good screening test for malingering; however, it should never be used as the only criterion for determining malingering because of its modest sensitivity and specificity (Pankratz & Binder, 1997). Another popular method for assessing malingering is forced-choice testing, which is most often used to assess malingered sensory and memory functions. Examples of such tests includes the *Digit Memory Test* (Hiscock & Hiscock, 1989) and the *Portland Digit Recognition Test* (PDRT; Binder, 1990). Patients are forced to choose one of two responses over many trials; patients who perform significantly below chance are most likely malingering. Many malingerers, however, do not score below chance; the development of cutoff scores has improved the clinical utility of this method (Pankratz & Binder).

Lastly, methods that are not specific to neuropsychology can be used to indicate malingering on neuropsychological tests. The validity scales of the MMPI are frequently used for this purpose. Although one should be cautious when interpreting the MMPI in a neurologically impaired population, it provides a good assessment of behavioral and personality characteristics, and can provide information about malingering when used in conjunction with neuropsychological measures (Zielinski, 1994). Structured interviews, such as the *Schedule of Affective Disorders and Schizophrenia* (SADS; Spitzer & Endicott, 1978) and the *Structured Interview of Reported Symptoms* (SIRS; Rogers, Bagby, & Dickens, 1992), provide an accuracy check of the patient's self-report of symptoms, and can be used in conjunction with a neuropsychological battery in the detection of malingering (Zielinski).

Clinical judgment alone is not sufficient to support the opinion that a patient is not malingering (Hart, 1995; Ruff et al., 1993). Thus, more formal measures of malingering should be employed. Because none of the methods described above provides conclusive evidence of malingering when used alone, the clinician should use a combination of these methods when determining if the patient put forth his or her best effort (Nies & Sweet, 1994). A thorough assessment for malingering should include a review of preinjury medical and school records, interviews with the patient and others about his or her functioning before and after injury, an examination of consistency of performance, and administration of specific tests of malingering and the MMPI–2 (Butcher, Dahlstrom, Graham, Tellegen, & Kaemmer, 1989). Evidence from all of these sources should be combined when making a determination of malingering. For a detailed list of potential indicators of malingering, see Ruff et al.

If a thorough evaluation for malingering is not performed, the opinion provided to the trier of fact will not be adequately supported by the facts. This situation is illustrated by the following testimony.

> Q: Let me ask you this, Doctor: Does neuropsychological testing, the various tests administered, take into account the possibility that a particular person might be faking or malingering?
>
> A: Yes, it does. You administer many tests that have embedded in them different objective measures to see whether or not you're consistent across the board. For example, you would administer a vocabulary test and another test that has a measure of vocabulary in it and see if the person's performance is similar between the two tests. So one of the things we look at in order to assess faking or malingering is whether the problems are consistent across all of the tests. We also look to see if the performance on the tests are consistent with what the patient is reporting. I'd have to say it's really virtually impossible to fake these kinds of problems.
>
> Q: In addition to looking at consistency of performance, did you assess for malingering in other ways? Did you administer the *Rey 15-Item Test,* the *Portland Digit Recognition Test,* or the MMPI?
>
> A: No.

As previously stated, litigation affects motivation during neuropsychological evaluations in a substantial percentage of cases. Thus, the possibility of malingering should be considered seriously and thoroughly evaluated. If a clinical neuropsychologist adequately assesses for malingering, the results can be explained so that the trier of fact can weigh the evidence.

Conclusions

As experts in mild brain injury litigation, clinical neuropsychologists provide a valuable service when they perform their duty adequately. When they perform their duties incorrectly or incompletely, however, clinical neuropsychologists can confuse, rather than clarify, complex neuropsychological issues. To ensure that this does not happen, clinical neuropsychologists should hold themselves to the highest ethical and professional standards when acting as experts in the courtroom. This chapter has attempted to summarize these standards and to illustrate the outcome when these standards are not maintained.

References

American Psychiatric Association. (1994). *Diagnostic and statistical manual of mental disorders* (4th ed.). Washington, DC: Author.

American Psychological Association. (1992). Ethical principles of psychologists and code of conduct. *American Psychologist, 47,* 1597–1611.

Anastasi, A., & Urbina, S. (1997). *Psycholgical testing* (7th ed.). Upper Saddle River, NJ: Prentice Hall.

Barona, A., & Chastain, R. L. (1986). An improved estimate of premorbid IQ for blacks and whites on the WAIS–R. *International Journal of Clinical Neuropsychology, 8,* 169–173.

Barona, A., Reynolds, C. R., & Chastain, R. L. (1984). A demographically based index of premorbid intelligence for the WAIS–R. *Journal of Consulting and Clinical Psychology, 52,* 885–887.

Barth, J. T., Ryan, T. V., & Hawk, G. L. (1991). Forensic neuropsychology: A reply to the method skeptics. *Neuropsychology Review, 2*(3), 251–266.

Berry, D. T., Carpenter, G. S., Campbell, D. A., Schmitt, F. A., Helton, K., & Lipke-Molby, T. (1994). The New Adult Reading Test–Revised: Accuracy in estimating WAIS–R IQ scores obtained 3.5 years earlier from normal older persons. *Archives of Clinical Neuropsychology, 9,* 239–250.

Binder, L. (1990). Malingering following minor head trauma. *The Clinical Neuropsychologist, 4*(1), 25–36.

Binder, L. M., Rohling, M. L., & Larrabee, G. J. (1997). A review of mild head trauma I: Meta-analytic review of neuropsychological studies. *Journal of Clinical and Experimental Neuropsychology, 19*(3), 421–431.

Blair, J., & Spreen, O. (1989). Predicting premorbid IQ: A revision of the National Adult Reading Test. *Clinical Neuropsychologist, 3,* 129–136.

Bolter, J., Gouvier, W., Veneklasen, J., & Long, C. J. (1982). Using demographic information to predict premorbid IQ: A test of clinical validity with head trauma patients. *Clinical Neuropsychology, 4,* 171–174.

Butcher, J. N., Dahlstrom, W. G., Graham, J. R., Tellegen, A. M., & Kaemmer, B. (1989). *MMPI–2: Minnesota Multiphasic Personality Inventory–2 manual for administration and scoring.* Minneapolis: University of Minnesota Press.

Chelune, G. J., & Moehle, K. A. (1986). Neuropsychological assessment and everyday functioning. In D. Wedding, A. M. Horton, & J. Webster (Eds.), *The neuropsychology handbook: Behavioral and clinical perspectives* (pp. 489–525). New York: Springer.

Committee on Ethical Guidelines for Forensic Psychologists. (1991). Specialty guidelines for forensic psychologists. *Law and Human Behavior, 15*(6), 655–665.

Crawford, J. R. (1989). Estimation of premorbid intelligence: A review of recent developments. In J. R. Crawford & D. M. Parker (Eds.), *Developments in clinical and experimental neuropsychology* (pp. 55–74). New York: Plenum.

Crawford, J. R., Cochrane, R. H. B., Besson, J. A. O., Parker, D. M., & Stewart, L. E. (1990). Premorbid IQ estimates obtained by combining the NART and demographic variables: Construct validity. *Personality and Individual Differences, 11,* 209–210.

Crawford, J. R., Parker, D. M., & Besson, J. A. O. (1988). Estimation of premorbid intelligence in organic conditions. *British Journal of Psychiatry, 153,* 178–181.

Crawford, J. R., Parker, D. M., Stewart, L. E., Besson, J. A. O., & DeLacey, G. (1989). Prediction of WAIS IQ with the National Adult Reading Test: Cross-validation and extension. *British Journal of Clinical Psychology, 28,* 267–273.

Crawford, J. R., Stewart, L. E., Parker, D. M., Besson, J. A. O., & Cochrane, R. H. B. (1989). Estimation of premorbid intelligence: Combining psychometric and demographic approaches improves predictive accuracy. *Personality and Individual Differences, 10,* 793–796.

Delis, D. C., Kramer, J. H., Kaplan, E., & Ober, B. A. (1987). *California Verbal Learning Test: Adult Version.* San Antonio, TX: The Psychological Corporation.

Dikmen, S., McLean, A., & Temkin, N. (1986). Neuropsychological and psychosocial consequences of minor head injury. *Journal of Neurology, Neurosurgery, and Psychiatry, 49*(11), 1227–1232.

Division 40 of the American Psychological Association. (1995). Definition of a clinical neuropsychologist [On-line]. Available Internet: http://www.div40.org/def.html.

Dodrill, C. B. (1997). Myths of neuropsychology. *The Clinical Neuropsychologist, 11*(1), 1–17.

Eppinger, M. G., Craig, P. L., Adams, R. L., & Parsons, O. A. (1987). The WAIS–R index for estimating premorbid intelligence: Cross-validation and clinical utility. *Journal of Consulting and Clinical Psychology, 55,* 86–90.

Faust, D., & Ziskin, J. (1988). The expert witness in psychology and psychiatry. *Science, 241,* 31–35.

Franzen, M. D., Iverson, G. L., & McCracken, L. M. (1990). The detection of malingering in neuropsychological assessment. *Neuropsychology Review, 1*(3), 247–279.

Giuliano, A. J., Barth, J. T., Hawk, G. L., & Ryan, T. V. (1997). The forensic neuropsychologist: Precedents, roles, and problems. In R. J. McCaffrey, A. D. Williams, J. M. Fisher, & L. C. Laing (Eds.), *The practice of forensic neuropsychology: Meeting challenges in the courtroom* (pp. 1–35). New York: Plenum.

Goldstein, F. C., Gary, H. E., & Levin, H. S. (1986). Assessment of the accuracy of regression equations proposed for estimating premorbid intellectual functioning on the Wechsler Adult Intelligence Scale. *Journal of Clinical and Experimental Neuropsychology, 8,* 405–412.

Gouvier, W., Uddo-Crane, M., & Brown, L. (1988). Base rates of post-concussional syndromes. *Archives of Clinical Neuropsychology, 3,* 273–278.

Guilmette, T. J., & Kastner, M. P. (1996). The prediction of vocational functioning from neuropsychological data. In R. J. Sbordone & C. J. Long (Eds.), *Ecological validity of neuropsychological testing* (pp. 387–411). Delray Beach, FL: GR Press/St. Lucie Press.

Hart, K. J. (1995). The assessment of malingering in neuropsychological evaluations: Research-based concepts and methods for consultants. *Consulting Psychology Journal Practice and Research, 47*(4), 246–254.

Hathaway, S. R., & McKinley, J. C. (1951). *The Minnesota Multiphasic Personality Inventory manual* (rev. ed.). New York: The Psychological Corporation.

Heaton, R. K., Grant, I., & Matthews, C. G. (1991). *Comprehensive norms for an expanded Halstead-Reitan battery: Demographic corrections, research findings, and clinicala.* Odessa, FL: Psychological Assessment Resources.

Heaton, R. K., & Pendleton, M. G. (1981). Use of neuropsychological tests to predict adult patients' everyday functioning. *Journal of Consulting and Clinical Psychology, 49*(6), 807–821.

Heilbronner, R. L., & Karavidas, T. (1997). Presenting neuropsychological evidence in traumatic brain injury litigation. *The Clinical Neuropsychologist, 11*(4), 445–453.

Heilbrun, K. (1992). The role of psychological testing in forensic assessment. *Law and Human Behavior, 16,* 257–272.

Hiscock, M., & Hiscock, C. K. (1989). Refining the forced-choice method for the detection of malingering. *Journal of Clinical and Experimental Neuropsychology, 11,* 967–974.

International Neuropsychology Task Force. (1981). Reports of the Task Force on Education, Accreditation, and Credentialing of the International Neuropsychological Society. *The INS Bulletin,* 5–10.

Jastak, S. & Wilkinson, G. S. (1984). *WRAT–R: Wide Range Achievement Test administration manual.* Los Angeles: Western Psychological Services.

Johnstone, B., Callahan, C. D., Kapila, C. J., & Bouman, D. E. (1996). The comparability of the WRAT–R Reading Test and NAART as estimates of premorbid intelligence in neurologically impaired patients. *Archives of Clinical Neuropsychology, 11*(6), 513–519.

Johnstone, B., & Wilhelm, K. L. (1996). The longitudinal stability of the WRAT–R reading subtest: Is it an appropriate estimate of premorbid intelligence? *Journal of the International Neuropsychological Society, 2,* 282–285.

Kane, R. (1991). Standardized and flexible batteries in neuropsychology: An assessment update. *Neuropsychology Review, 2,* 281–339.

Kaplan, R. M., & Saccuzzo, D. P. (1993). *Psychological testing.* Pacific Grove, CA: Brooks/Cole.

Karzmark, P., Heaton, R. K., Grant, I., & Matthews, C. G. (1985). Use of demographic variables to predict full scale IQ: A replication and extension. *Journal of Clinical and Experimental Neuropsychology, 7,* 412–420.

Kaufman, A. S. (1990). *Assessing adolescent and adult intelligence.* Boston: Allyn and Bacon.

Kertesz, A. (1982). *Western Aphasia Battery.* San Antonio, TX: The Psychological Corporation.

Klesges, R. C. (1982). Establishing premorbid level of intellectual functioning in children: An empirical investigation. *Clinical Neuropsychology, 4,* 15–17.

Klesges, R. C., & Sanchez, V. C. (1981). Cross-validation of an index for premorbid functioning in children. *Journal of Consulting and Clinical Psychology, 49,* 141.

Klesges, R. C., Sanchez, V. C., & Stanton, A. L. (1981). Cross validation of an adult premorbid functioning index. *Clinical Neuropsychology, 3,* 13–15.

Krull, K. R., Scott, J. G., & Sherer, M. (1995). Estimation of premorbid intelligence from combined performance and demographic variables. *The Clinical Neuropsychologist, 9*(1), 83–88.

Lezak, M. (1983). *Neuropsychological assessment* (2nd ed.). London: Oxford University Press.

Lezak, M. (1995). *Neuropsychological assessment* (3rd. ed.). London: Oxford University Press.

Long, C. J., & Collins, L. F. (1997). Ecological validity and forensic neuropsychological assessment. In R. J. McCaffrey, A. D. Williams, J. M. Fisher, & L. C. Laing (Eds.), *The practice of forensic neuropsychology: Meeting challenges in the courtroom* (pp. 153–164). New York: Plenum.

Long, C. J., & Schmitter, M. E. (1992). Cognitive sequelae in closed head injury. In C. J. Long & L. K. Ross (Eds.), *Handbook of head trauma: Acute care to recovery* (pp. 107–122). New York: Plenum.

Lynch, J. K., & McCaffrey, R. J. (1997). Premorbid intellectual functioning and the determination of cognitive loss. In R. J. McCaffrey, A. D. Williams, J. M. Fisher, & L. C. Laing (Eds.), *The practice of forensic neuropsychology: Meeting challenges in the courtroom* (pp. 91–115). New York: Plenum.

Matarazzo, J. D. (1972). *Wechsler's measurement and appraisal of adult intelligence* (5th ed.). Baltimore: Williams & Wilkins.

Matarazzo, J. D., & Herman, D. O. (1984). Relationship of education and IQ in the WAIS–R standardization sample. *Journal of Consulting and Clinical Psychology, 52,* 631–634.

Matarazzo, J. D., & Herman, D. O. (1985). Clinical uses of the WAIS–R: Base rates of differences between VIQ and PIQ in the WAIS–R standardization sample. In B. B. Wolman (Ed.), *Handbook of intelligence: Theories, measurements, and applications*. New York: Wiley.

McCaffrey, R. J., & Westervelt, H. J. (1995). Issues associated with repeated neuropsychological assessments. *Neuropsychology Review, 5*, 203–221.

McCaffrey, R. J., Williams, A. D., Fisher, J. M., & Laing, L. C. (1993). Forensic issues in mild head injury. *The Journal of Head Trauma Rehabilitation, 8*(3), 38–47.

Meier, M. J. (1981). Education competency assurance in human neuropsychology: Antecedents, models, and directions. In S. B. Filskov & T. J. Boll (Eds.), *Handbook of clinical neuropsychology* (pp. 754–781). New York: Wiley.

Mild Traumatic Brain Injury Committee of the Head Injury Interdisciplinary Special Interest Group of the American Congress of Rehabilitation Medicine. (1993). Definition of mild traumatic brain injury. *The Journal of Head Trauma Rehabilitation, 8*(3), 86–87.

Moore, J. W. (1985). *Moore's federal practice: Federal rules of evidence.* New York: Matthew Bender.

Nelson, H. E. (1982). *National Adult Reading Test (NART): Test manual.* Windsor, England: NFER Nelson.

Newcombe, F. (1987). Psychometric and behavioral evidence: Scope, limitations, and ecological validity. In H. S. Levin, J. Grafman, & H. M. Eisenberg (Eds.), *Neurobehavioral recovery from head injury* (pp. 129–145). New York: Oxford University Press.

Newman, R. (1991). The role of the psychologist expert witness: Provider of perspective and input. *Neuropsychology Review, 2*(3), 241–249.

Nies, K. J., & Sweet, J. J. (1994). Neuropsychological assessment and malingering: A critical review of past and present strategies. *Archives of Clinical Neuropsychology, 9*(6), 501–552.

Pankratz, L., & Binder, L. M. (1997). Malingering on intellectual and neuropsychological measures. In R. Rogers (Ed.), *Clinical assessment of malingering and deception* (2nd ed., pp. 223–236). New York: Guilford.

Paolo, A. M., & Ryan, J. J. (1992). Generalizability of two methods of estimating premorbid intelligence in the elderly. *Archives of Clinical Neuropsychology, 7,* 135–143.

Paolo, A. M., Ryan, J. J., Troster, A. I., & Hilmer, C. D. (1996). Utility of the Barona demographic equations to estimate premorbid intelligence: Information from the WAIS–R standardization sample. *Journal of Clinical Psychology, 52*(3), 335–343.

Parker, R. S., & Rosenblum, A. (1996). IQ loss and emotional dysfunctions after mild head injury in a motor vehicle accident. *Journal of Clinical Psychology, 52*(1), 32–43.

Reitan, R. M., & Wolfson, D. (1993). *The Halstead-Reitan Neuropsychological Test Battery: Theory and clinical interpretation* (2nd ed.). Tuscon, AZ: Neuropsychology Press.

Reitan, R. M., & Wolfson, D. (1997). *Detection of malingering and invalid test scores.* Tucson, AZ: Neuropsychology Press.

Rey, A. (1964). *L'examen clinique en psychologie* [The clinical examination in psychology]. Paris: Presse Universitaires de France.

Reynolds, C. R., Chastain, R. L., Kaufman, A. S., & McLean, J. E. (1987). Demographic characteristics and IQ among adults: Analysis of the WAIS–R standardization sample as a function of the stratification variables. *Journal of School Psychology, 25,* 323–342.

Reynolds, C. R., & Gutkin, T. B. (1979). Predicting the premorbid intellectual status of children using demographic data. *The Clinical Neuropsychologist, 1,* 36–38.

Richardson, J. T. E. (1990). *Clinical and neuropsychological aspects of closed head injury.* New York: Taylor & Francis.

Richardson, R. E. L., & Adams, R. L. (1992). Neuropsychologists as expert witnesses: Issues of admissibility. *The Clinical Neuropsychologist, 6,* 295–308.

Rogers, R., Bagby, R. M., & Dickens, S. E. (1992). *SIRS Structured Interview of Reported Symptoms professional manual.* Odessa, FL: Psychological Assessment Resources.

Ruff, R. M., Wylie, T., & Tennant, W. (1993). Malingering and malingering-like aspects of mild closed head injury. *Journal of Head Trauma Rehabilitation, 8*(3), 60–73.

Russell, E. W. (1972). WAIS factor analysis with brain-damaged subjects using criterion measures. *Journal of Consulting and Clinical Psychology, 39,* 133–139.

Ryan, J. J., & Sattler, J. M. (1988). Wechsler Adult Intelligence Scale–Revised (WAIS–R). In J. M. Sattler (Ed.), *Assessment of children* (3rd. ed., pp. 219–244). San Diego: Sattler.

Saks, M. J. (1990). Expert witnesses, nonexpert witnesses, and nonwitness experts. *Law and Human Behavior, 14,* 291–313.

Saks, M. (1992). Normative and empirical issues about the role of expert witnesses. In D. Kagehiro & W. Laufer (Eds.), *Handbook of psychology and law.* Berlin: Springer-Verlag.

Silverstein, A. B. (1987). Accuracy of estimates of premorbid intelligence based on demographic variables. *Journal of Clinical Psychology, 43,* 493–495.

Smith, A. (1994). Critical clinical considerations in neuropsychological assessments of closed head injury and traumatic brain injury. In C. N. Simkins (Ed.), *Analysis, understanding, and presentation of cases involving traumatic brain injury* (pp. 1–14). Washington, DC: National Head Injury Foundation.

Spitzer, R. L., & Endicott, J. (1978). *Schedule of Affective Disorders and Schizophrenia.* New York: Biometric Research.

Standards for educational and psychological testing. (1985). Washington, DC: American Psychological Association.

Stebbins, G. T., Gilley, D. W., Wilson, R. S., Bernard, B. A., & Fox, J. H. (1990). Effects of language disturbances on premorbid estimates of IQ in mild dementia. *The Clinical Neuropsychologist, 4,* 64–68.

Vogt, A. T., & Heaton, R. K. (1977). Comparison of Wechsler Adult Intelligence Scale indices of cerebral dysfunction. *Perceptual and Motor Skills, 45,* 607–615.

Wechsler, D. (1955). *Manual for the Wechsler Adult Intelligence Scale.* New York: The Psychological Corporation.

Wechsler, D. (1981). *WAIS–R manual: Wechsler Adult Intelligence Scale–Revised.* San Antonio, TX: The Psychological Corporation.

Wechsler, D. (1987). *WMS–R manual: Wechsler Memory Scale–Revised.* San Antonio, TX: The Psychological Corporation.

Wedding, D. (1991). Clinical judgment in forensic neuropsychology: A comment on the risks of claiming more than can be delivered. *Neuropsychology Review, 2*(3), 233–239.

Wiens, A. N., Bryan, J. E., & Crossen, J. R. (1993). Estimating WAIS–R FSIQ from National Adult Reading Test–Revised in normal subjects. *The Clinical Neuropsychologist, 7,* 70–84.

Williams, A. D. (1997). The forensic evaluation of adult traumatic brain injury. In R. J. McCaffrey, A. D. Williams, J. M. Fisher, & L. C. Laing (Eds.), *The practice of forensic neuropsychology: Meeting challenges in the courtroom* (pp. 37–56). New York: Plenum.

Williams, J. (1991). *Memory Assessment Scales.* Odessa, FL: Psychological Assessment Resources.

Wilshire, D., Kinsella, G., & Prior, M. (1991). Estimating WAIS–R IQ from the National Adult Reading Test: A cross validation. *Journal of Clinical and Experimental Neuropsychology, 13,* 204–216.

Wilson, B. A. (1993). Ecological validity of neuropsychological assessment: Do neuropsychological indexes predict performance in everyday activities? *Applied and Preventive Psychology, 2,* 209–215.

Wilson, R. S., Rosenbaum, G., & Brown, G. (1979). The problem of premorbid intelligence in neuropsychological assessment. *Journal of Clinical Neuropsychology, 1,* 49–53.

Wilson, R. S., Rosenbaum, G., Brown, G., Rourke, D., Whitman, D., & Grisell, J. (1978). An index of premorbid intelligence. *Journal of Consulting and Clinical Psychology, 46,* 1554–1555.

Zielinski, J. J. (1994). Malingering and defensiveness in the neuropsychological assessment of mild traumatic brain injury. *Clinical Psychology Science and Practice, 1,* 169–184.

Social and Legal Impact of Malingered Mild Traumatic Brain Injury

10

Kay B. Stevens
and J. Randall Price

Introduction

The seriousness of traumatic head injuries is difficult to overestimate. Lives are shattered; families are changed forever. Traumatic head injury is the leading cause of death in young males, and the cost to an overburdened health care system is staggering. The problems of assessing and treating head trauma are difficult enough without the complicated psycholegal and societal overlay of symptom exaggeration and malingering. This chapter examines the implications of invalid traumatic head injury claims by describing the roles of the participants in both the psychological health care system and the legal system. The role of the neuropsychologist is specifically emphasized.

The detection of valid and invalid symptoms related to mild head trauma is often the responsibility of a neuropsychologist. Although there are a variety of diagnostic techniques, none are foolproof. On a trip to Havana to study the health care system, the second author asked the chief psychologist of the Psychiatric Hospital of Havana if malingering was a problem, especially during what Fidel Castro called the "special period" following the fall of the Soviet Union and the economic blockade by the United States. It is speculated that severe economic shortages might increase the motivation for the relative comforts of hospitalization ("three hots and a cot"). Indeed, the doctor reported that more Cuban citizens than ever attempted to feign a mental disorder to gain admission to the hospital. Even more interesting was one of the techniques used by the doctor to identify malingerers. He asked the patient to hold a burning match or piece of paper. His theory was that

---

Reprinted, with changes, from "Psycholegal Implications of Malingered Head Trauma," by J. Randall Price and Kay B. Stevens, 1997, *Applied Neuropsychology, 4*(1), pp. 75–83. Copyright 1997 by Lawrence Erlbaum Associates, Inc.

only the malingerers would let it burn their hand to "prove" they were mentally ill. Of course, such societal conditions or examination techniques are not directly applicable to the United States, but the problem of diagnosing malingering and symptom exaggeration is well illustrated by the Cuban doctor's technique. The diagnosis of malingering can be extremely difficult.

Roles of the Neuropsychologist

The neuropsychologist typically provides one or more of the following services related to a case of malingered traumatic head injury: (a) diagnostician, (b) therapist, (c) expert witness, (d) consultant. Each of these roles will be generally described, as will the relationship of the roles.

Neuropsychologist as Diagnostician

As diagnostician, the neuropsychologist is generally guided by the *Diagnostic and Statistical Manual of Mental Disorders* (*DSM–IV;* American Psychiatric Association, 1994) or the *International Classification of Disease, Ninth Revision, Clinical Modification* (*ICD–9–CM*; MEDICODE, 1995). Although both manuals can be helpful, neither is conclusive. The *DSM–IV* does not have one clear and distinct category for brain injury resulting from head trauma. However, it does include categories to describe mental problems that might result from head trauma, such as Dementia, Amnestic Disorders, and Cognitive Disorder, Not Otherwise Specified. The *ICD–9–CM* provides a more useful set of criteria for brain injury resulting from head trauma, including a description of postconcussive syndrome (PCS).

A general definition of malingering is included in both manuals. According to the *DSM–IV* malingering is the "intentional production of false or grossly exaggerated physical or psychological symptoms motivated by external incentives" (American Psychiatric Association, 1994, p. 683). Further, it states that malingering should be suspected if any combination of the following are observed:

1. Medicolegal context of presentation
2. Marked discrepancy between the person's claimed stress or disability and the objective findings
3. Lack of cooperation during the diagnostic evaluation and in complying with the prescribed treatment regimen
4. The presence of Antisocial Personality Disorder (p. 683)

The *ICD–9–CM* defines malingering as follows:

> A clinical picture in which the predominant feature is the presentation of fake or grossly exaggerated physical or psychiatric illness apparently under voluntary control. . . . the symptoms produced in malingering are in pursuit of a goal which when known, is recognizable and obviously understandable in light of knowledge of the individual's circumstances. (MEDICODE, 1995, p. 236)

Ruff, Wylie, and Tennant (1993) criticized the American Psychiatric Association criteria for being overly inclusive. They specifically pointed out that many mild head traumas are sustained in motor vehicle accidents, involve litigation, result in a lack of objective neuroimaging results, involve deficits (including denial) that lead to diminished cooperation, and occur in young, risk-taking males (often positive for an antisocial history). This response provides a good example of the difficulty related to an accurate diagnosis.

Using the guidelines available and his or her experience and expertise, the neuropsychologist must determine the presence or absence of neuropsychological impairment. One of the most difficult tasks is to differentiate valid from invalid complaints. Whereas the *DSM–IV* and *ICD–9–CM* definitions imply that malingering is a distinct entity, in fact, malingering is best defined as falling on a continuum from pure malingering, the faking of invented symptoms, to partial malingering, the exaggeration of actual symptoms. First the neuropsychologist must determine if malingering is present and, if so, where on the continuum the malingering falls.

To make things more difficult, the patient's motivation also must be assessed. Intentionality refers to the patient's conscious awareness of symptom exaggeration. Some individuals are unaware of the exaggeration of their symptoms. Others consciously and intentionally fake symptoms for external gain. Many fall in between these two extremes. Ruff et al. (1993) concluded that when evaluating for conscious and unconscious motivation, neuropsychologists "may have reached the limits of science only to enter into the realm of metaphysics" (p. 64).

A review of strategies for detecting malingering and symptom exaggeration is beyond the scope and purpose of this chapter (see Miller & Miller, 1992; Nies & Sweet, 1994); however, the theoretical foundations for such psychological opinions have been established in works by Resnick (1984) and Rogers (1997). These were followed by works from neuropsychological investigators such as Franzen, Iversin, & McCracken (1990), Binder (1993), Trueblood and Schmidt (1993), and Mittenberg, Rotholc, Russell, & Heilbronner (1996). Although methods for detecting malingering and symptom exaggeration are not foolproof, specific procedures have been developed and researched during the last decade. This development and research has resulted in recommendations and guidelines for the practicing neuropsychologist. Nies and

Sweet described the following six strategies to assist in the identification of malingering:

1. Use specific tests of malingering such as the *Portland Digit Recognition Test* and the *Rey 15-Item Test.*
2. Evaluate patterns of performance on common neuropsychological tests that are forced-choice and for which a below-chance level of performance can be computed.
3. Examine nonsensical test patterns that have not been found to occur in real psychiatric or neurological patients.
4. Examine excessive inconsistency of test scores within and across test sessions.
5. Seek independent information that confirms or refutes the patient's self-report of limited success in coping with everyday living and work activities.
6. Verify preinjury ability levels, attainments, and losses through objective, independent sources such as school and employment records.

Clinically, neuropsychologists attempt to obtain a picture of the patient's life history and current situation by (a) gathering background factors during interviews and review of records, (b) conducting behavioral observations during the examination, and (c) analyzing reported activities of daily life. Most importantly, the well trained and experienced neuropsychologist is aware of the characteristics and course of valid brain injuries, and therefore is in an excellent position to assess the validity of alleged symptoms of mild head trauma.

Neuropsychologist as Therapist

Neuropsychologists, as well as psychiatrists and other physicians who are involved in the treatment of the patient, are referred to as the "treating doctors" within the legal system. This is important because it differs from the psychological or medical professionals who are retained as consultants or expert witnesses. Typically, the patient seeks or is referred to the treating doctor to receive medical or psychological intervention in the course of recovery. When a treating doctor provides legal testimony, it should focus on the diagnosis and treatment procedures rather than complex legal issues (e.g., competency to manage one's affairs, criminal responsibility, malingering).

Neuropsychologists who serve as treating doctors for persons with head trauma typically work in an inpatient or outpatient rehabilitation setting or as independent practitioners. When working in a rehabilitation setting, the treating neuropsychologist typically is a member of a team of treatment personnel. This team provides a multidisciplinary perspective on the patient's condition, thus making it more difficult for malingering to escape detection. Although symptom exaggeration does occur in such settings, the team approach and the team members' knowledge of head trauma and malingering assists in the diagnosis of valid injuries. This is not the case for treating doctors working as independent practitioners. These neuropsychologists often work alone. In addition, they usually see patients whose symptoms are less overt and/or severe, thus more difficult to diagnose. However, they may be the most qualified among the health care professionals who treat the patient, to detect malingering. They should be knowledgeable about the assessment of malingering so as to detect it when it occurs, thus avoiding the waste of treatment resources and invalid litigation.

Neuropsychologist as Expert Witness

Increasingly, neuropsychologists are retained by defense and plaintiff attorneys to conduct an evaluation of an individual who is alleging a brain injury and provide expert testimony regarding their findings. This evaluation may include a face-to-face evaluation of the plaintiff and/or a comprehensive review of all records discovered by the attorneys. The neuropsychologist also may request that additional records be discovered. The plaintiff may be sent to the neuropsychologist by his or her own attorney, or the court may order the individual to go for an independent evaluation at the request of the defense attorney. Regardless of the referral source, the purpose of this evaluation is not only to determine the presence or absence of brain injury, but also, if an injury is present, to arrive at an opinion regarding the etiology and extent of the injury and prognosis for recovery. Attorneys may request that the neuropsychologist provide other complex legal opinions (e. g., competency to manage affairs, the capacity to engage in gainful employment). When the referral has a medicolegal basis, the neuropsychologist should be alert to the possibility of malingering. This is critical to avoid external gain for those who are malingering, and to validate the claims of credible plaintiffs and assist in their just compensation.

Testimony concerning malingering (as with all testimony) must be admissible under rules of evidence. An excellent overview of the relevant issues is covered in Ogloff (1990). Basically, the Federal Rules of Evidence (FRE) provide the framework for admissibility of all testimony, including expert testimony. Ogloff noted that the substantive provisions of the FRE governing expert testimony include (a) opinion testimony by lay witnesses (FRE 701), (b) testimony by experts (FRE 702), (c) basis of opinion testimony by experts (FRE 703), (d) opinion on ultimate issue (FRE 704), and (e) disclosure of facts or data underlying expert opinion (FRE 705).

Basically, the guidelines for determining the admissibility of expert testimony regarding malingering and symptom exaggeration are:

1. The expert's testimony must be relevant to the case.
2. The witness must be qualified as an expert.
3. The expert's testimony must be necessary to assist the trier of fact in a determination.
4. The probative value of the testimony must not be outweighed by its prejudicial impact.
5. The Daubert test must be satisfied.

Ogloff (1990) discussed all of the above with the exception of the Daubert test. *Daubert v. Merrell Dow Chemical Co.* (1993) is a case that replaced the standard of *Frye v. United States* (1923). The long-standing Frye test required that any scientific expert testimony, including that regarding malingering and symptom exaggeration, be generally accepted in the related field. *Daubert v. Merrell Dow Chemical Co.* supersedes this test with the requirement that the trial judge be satisfied that the expert's testimony rests on reliable foundation and is relevant to the task at hand. What this means to the expert is not exactly clear at this time, but it appears that expert testimony will require good science rather than peer acceptance. Exactly how judges will assess the scientific validity of the expert's testimony likely will vary from judge to judge, depending on the judge's scientific background and evidentiary philosophy.

Being retained on numerous cases involving issues of symptom exaggeration or malingering has further implications for the expert witness's objectivity. Experts who align themselves exclusively with either the plaintiff or defense may become ego-involved in supporting the claims of symptom exaggerators or in developing a cynical attitude toward any plaintiff's report of symptoms. Neuropsychologists might do well to balance plaintiff and defense consultations. Involvement in other types of clinical work, research projects, or teaching also helps to avoid opinion bias. A late 19th-century French medico-legalist, P. C. H. Brouardel, said, "If the law has made you a witness, remain a man of science. You have no victim to avenge, no guilty or innocent person to convince or save—you must bear testimony within the limits of science" (P. J. Resnick, personal communication, December, 1989).

Neuropsychologist as Consultant

The neuropsychologist as consultant in legal matters is retained to assist the attorney in understanding the technical information contained in the records concerning an alleged brain injury. The consultant's major responsibility is to comprehensively review the records, including rescoring and interpreting raw test data, reviewing related research and its application to the case, and preparing questions for cross-examination of opposing counsel's expert witness. The consultant's responsibilities are different from those of the expert witness in that (a) the consultant does not provide testimony, (b) the consultant works behind the scenes with the attorney, (c) the consultant does not have face-to-face contact with the plaintiff, (d) the identity and work product of the consultant is privileged (not discoverable), and (e) the consultant is an advisor to an adversarial team. As advisor to the attorney, the consultant can freely generate ideas and suggest procedures for gathering and presenting information that assist in validating or invalidating the plaintiff's injury. The ultimate goal of the neuropsychological consultant is providing objective and scientifically sound advice that leads to just compensation for valid head injuries.

Role of the Plaintiff

As discussed previously, the plaintiff who is presenting an invalid claim may be intentionally malingering or unintentionally exaggerating symptoms. There is not a definitive profile for either type. However, certain clinical indicators have been identified to assist neuropsychologists in the detection of each (Resnick, 1984; Rogers, 1997).

Intentional Malingering

In addition to the testing patterns demonstrated by malingerers (Nies & Sweet, 1994; Mittenberg et al., 1996), the plaintiff may exhibit certain other behaviors that indicate malingering. The neuropsychologist should examine the plaintiff's background, response style, and clinical signs and symptoms to determine if he or she is malingering.

There are several general background factors that may alert the neuropsychologist to intentional malingering or symptom exaggeration. They include (a) recognizable external incentives for malingering, (b) a history of spotty employment, incapacitating injuries, and/or excessive absences from work, (c) a well ingrained capacity for dishonesty, (d) knowledge of relevant legal standards for his or her case, (e) exposure to the litigation process, (f) experience with a health care field or perhaps the insurance industry, and (g) a disability role model in the family.

Various response styles exhibited during the examination or treatment may indicate malingering or the conscious exaggeration of symptoms. Possibly the most common response style involves a lack of cooperation with the diagnostic and treatment process. This lack of cooperation may be manifested in a variety of ways, such as (a) attempting to take control of the interview and behaving in an intimidating or bizarre manner, (b) being unwilling to submit to treatment because it is inconvenient (e.g., hospitalization) or because it "will not work," (c) refusing to complete an evaluation task, (d) providing approximate answers to problems that are "near misses," and (e) missing or arriving late for evaluation or treatment appointments. Another malingering response style involves using every opportunity to enhance present credibility and preinjury functioning (e.g., magnifying his or her position in society, affirming complete honesty and total self-disclosure, depicting prior functioning in exclusively complimentary terms). Finally, the malingerer's response style can be affected by the length of the diagnostic process. If the examination is short, the malingerer may be able to maintain the simulation of a brain injury, but with a longer examination, fatigue can create a "pull of reality." The same theory can be applied to the length of the litigation process; continual observation and documentation of the plaintiff's behavior during the entire litigation process, especially during daily living routines, may uncover behavior that is inconsistent with the symptoms of brain injury.

In addition to response styles, other specific signs and symptoms presented by a plaintiff during a clinical examination may indicate malingering. Clinical signs and symptoms of malingering include (a) an eagerness to discuss or call attention to symptoms in an overly dramatic manner, (b) making false imputations about valid symptoms, (c) endorsing symptoms rarely found in credible head trauma patients and reporting improbable numbers of symptoms, (d) simulating positive symptoms more often than negative symptoms (positive symptoms signify a brain injury, whereas negative symptoms are those whose absence is characteristic of a brain injury), (e) endorsing more blatant than subtle brain injury symptoms, (f) endorsing symptoms that are of unusually extreme severity, even if bizarre and ridiculous, (g) reporting symptoms or performing tasks that are inconsistent with previous self-reports, reports from others, or observations of the person's behavior in other situations, (h) presenting a constellation of signs and symptoms that are inconsistent with a recognizable brain injury, and demonstrating a course of the alleged injury that is contrary to the development of actual injuries, (i) an eagerness to endorse new symptoms suggested by the neuropsychologist, and (j) focusing on his or her perceived disability (e.g., cannot work) rather than on the alleged injury, and rarely mentioning or acknowledging his or her abilities or capacity.

A careful analysis of response types and patterns during testing, background factors, response styles, and clinical signs and symptoms is beneficial in the detection of intentional malingering and symptom exaggeration. The more of these factors that are observed or documented, the stronger the probability that the plaintiff is malingering or exaggerating symptoms. The relative absence of these factors should support the opinion that the brain injury is valid.

Unintentional Symptom Exaggeration

Unconscious or unintentional symptom exaggeration is thought by many to be more common than intentional malingering or exaggeration. Unconscious symptom exaggeration often is an extension of an actual injury. As expressed previously, it is difficult to differentiate persons who are intentionally malingering from those who are unintentionally exaggerating because many of the factors and characteristics are the same. Although patients who unintentionally exaggerate symptoms may be focused on external gain or avoiding a dreaded or unpleasant event (e.g., work, school), there may be other reasons for the exaggeration. According to Matheson (1987), some patients exaggerate or magnify existing symptoms to the point of becoming dysfunctional. This dysfunction becomes a separate problem from the originally alleged injury. Their continued symptom exaggeration may be focused on alerting others that they are in trouble and need help rather than on obtaining an external goal. In addition, a dependent person who suffers an actual injury may be led by an authority figure and/or significant other to maintain his or her symptoms and avoid recovery in order to reap maximum benefit from the injury. Regardless of the source, when actual head trauma results in neuropsychological injury, unconscious symptom exaggeration complicates the diagnostic process. Unconscious symptom exaggeration almost always prolongs recovery and increases health care costs.

Implications for the Legal System

The courts (judges or juries) frequently are asked to decide the genuineness of brain injury caused by head trauma. The implications of these decisions often are extreme for the plaintiff, the defendant, and the attorneys. Although not directly implicated in the decision, the jurors and judges may pay a toll due to making fair decisions with less than clear criteria and facts. These decisions often are based on the testimony of neuropsychologists who serve as expert witnesses.

Implications for Attorneys

Plaintiff attorneys evaluate their clients and formulate a theory to guide their litigation plan including discovery of evidence, witness selection and examination, opening statements, and closing arguments. The role of the plaintiff's attorney is to present the case in a way that will most benefit the plaintiff's legal recovery or compensation. The American legal system is set up so that plaintiff attorneys are compensated by a contingency fee (a percentage of the plaintiff's award goes to the attorney); therefore, plaintiff attorneys typically benefit from zealously representing their clients. There are at least three potential problems with this system for compensating plaintiff attorneys. First, the relaxation of certain ethical guidelines for attorneys several years ago resulted in a proliferation of advertising by plaintiff attorneys. Individuals who have not actually been injured may be encouraged by these advertisements to become involved in litigation. Second, attorneys can misevaluate plaintiff cases if they do not regard the possibility of malingering or symptom exaggeration. No attorney likes to be surprised at trial by an invalid claim; however, naive attitudes and practices by plaintiff attorneys may lead to just that. In addition, invalid claims that go to trial clog already overcrowded court dockets. The use of a neuropsychological consultant by the plaintiff attorney at the case evaluation stage is a strategy for avoiding misevaluation of the plaintiff's mental status and probable cause of any impairments (Taylor, 1995). Third, the attorney may coach or prepare a plaintiff for an evaluation by a mental health professional. This preparation may range from simply describing the evaluation process to telling the plaintiff how to respond to certain questions or tests. In a survey by Wetter and Corrigan (1995), the majority of law students and practicing attorneys reported that they would engage in some form of coaching with their clients. Youngjohn (1995) reported a confirmed case in which an attorney admitted to an administrative law judge that he had coached his client prior to examination. Youngjohn's article includes strategies for reducing the effects of attorney coaching, thereby increasing the validity of neuropsychological test results.

The defense attorney in civil litigation has a different set of responsibilities and operates under a different compensation system than the plaintiff attorney. The defense attorney formulates a theory in response to the plaintiff's claims. Like the plaintiff attorney, the defense attorney discovers evidence, selects and examines witnesses, and presents opening statements and closing arguments. However, the defense attorney's primary goal in a head trauma claim is to prove that the plaintiff (a) does not have a brain injury, (b) has recovered from a brain injury, (c) has a brain injury caused by some action other than that of the defendant, or (d) deserves no more than a specified amount of damages due to a brain injury. As can be surmised, malingering often is considered in the defense theory of head trauma claims. Malingering is considered more when symptoms are mild than when the injury is moderate or severe and the etiology is clear. When there is a possibility of great external gain for the plaintiff, mild symptoms should be investigated carefully. The potential problem in these circumstances is the denial of a valid claim of brain injury. One of the major responsibilities of the neuropsychologist is to assist the defense attorney in preparing an accurate and fair defense based on the actual condition of the plaintiff, attempting to ensure that fair settlements are made and trial is avoided when possible.

The defense attorney is compensated on a hourly basis, commonly referred to as "billable hours." Typically, neuropsychologists who serve as expert witnesses or consultants also bill by the hour. The abuse of an hourly billing system by attorneys, consultants, or expert witnesses leads to increased cost of litigation, increased insurance premiums, and delays in the litigation process. Although thorough and comprehensive case preparation is the primary goal of the defense team, and is necessary to avoid the awarding of spurious damages, completing the work expeditiously should be a parallel goal.

Implications for the Defendant

The defendant and the defendant's insurance company clearly have the most to lose in an invalid injury claim. The idea of insurance companies as "big brother" has been used as justification for fraudulent and exaggerated claims, even by otherwise honest citizens. The effect of this type of thinking on individuals who are predisposed to malinger is unknown but possibly quite significant. The belief is that financial compensation from any large corporation, especially an insurance company, has no consequences for either society or any individual. Many states even prohibit the mention of insurance in civil suits (see *Texas Rules of Civil Procedures,* 1993, 226a, for example). The mention of "insurance company" by any witness, including an expert witness, may result in a mistrial.

However, "lawsuit abuse" has been publicized through explanations of the shared-risk concept that underlies the insurance industry: all premiums are raised to cover unexpected claims. When the plaintiff prevails in an invalid or inflated claim, the defendant takes the most direct hit on premium increases; but ultimately all policy holders pay the tab. In our litigious society, it is becoming more and more justifiable to protect "big brother" from invalid claims in order to protect individuals who pay insurance premiums, health care costs, and taxes. The neuropsychologist can play an important role in accomplishing this when he or she detects fraudulant claims of head trauma.

Implications for the Trier of Fact

After a lawsuit pertaining to an alleged brain injury has been filed, both sides aim their efforts toward a settlement. Records are discovered and analyzed, depositions are taken, and negotiation conferences and mediation are completed. Nevertheless, some cases of alleged brain injury go to trial, where a trier of fact hears the evidence and reaches a verdict. The trier of fact can be a jury or a judge, depending on jurisdiction matters and the preferences of the lawsuit participants. In brain injury cases the judge or jury typically decides three issues. First, the verdict must address whether or not the plaintiff suffered a brain injury. Second, the probable cause of the injury, if any, must be determined. This allows the assignment of liability or fault. Third, the amount of damages, if any, to be awarded to the plaintiff must be decided. As can be seen, the role of the jury or judge is critical in such cases.

According to Wrightsman (1991), the experience of serving on a jury demands sacrifices of income, time, and energy for a great many citizens in the United States. More than 300,000 jury trials are held annually. Three million citizens receive jury summons each year, and more than one fourth of all Americans will serve on a jury at some time in their lives. Trials involving allegations of brain injury often involve millions of dollars and can affect the parties for years to come. These factors put a great responsibility on a juror. We should not be surprised that many people are reluctant, anxious, and sometimes even hostile about serving on a jury. We also should not be surprised that evidence of malingering may result in increased juror hostility. The neuropsychologist appearing as an expert witness is advised that clear, objective testimony presented in a "user-friendly" fashion will be best received by and most useful to the jury.

Wrightsman (1991) also reviewed research that calls into question commonly held assumptions about jurors and juries. These include the assumptions that (a) jurors enter the trial free of overwhelming biases, (b) jurors use only the evidence presented in court to arrive at their decisions, (c) jurors are able to understand and retain all important information in a case necessary to deliberate their decisions, (d) jurors withhold judgment until the trial is over and all the evidence is presented, and (e) jury deliberations are unaffected by either group pressures or the personal wishes of the jurors. Each of these assumptions is likely false concerning brain injury trials. Jurors do not enter a head injury trial without some experience of what a brain injury does to people—even if their experiences come from movies, television, or the popular press. Similarly, jurors frequently have information and opinions about fraud and deceit in legal cases before they are ever selected to serve on a jury. Evidence presented via a "battle of the experts" can be confusing rather than helpful to a jury in a brain injury trial. The evidence presented early in such a trial is frequently very dramatic (e.g., "day in the life of" video) and may lead jurors to a decision before all the evidence is presented. Just as in other trials, the group and personality dynamics involved in jury deliberations may be equally as important in the ultimate decision as the evidence presented in court. The implications for the testifying neuropsychologist are clear: testimony must be educational and presented in an objective and helpful fashion. Testimony laden with jargon and delivered in a condescending tone will only confuse and frustrate jurors.

A bench trial is one where a judge rather than a jury evaluates the evidence and arrives at a decision. A critical question is how evidence pertaining to symptom exaggeration or malingering might affect the judge's decision as opposed to a jury's decision. Kalven and Zeisel (1966) compared the decisions of juries and judges in approximately 3,500 trials. Overall, the judges and juries agreed in their verdicts in approximately 75% of the cases.

Analysis of the discrepancies suggests that juries and judges differed in cases where the evidence was close. In most of these cases, the jury was thought to rely more on emotion than on evidence, which is referred to as jury sentiment. In other instances, the jury completely ignored requirements of the law and the instructions from the judge, which is referred to as jury nullification. Based on these concepts, it would be reasonable to conclude that a trial by judge would more likely be decided on the weight of the evidence and the requirements of the law, and a trial by jury would more likely be decided on extraneous factors, such as the appearance and demeanor of the plaintiff.

Conclusions

Whether the trier of fact is a judge or jury, the overall psycholegal and societal importance of the decision cannot be overemphasized. Better legal outcomes promote better clinical outcomes in brain injury cases (Taylor, 1995). When a favorable plaintiff verdict is handed down in a valid head trauma case, the plaintiff's future is secured. Rehabilitation is planned, and the plaintiff's family is relieved of the financial burden of health care and lost earnings. When a jury or judge rejects a malingered head trauma case and the defense prevails, the defendant is free to carry on business as usual, providing jobs for the national economy and conserving financial resources. Moreover, the malingering plaintiff is hopefully forced to be self-sufficient and contribute to society in a meaningful way.

References

American Psychiatric Association. (1994). *Diagnostic and statistical manual of mental disorders* (4th ed.). Washington, DC: Author.

Binder, L. M. (1993). Assessment of malingering after mild head trauma with the Portland Digit Recognition Test. *Journal of Clinical and Experimental Neuropsychology, 15,* 170–182.

Daubert v. Merrell Dow Chemical Co., 509 U.S., 113 S.Ct. 2786, 125 Ed.2d 469 (1993).

Franzen, M. D., Iversin, G. L., & McCracken, L. M. (1990). The detection of malingering in neuropsychological assessment. *Neuropsychology Review, 1,* 247–279.

Frye v. United States, 293 F. 1013 (D.C. Cir. 1923).

Kalven, H., & Zeisel, H. (1966). *The American jury.* Boston: Little, Brown.

Matheson, L. N. (1987). *Work capacity evaluation: Systematic approach to industrial rehabilitation.* Anaheim, CA: E. R. I. C.

MEDICODE, Inc. (1995). *International classification of diseases, ninth revision, clinical modification* (5th ed.). Salt Lake City, UT: Author.

Miller, W. G., & Miller, E. S. (1992). Malingering and neuropsychological assessment. *Physical Medicine and Rehabilitation, 6,* 547–563.

Mittenberg, W., Rotholc, A., Russell, E., & Heilbronner, R. (1996). Identification of malingered head injury on the Halstead-Reitan battery. *Archives of Clinical Neuropsychology, 11,* 271–281.

Nies, K. J., & Sweet, J. J. (1994). Neuropsychological assessment and malingering: A critical review of past and present strategies. *Archives of Clinical Neuropsychology, 9,* 501–522.

Ogloff, J. R. P. (1990). The admissibility of expert testimony regarding malingering and deception. *Behavioral Sciences and the Law, 8,* 27–43.

Resnick, P. J. (1984). The detection of malingered mental illness. *Behavioral Sciences and the Law, 2,* 21–37.

Rogers, R. (Ed.). (1997). *Clinical assessment of malingering and deception* (2nd ed.). New York: Guilford.

Ruff, R. M., Wylie, T., & Tennant, W. (1993). Malingering and malingering-like aspects of mild closed head injury. *Journal of Head Trauma Rehabilitation, 8,* 60–73.

Taylor, S. J. (1995). Neurolaw: Towards a new medical jurisprudence. *Brain Injury, 9,* 745–751.

Texas rules of civil procedures. (1993). Saint Paul, MN: West Publishing Co.

Trueblood, W., & Schmidt, M. (1993). Malingering and other validity considerations in the neurological evaluation of mild head injury. *Journal of Clinical and Experimental Neuropsychology, 15,* 578–590.

Wetter, M. W., & Corrigan, S. K. (1995). Providing information to clients about psychological tests: A survey of attorneys' and law students' attitudes. *Professional Psychology: Research and Practice, 26,* 474–477.

Wrightsman, L. S. (1991). *Psychology and the legal system.* Pacific Grove, CA: Brooks Cole.

Youngjohn, J. R. (1995). Confirmed attorney coaching prior to neuropsychological evaluation. *Assessment, 2,* 279–283.

III

Treatment and Rehabilitation Issues

Effective Treatment of Mild Traumatic Brain Injury and Understanding its Neurological Consequences

11

Michelle Kibby
and Charles J. Long

Although most inpatient treatment is directed at more severe brain injuries, there remains a large population of head injury survivors whose injury is less severe and referred to as mild TBI. These individuals should fully recover from the neurological consequences of their trauma, but they often have persistent symptoms that must be understood if effective treatment is to be provided.

Defining Mild TBI

Upper Limits

Mild TBI is generally defined as TBI resulting in (a) coma of less than 30 minutes, (b) posttraumatic amnesia (PTA) that dissipates within 24 hours, (c) a Glasgow Coma Scale (GCS) score of 13 or higher on admission, and (d) hospitalization of less than 48 hours (Rimel, Giordani, Barth, Boll, & Jane, 1981). In Russell's (1932) scale of head injury severity, PTA of under 24 hours is an indicator of both mild and moderate brain injury.

Lower Limits

Whereas the upper limits of mild TBI are vaguely defined, no lower limits of mild head injury have been set. Thus, the present definition includes moderate to minimal brain injury, and even no brain injury.

Reprinted, with changes, from "Effective Treatment of Minor Head Injury and Understanding Its Neurological Consequences," by Michelle Y. Kibby and Charles J. Long, 1997, *Applied Neuropsychology, 4*(1), pp. 34–42. Copyright 1997 by Lawrence Erlbaum Associates, Inc.

The important question is, How severe can the brain injury be and still leave no persistent, residual damage? Clearly there is a need for the establishment of lower limits of brain injury. With the definition as it is, anyone who has sustained the slightest bump to the head could say he or she has a mild brain injury. Dicker (1989) declared a need for more reproducible and restrictive lower limits of brain injury and stated that a lower limit could be established by requiring the presence of headache, neurological problems, or the act of seeking medical care within 24 hours of injury. This definition is a step in the right direction, but the true lower limit should include other factors as well (for a more detailed review, see Kibby & Long, 1996).

Determination of Brain Injury Severity

Coma Versus PTA

Severity of brain injury cannot be determined by the extent of impairment on neuropsychological tests alone, because these tests are sensitive to many factors that may predate or interact with the injury (e.g., age, education, emotional adjustment, situational stress, other system injuries, pain). Determination of presence and severity of brain injury must be based on external factors. Duration of coma and/or duration of PTA have been used as determining factors. However, in persons with mild brain injury, coma tends to be brief, and the researcher often is unable to reliably measure how long the person was unconscious and what depth of coma the person reached. In contrast, PTA duration is considered to be the best measure of injury severity because it is longer, can be established retrospectively when taking the history, and occurs later in the recovery process—closer to the end-point (Lidvall, Linderoth, & Norlin, 1974).

Russell (1932) provided the following scale of head injury severity based on PTA duration. Mild head injury is indicated by PTA of less than 1 hour; moderate, by PTA of 1 to 24 hours; severe, by PTA of 1 to 7 days; and very severe, by PTA of more than 7 days.

PTA

Severity of injury increases in proportion to the duration of coma and PTA (Bond, 1983; Russell, 1932). PTA is defined as the time from injury until the return of continuous memory (Wrightson & Gronwall, 1981), and has been found to hold the highest correlation with recovery of function. Generally, the longer the period of PTA, the slower the return to work and the greater the likelihood of prolonged disability (Guthkelch, 1979). PTA is also a global indicator of injury severity because length of PTA is related to severity of brain injury across minimal to severe cases (Crovitz, Horn, & Daniel, 1983), and is highly correlated with the length of time required to reach maximum recovery (Jones & Long, 1990).

Findings vary regarding the relationship between duration of PTA and recovery of function. A general guideline is that mildly impaired individuals recover within 3 months, moderately impaired individuals recover in 3 to 12 months, severely impaired persons recover within 1 to 2 years, and very severely impaired individuals recover for up to approximately 2 years. Both severely and very severely injured individuals are likely to have residual deficits (Bond, 1983; Dikmen, Reitan, & Temkin, 1983). This model demonstrates the strong relationship between severity of injury and time of recovery (see Table 11.1).

Mild Brain Injury

It is likely that even an injury of mild severity (PTA under 1 hour) may cause some cognitive weakness for a brief time. However, these deficits are transient and should be resolved within a few months. One study found that 3 months postinjury, only 2% of the persons with minor head injury showed more permanent intellectual impairment (Ruesch & Bowman, 1945). Levin et al. (1987) found that within 3 months of injury, patients with mild head injury were performing at the same level of cognitive functioning as control subjects. These findings suggest that although there may be some cognitive weaknesses early in the course of recovery, mild brain damage alone should not cause permanent cognitive impairment or symptoms lasting more than

Table 11.1

Modification of Russell's Severity Classification with Associated Cognitive Functioning Outcomes

Estimated severity	Duration of PTA	Time to cognitive recovery	Residual cognitive deficits
Minimal	0–5 min.	1–2 weeks	none
Mild	5–60 min.	2 weeks–3 months	none
Moderate	1–24 hours	3–12 months	some
Severe	1–7 days	12–24 months	most
Very Severe	7+ days	24+ months	most

a few months. However, not all researchers agree that full recovery should occur within 3 months. Neuropsychological impairment has been recorded up to 22 months postinjury in some patients with mild brain injury (Leininger, Gramling, Farrell, Kreutzer, & Peck, 1990), and a large number of patients with minor head injuries have mild neuropsychological impairment at 3 months postinjury (Rimel et al., 1981). These studies should be interpreted with caution, however, as many nonneurological factors were not taken into account.

It is clear from a review of much of the literature that minimal to mild brain injury should not cause significant or prolonged cognitive impairment (Kibby & Long, 1996). Although neurons are not replaced, cognitive and behavioral functions appear to recover to their preinjury levels. In cases where this does not occur, nonneurological factors must be investigated.

Moderate Brain Injury

It appears clear that individuals with brain injury that is less than moderately severe (PTA of less than 1 hour) recover within 3 months without significant residual impairment. In contrast, individuals with moderate brain injury (PTA of 1 to 24 hours) require longer recovery times. Levin, Amparo, et al. (1987) found that 45% of patients with moderate head injury continued to have cognitive problems and disability 3 months postinjury; all those with mild head injury demonstrated good recovery. However, another study (Dikmen, Temkin, McLean, Wyler, & Machamer, 1987) found that adults with moderate and mild head injury did not perform significantly differently than control subjects on two memory measures at 1 year postinjury. Thus, it appears that patients with mild brain injury recover within 3 months, but individuals with moderate brain injury can take up to 1 year to recover.

The question remains as to what point in the continuum of brain injury severity does one suffer brain injury, and at what point does one suffer residual cognitive (neurological) impairment? It is important for researchers and clinicians to differentiate between deficits in cognitive functioning that can be related directly to brain injury and those changes that relate to nonneurological factors.

Factors Confounding the Study of Outcome

The primary source of confusion in the literature relates to the failure to differentiate between cognitive impairment resulting directly from brain injury and cognitive impairment resulting from other factors. More specifically, the confusion relates to the failure to differentiate between postconcussive symptoms and cognitive impairment when measuring recovery from minor head injury. Postconcussive symptoms reflect stress, poor stress management, or the interaction of cognitive weaknesses with situational stress. They do not reflect brain impairment alone and are not good measures of cognitive recovery from brain injury, although they do reflect the individual's ability to cope with stress following the injury.

TBI can cause cognitive impairment or postconcussive symptoms, and these consequences are reflected in the observable behavior that is measured when assessing outcome. However, cognitive impairment and postconcussive symptoms, especially the latter, are influenced by preexisting factors. Much of the remaining discussion will focus on noncognitive factors that influence recovery.

Postconcussive Symptoms

Postconcussive symptoms refers to a collection of symptoms, including headache, dizziness, fatigue, irritability, memory weakness, impaired concentration, alcohol intolerance, and so on, that are often observed following brain injury. The majority of postconcussive symptoms do not relate to cognitive impairment alone; they are often observed in individuals without brain injury when they are under stress. Postconcussive symptoms have an inverse correlation with severity of injury, and are often more pronounced in less severely impaired individuals (Lidvall et al., 1974). They occur at the point in recovery when the patient is attempting to resume social, work, and/or academic duties (Long & Haban, 1986). Hence, it is when life events are particularly stressful that postconcussive symptoms are likely to appear. Postconcussive symptoms appear to relate to interactions among the individual's brain function, stress management abilities, and perceived stress (Novack, Daniel, & Long, 1983). Several authors state that postconcussive syndrome (PCS) is due to a combination of organic and psychological factors (Dacey et al., 1991; Dikmen, McLean, & Temkin, 1986; Dikmen et al., 1983; Gronwall & Wrightson, 1974; Nemeth, 1991; Ruesch & Bowman, 1945).

In studies where the authors refer to postconcussive symptoms as the primary reason for individuals having residual deficits despite no measured cognitive deficits, the possibility remains that stress and/or poor stress management may be the predominant factor. In addition, there is a high probability that postconcussive symptoms interact with performance on neuropsychological assessments and contribute to the appearance of impaired congnitive functioning. Mild concussions can cause persistent postconcussive symptoms that last for more than 3 months after injury in some cases (Hugenholtz, Stuss, Stethem, & Richard, 1988).

Confounding Factors

Much of the research on mild brain injury suggests that patients experience full recovery within 3 months, although other researchers find residual impairment months later on neuropsychological test performance. Although the reasons for referral, the comparison groups, and the tests used vary across studies, much of the variability may relate to the criteria for recovery of function and the extent to which other factors contribute to the impaired test performance.

When recovery does not occur within 1 to 3 months in mild brain injury, one must look for other contributing factors. There appear to be three categories of factors to account for this outcome. First, the individuals may have a brain injury of moderate severity (PTA of 1 to 24 hours) and need more time to recover. Second, the delayed recovery may be due to the presence of postconcussive symptoms and/or emotional distress rather than cognitive deficits. Third, factors not directly resulting from, but possibly interacting with the trauma may be primary contributors. Preexisting factors such as past injuries, neurological disorders, disease, limited education, genetics, age, education, and emotional adjustment, as well as postinjury and injury-related factors can all influence both neuropsychological test performance and postinjury recovery.

Preinjury Factors

Preinjury factors play a significant role in outcome (Dikmen et al., 1983). Certain reports in the literature may overestimate brain injury–related losses due to lack of control for the effects of preinjury characteristics and other system injuries (Dikmen et al., 1986). Both preinjury cognitive functioning and personality characteristics influence outcome (Dikmen et al., 1986; Jones & Long, 1990). Several preinjury factors can influence recovery. These include personality, alcohol abuse, neuropsychiatric history, level of education, and occupation.

Alcohol and Drug Abuse

Mild brain injury occurrence is highly associated with alcohol use (Dicker, 1989), and abusers of alcohol and/or drugs are overrepresented in the head injury population (Levin, Amparo, et al., 1987). In fact, alcoholism is an important determinant for predicting poor recovery (Levine, 1988).

Age

Age and length of PTA interact so that taking into account both age and severity of brain injury in predicting recovery is more reliable than making predictions based upon only one of the two factors. Russell and Smith (1961) found the number of postconcussive symptoms (motor disorders, anosmia, dysphasia, memory or calculation defects) increased with increased duration of PTA and with advancing age. Other studies have also found a positive relationship between increasing age and poorer outcome. Denker (1944) found that patients over 40 years old were 2 times as likely to have persistent sequelae as those under 30. Using the Halstead-Reitan Impairment Index as their external criteria, Jones, Fahy, and Long (1989) demonstrated that age accounted for more of the variance in the recovery process than did PTA duration and time since injury, combined.

Education and Occupation

Education and occupation are also related to the time needed for recovery. Individuals with brain injury who hadn't returned to work by 1 year postinjury had lower WAIS IQ scores at 1 month postinjury (Fraser, Dikmen, McLean, Miller, & Temkin, 1988). In addition, lower levels of preinjury education are related to a higher number of reported postconcussive symptoms. Individuals who report more than six postconcussive symptoms tend to be older, be less educated, and have lower occupational status (Dikmen, Temkin, & Armsden, 1989). A high preinjury occupational status is also related to poorer outcome. Higher levels of occupation require higher level cognitive skills and the ability to work under pressure, which may be impaired by the head injury (Lees-Haley, 1987).

Personality Characteristics

An individual's personality influences how he or she copes with situational stress. Preinjury personality traits may exacerbate postconcussive symptoms (Ruff, Levin, & Marshall, 1986), and preinjury personality deviations in patients with head injury have been found to exceed the number predicted by population base rate. These deviations were essentially confined to somatic concerns and anxiety (Levin & Grossman, 1978). Preinjury personality qualities and psychosocial adjustment play an important role in how well the patient copes with the concussion-induced anxiety (Nemeth, 1991). Brain injury is liable to tap personality resources during convalescence; thus, preinjury personality difficulties are accentuated in the presence of brain damage. Persons with prior emotional instability are likely to have prolonged disability, and may never fully recover. The longer the postconcussive symptoms last, the less likely they are to be an expression of brain damage; by 1 year postinjury, most postconcussive symptoms constitute personality problems (Reusch & Bowman, 1945). Hence, preinjury personality is often a determining factor for delayed recovery following head injury.

Emotional Adjustment

Poor emotional adjustment can also significantly impair recovery. Preexisting emotional factors can be significantly augmented by or interact with the transient effects of brain injury, or emotional factors may evolve in the process of recovery. Emotional sequelae may take the form of denial, defensiveness, aggression, dependency, and/or anger (O'Hara, 1988). They may also take the form of postconcussive symptoms including depression, anxiety, and somatic concerns (Smith, 1989), especially when they occur later in recovery. These emotional sequelae adversely affect recovery. Long-term memory, attention, concentration, and reasoning difficulties may be associated with an emotional reaction to the injury and influenced by preinjury and postinjury psychological factors, including personality and psychosocial factors (Davidoff, Kessler, Laibstain, & Mark, 1988). Postconcussive symptoms were found to be significantly correlated with MMPI elevations, suggesting that the number of symptoms may roughly indicate the adequacy of emotional adjustment after head trauma (Novack et al., 1983). Even if neuropsychological impairments are established, this does not necessarily mean that the head injury produced them or caused the postconcussive symptoms. In some cases, the most prominent and disabling difficulties are emotional in nature (Dikmen et al., 1989).

Neurological and Psychiatric History

Neuropsychiatric history is associated with level of recovery. Studies that exclude patients based on history of alcohol or drug abuse, previous head injury, or other neuropsychiatric disorders demonstrate better recovery rates from minor head injury (Ruff et al., 1986). Prior head injuries are reported by 21% of the head injury population, compared to 5% of the general population. This may be due to personality factors or prior cognitive status (poor judgment, impulsivity) (Dicker, 1989). Previous psychiatric and neurological history influences the level to which one can recover. Successive head injuries may have a cumulative effect, making it harder to recover to preinjury functioning after each successive head injury (Gronwall & Wrightson, 1975; Levin, Gary, et al., 1987; Levine, 1988). Previous psychiatric history and certain preinjury personalities may accentuate the number of postconcussive symptoms and make recovery more difficult (Lishman, 1973; Ruff et al., 1986).

Posttraumatic, Noncognitive Factors

Stress

Excess stress can play an important role in lengthening the recovery process. When patients with head injury who complained of postconcussive symptoms were compared with patients without these symptoms, those with postconcussive symptoms reported significantly higher stress at work and had difficulties in the home at the time of the accident or later during the recovery period (Lidvall et al., 1974). Stress can develop when the person rapidly tries to resume preinjury activities with decreased cognitive capacity. For example, an individual can no longer meet job demands soon after returning to work and does not understand why. He was not informed of the initial effects of minor head injury. As he tries to keep up and is not successful, postconcussive symptoms develop and increase (Gronwall & Wrightson, 1974). Stress level and coping capacity interact during recovery. Also, not everyone with a head injury has to deal with the same amount of stress. A number of factors determine the individual's stress level, such as circumstances surrounding the accident (Long, 1991).

Medical Acknowledgment

Individuals with minor head injury often do not receive medical acknowledgment of their condition. The effects of a mildly altered state of consciousness on the individual's mental and emotional functioning are virtually never recognized by the medical practitioner. Deficits encountered after minor head injury are unexpected and not readily apparent to others; yet the individual knows he or she is not functioning as well as before (Nemeth, 1991). Having unexplained and unacknowledged cognitive difficulties early on can lead to enduring emotional problems after cognitive deficits have been resolved. These emotional problems can cause a neurotic reaction and lead to the development of postconcussive symptoms (Gronwall & Wrightson, 1974).

Expectations

Mittenberg, DiGiulio, Perrin, and Bass (1992) proposed an alternative hypothesis. They noted that postconcussive symptoms occur frequently in individuals without injury, and at a rate nearly equal to that in individuals with minor head injury. They suggested that this could be due to the fact that people expect certain symptoms of a head injury. Such expectations could result in attribution of preexisting symptoms to trauma, selective attention to symptoms, and anxiety about their significance. Selective attention and anxiety both increase the subjective intensity of symptoms, eliciting further anxiety. This circular reinforcement may explain why postconcussive symptoms persist in the absence of impairment on neuropsychological exams, and why PCS appears to be inversely related or unrelated to severity of trauma.

Regardless of their cause, it is clear that postconcussive symptoms are significantly different from cognitive dysfunction directly obtained from brain injury. Unless outcome studies carefully separate cognitive and noncognitive symptoms, there will be little clarification as to the relationship between severity of brain injury and recovery.

Other postinjury factors need to be considered when assessing recovery of function. Factors such as other system injuries, neurological complications, family functioning, malingering, stress, medical acknowledgment, and the individual's expectations influence the recovery process. Methodological issues contribute to the variety of findings regarding recovery from minor head injury. All these factors need to be considered when looking at the literature and forming conclusions about the nature of recovery from minor head injury.

Other system injuries obtained simultaneously with the brain injury affect the recovery process as well, especially when pain is involved. Neck injuries often accompany head injuries in the case of whiplash. Whiplash severe enough to cause concussion could cause neck stiffness and reflex myodystonia. Brain injury severity is closely related to overall injury severity and neck injury severity (Fife & Jagger, 1984). Nonneurological injuries are among factors that predict brain injury recovery (Levine, 1988). Physical difficulties are associated with lower postinjury vocational status (Stambrook, Moore, Peters, Deviaene, & Hawryluk, 1990). At 1 month postinjury, other system injuries sustained in the same accident appear to have a strong detrimental effect on work and leisure. Nonneurological injuries were a better predictor of who would return to work and who would have psychosocial deficits than was neuropsychological functioning (Dikmen et al., 1989). In contrast, neuropsychological or cognitive outcome was better predicted by the severity of the patient's brain injury (Dacey et al., 1991). These relations are particularly true for mild to moderate brain injury. In a study by Lidvall et al. (1974), which focused on individuals with mild and moderate brain injury, those with postconcussive symptoms worried significantly more than did control subjects about symptoms in other parts of the body, including back pain, wounds and fractures, scars on the face, abdominal disturbances, and so on.

Neurological Complications

Neurological complications also influence recovery. Certain types of neurological sequelae, such as persistent focal neurological signs, are predictive of poorer outcome (Dikmen & Reitan, 1976). Global outcome at 6 months was better in patients with uncomplicated mild head injury than in patients with complicated mild and moderate injuries (Williams, Levin, & Eisenberg, 1990). Complicated minor head injury included brain lesions or skull fractures. Neurobehavioral functioning was impaired in the groups with complicated mild and moderate brain injury, as compared to the group with uncomplicated mild brain injury. Analysis of the various complications revealed that the presence of an intracranial lesion was related to more severe neurobehavioral sequelae than were injuries complicated by a depressed fracture. Hence, the presence of contusions predicts poorer outcome. Neuroradiological evidence indicates that patients with diffuse axonal injury and patients with extensive contusional injuries have distinctive characteristics on MRI scans. Both diffuse white matter damage and extensive frontotemporal lobe injuries may predict poor outcome, but only the former may be marked by low GCS scores on admission. This view is consistent with the concept that depth and duration of coma reflect the degree of diffuse white matter damage, rather than the extent of cortical contusion or other frontal injuries (Wilson, 1990). Therefore, scales based on coma or PTA duration may not be good indicators of injury severity for those with contusions, which may confound the prediction of recovery and the study of outcome.

Some researchers separate contusion and diffuse axonal injury. Diffuse axonal injury is associated with high velocity injuries such as those sustained in motor vehicle accidents, whereas contusions are associated with falls and direct blows to the head (Abrams et al., 1989; Graham, Adams, & Gennarelli, 1988). The problem is, many studies combine brain injuries from falls and motor vehicle accidents when researching the effects of mild head injury. As a result, these studies may have participants with contusions and minor diffuse axonal injury. Not enough is known about how contusions complicate recovery from mild brain injury and how much longer it takes to recover because of them. Including those individuals with injuries from falls or blows to the head in a mild brain injury sample could extend the recovery time, making it appear that it takes longer than 3 to 12 months to recover from mild brain injury.

Compensation

Compensation claims have been noted to affect the recovery process. Miller (1966) estimated that the compensation issue contributes to disability in one fourth to one third of all patients when the accident has fulfilled two criteria: (a) someone else is at fault in the patient's view, and (b) financial compensation is at least a possibility. Prolonged legal negotiation often aggravates the situation. Individuals with brain injury who blamed employers or large organizations tended to report two or more symptoms at 6-week follow-up, compared to those who were not litigating, who averaged one or no symptoms (Rutherford, Merrett, & McDonald, 1977). Cook (1972) conducted a survey on compensation issues. He found that the group of patients with brain injury who did not consider compensation claims were off work an average of 23.9 days, whereas those who did consider claims were off an average of 87.9 days.

Family Support

The family can play an important role in the recovery process through four mechanisms. First, domestic troubles, such as threat to the family or personal security, assume crucial importance in the development of postconcussive symptoms in individuals with head injury (Lishman, 1973). Second, the family's expectations have a strong influence on recovery. When the family expects more than what the individual can live up to, many problems can result, especially early in the recovery process (Long, 1991). Gronwall (1989) noted that if individuals with mild TBI are expected to perform at their preinjury level with reduced information-processing capacity, their cognitive skills will not improve at the expected rate. Third, families influence recovery by how they respond to the individual with brain injury. If they respond with rejection or avoidance, the individual will recognize this as an adjustment failure and can develop a secondary reaction to the changes in his coping capacity (Ruff et al., 1986). Finally, the head injury also affects the family's financial security. When the breadwinner is injured, financial strain is a significant predictor of adjustment. The impact of head injury on employment and financial concerns may be one of the major stressors on the family system (Stambrook et al., 1990).

Conclusions

Although considerable research has been conducted on mild TBI, several critical issues still require resolution. First, one of the more noticeable problems relates to the fact that mild brain injury does not have well defined lower limits (in some cases no limits at all). This lack of a lower limit can lead to individuals being categorized as having a mild brain injury despite never enduring trauma to the brain. Mild brain injury is typically associated with coma and PTA of short duration. Although some cognitive deficits may occur following an injury severe enough to cause alterations in consciousness (PTA or coma), they tend to be brief in duration, and full recovery is expected in most patients with mild brain injury. Clearly, individuals with no PTA should recover cognitive functions very quickly if, in fact, they are impaired at all. Hence, future researchers must include lower limits of mild head injury as well as upper limits, to avoid misinterpretation of their findings (for a review on the topic, see Kibby & Long, 1996).

The second problem relates to the failure of researchers to differentiate between cognitive deficits and postconcussive symptoms when assessing outcome. Because postconcussive symptoms can occur in the absence of TBI and are often present beyond the period of cognitive recovery from mild brain injury, the two clearly result from different factors. Because recovery time is related to severity of injury, PTA of less than 1 hour should be associated with cognitive recovery within 1 to 3 months. With PTA of 1 to 24 hours, full cognitive recovery should occur within 3 to 12 months. If full cognitive recovery from mild TBI does not occur within 12 months, other factors must be considered, such as age, preinjury level of functioning, personality, postinjury factors, and so on. These apparent residual deficits may be due to the presence of postconcussive symptoms or preexisting conditions that are misinterpreted as cognitive deficits resulting from the injury. Care should be taken to separate postconcussive symptoms from cognitive deficits, and a careful history is necessary to clarify the extent to which preexisting factors are contributing to current functioning. Only by carefully identifying the critical factors contributing to the postinjury symptoms can effective treatment be implemented. Providing education on the effects of mild head injury, and counseling as needed early in the recovery process, may avoid the development of postconcussive symptoms and augment the recovery process.

Finally, many preinjury factors (age, personality) and postinjury factors (stress, neurological complications) interact with cognitive functioning. Not only do these factors significantly affect recovery, but unless they are evaluated, may also confound the study of outcome.

References

Adams, J. H., Doyle, D., Ford, I., Gennarelli, T. A., Graham, D. I., & McLellan, D. R. (1989). Diffuse axonal injury in head injury: Definition, diagnosis and grading. *Histopathology, 15,* 49–59.

Bond, M. R. (1983). Standardized methods of assessing and predicting outcome. In M. Rosentahl, E. Griffith, M. Bond, & J. Miller (Eds.), *Rehabilitation of the head injured adult* (pp. 97–113). Philadelphia: Davis.

Cook, J. B. (1972). The post-concussional syndrome and factors influencing recovery after minor head injury admitted to hospital. *Scand J Rehab, 4,* 27–30.

Crovitz, H. F., Horn, R. W., & Daniel, W. F. (1983). Inter-relationships among retrograde amnesia, post-traumatic amnesia, and time since head injury: A retrospective study. *Cortex, 19,* 407–412.

Dacey, R., Dikmen, S., Temkin, N., McLean, A., Armsden, G., & Winn, H. R. (1991). Relative effects of brain and non-brain injuries on neuropsychological and psychosocial outcome. *The Journal of Trauma, 3*(2), 217–222.

Davidoff, D. A., Kessler, H. R., Laibstain, D. F., & Mark, V. H. (1988). Neurobehavioral sequelae of minor head injury: A consideration of post-concussive syndrome versus post-traumatic stress disorder. *Cognitive-Rehabilitation, 6,* 8–13.

Denker, P. G. (1994, February 15). Postconcussion syndrome: Prognosis and evaluation of the organic factors. *New York State Journal of Medicine,* 379–384.

Dicker, B. G. (1989). Preinjury and recovery after a minor head injury: A review of the literature. *Journal of Head Trauma Rehabilitation, 4*(4), 73–81.

Dikmen, S., McLean, A., & Temkin, N. (1986). Neuropsychological and psychosocial consequences of minor head injury. *Journal of Neurology, Neurosurgery, and Psychiatry, 49,* 1227–1232.

Dikmen, S., & Reitan, R. M. (1976). Psychological deficits and recovery of functions after head injury. *Transactions of the American Neurological Association, 101,* 72–77.

Dikmen, S., Reitan, R. M., & Temkin, N. R. (1983). Neuropsychological recovery in head injury. *Archives of Neurology, 40,* 333–338.

Dikmen, S., Temkin, N., & Armsden, G. (1989). Neuropsychological recovery: Relationship to psychosocial functioning and postconcussional complaints. In H. S. Levin, H. M. Eisenberg, & A. L. Benton (Eds.), *Mild head injury* (pp. 229–241). New York: Oxford University Press.

Dikmen, S., Temkin, N., McLean, A., Wyler, A., & Machamer, J. (1987). Memory and head injury severity. *Journal of Neurology, Neurosurgery, and Psychiatry, 50,* 1613–1618.

Fife, D., & Jagger, J. (1984). The contribution of brain injury to the overall injury severity of brain-injured patients. *Journal of Neurosurgery, 60,* 39–45.

Fraser, R., Dikmen, S., McLean, A., Miller, B., & Temkin, N. (1988). Employability of head injury survivors: First year post-injury. *Rehabilitation Counseling Bulletin, 31,* 276–289.

Graham, D. I., Adams, J. H., & Gennarelli, T. A. (1988). Mechanisms of non-penetrating head injury. *Perspectives in Shock Research,* 159–168.

Gronwall, D. (1989). Cumulative and persisting effects of concussion on attention and cognition. In H. S. Levin, H. M. Eisenberg, & A. L. Benton (Eds.), *Mild head injury* (pp. 153–162). New York: Oxford University Press.

Gronwall, D., & Wrightson, P. (1974). Delayed recovery of intellectual function after minor head injury. *Lancet, 2,* 605–609.

Gronwall, D., & Wrightson, P. (1975). Cumulative effect of concussion. *Lancet, 2,* 995–997.

Guthkelch, A. N. (1979). Assessment of outcome: Post-traumatic amnesia, post concussional symptoms, and accident neurosis. *Acta Neurochirurgica,* (Suppl. 28), 120–123.

Hugenholtz, H., Stuss, D. T., Stethem, L. L., & Richard, M. T. (1988). How long does it take to recover from a mild concussion? *Neurosurgery, 22,* 853–858.

Jones, C. L., Fahy, J. F., & Long, C. J. (1989, June). *Quantification of recovery of cognitive skills following head trauma as a function of severity of injury and age.* Poster session presented at the Traumatic Brain Injury Rehabilitation Research and Training Center, Richmond, VA.

Jones, C. L., & Long, C. J. (1990). Outcome following head trauma: A million dollar question. *The Journal of Head Injury, 1,* 12–15.

Kibby, M. Y., & Long, C. J. (1996). Minor head injury: Attempts at clarifying the confusion. *Brain Injury, 10,* 159–186.

Lees-Haley, P. (1987, November). Mild brain injury. *Trial,* 83–86.

Leininger, B. E., Gramling, S. E., Farrell, A. D., Kreutzer, J. S., & Peck, E. A. (1990). Neuropsychological deficits in symptomatic minor head injury patients after concussion and mild concussion. *Journal of Neurology, Neurosurgery, and Psychiatry, 53,* 293–296.

Levin, H. S., Amparo, E., Eisenberg, H. M., Williams, D. H., High, W. M., McArdle, C. B., & Weiner, R. L. (1987). Magnetic resonance imaging and computerized tomography in relation to the neurobehavioral sequelae of mild and moderate head injuries. *Journal of Neurosurgery, 66,* 706–713.

Levin, H. S., Gary, H. E., Jr., High, W. M., Jr., Mattis, S., Ruff, R. M., Eisenberg, H. M., Marshall, L. F., & Tabaddor, K. (1987). Minor head injury and the postconcussive syndrome: Methodological issues in outcome studies. In H. S. Levin, J. Grafman, & H. M. Eisenberg (Eds.), *Neurobehavioral recovery from head injury* (pp. 262–275). New York: Oxford University Press.

Levin, H. S., & Grossman, R. G. (1978). Behavioral sequelae of closed head injury. *Archives of Neurology, 35,* 720–727.

Levin, H. S., Mattis, S., Ruff, R. M., Eisenberg, H. M., Marshall, L. F., Tabaddor, K., High, W. M., & Frankowski, R. F. (1987). Neurobehavioral outcome following minor head injury: A three-center study. *Journal of Neurosurgery, 66,* 234–243.

Levine, M. J. (1988). Issues in neurobehavioral assessment of mild head injury. *Cognitive Rehabilitation, 6,* 14–20.

Lidvall, H. F., Linderoth, B., & Norlin, B. (1974). Causes of the post-concussional syndrome. *Acta Neurologica Scandinavica, 50* (Suppl. 56), 3–144.

Lishman, W. A. (1973). The psychiatric sequelae of head injury: A review. *Psychological Medicine, 3,* 304–318.

Long, C. J. (1991). A model of recovery to maximize the rehabilitation of individuals with head trauma. *The Journal of Head Injury, 2,* 18–28.

Long, C. J., & Haban, G. (1986). Strategies for developing a plan of intervention for head trauma patients. *Psychotherapy in Private Practice, 4,* 71–80.

Miller, H. (1966). Mental after-effects of head injury. *Proceedings of the Royal Society of Medicine, 59,* 257–261.

Mittenberg, W., DiGiulio, D. V., Perrin, S., & Bass, A. E. (1992). Symptoms following mild head injury: Expectation as aetiology. *Journal of Neurology, Neurosurgery, and Psychiatry, 55,* 200–204.

Nemeth, A. J. (1991). Blind spots in the diagnosis and management of minor brain trauma. *Medical Trial Technique Quarterly, 37,* 478–495.

Novack, T. A., Daniel, M. S., & Long, C. J. (1983). The relationship between MMPI scores, post-concussion symptoms, neuropsychological performance, and severity of head injury. *Clinical Neuropsychology, 6,* 139–142.

O'Hara, C. (1988). Emotional adjustment following minor head injury. *Cognitive Rehabilitation, 6,* 26–33.

Rimel, R. W., Giordani, B., Barth, J. T., Boll, T. J., & Jane, J. A. (1981). Disability caused by minor head injury. *Neurosurgery, 9*(3), 274–281.

Ruesch, J., & Bowman, K. M. (1945). Prolonged post-traumatic syndromes following head injury. *American Journal of Psychiatry, 102,* 145–163.

Ruff, R. M., Levin, H. S., & Marshall, L. F. (1986). Neurobehavioral methods of assessment and the study of outcome in minor head injury. *Journal of Head Trauma Rehabilitation, 1,* 43–52.

Russell, W. R. (1932). Cerebral involvement in head injury: A study based on the examination of 200 cases. *Brain, 35,* 549–603.

Russel, W. R., & Smith, A. (1961). PTA in closed head injury. *Archives of Neurology, 5,* 16–29.

Rutherford, W. H., Merrett, H. D., & McDonald, J. R. (1977). Sequelae of concussion caused by minor head injuries. *The Lancet, 1,* 1–4.

Smith, R. S. (1989). Psychological trauma following automobile accidents: A review of literature. *American Journal of Forensic Psychology, 7,* 5–20.

Stambrook, M., Moore, A. D., Peters, L. C., Deviaene, C., & Hawryluk, G. A. (1990). Effects of mild, moderate and severe closed head injury on long-term vocational status. *Brain Injury, 4*(2), 183–190.

Williams, D. H., Levin, H. S., & Eisenberg, H. M. (1990). Mild head injury classification. *Neurosurgery, 27*(3), 422–428.

Wilson, J. T. L. (1990). Significance of MRI in clarifying whether neuropsychological deficits after head injury are organically based. *Neuropsychology, 4,* 261–269.

Wrightson, P., & Gronwall, D. (1981). Time off work and symptoms after minor head injury. *Injury, 12,* 445–454.

who had less stability in their lives. Individuals who were in higher level occupations will often show less emotionality because they can defer challenges to coworkers whom they supervise, whereas individuals in less skilled occupations typically have to deal with all the demands that they experienced prior to the injury. The degree of support from family and significant others can also affect an individual's level of adjustment after the accident (Miller, 1993).

According to Dicker (1992), who has examined the effects of preinjury behavior on the recovery of individuals with mild brain injury, adults were more susceptible to mild brain injury if they had previously sustained a brain injury or been diagnosed with a learning disability. As noted in Table 12.2, a number of variables are considered predictors of mild brain injury.

Thus, it appears that the recovery curve is fastest for individuals who are young and well educated; have experienced no postinjury medical complications; have had no history of previous brain injury, learning disability, or illness; have good familial/social support; and have been educated on the medical and emotional aspects of brain injury.

As can be seen, a number of factors can contribute to difficulty in emotional adjustment after brain injury. The basis for the changes is not always clear, but it is clear that individuals will need emotional support to help them deal with the challenges they will face secondary to their cognitive problems. Indeed, some individuals with brain injury may need more help dealing with the emotional consequences than they will need dealing with the cognitive difficulties. Certainly, we also see patients who have very little emotional disturbance following a brain injury, but even these individuals would benefit greatly from learning about the effects of brain injury and techniques for coping with their altered level of functioning.

Table 12.2

Predictors of Mild Brain Injury

1. Age
2. Education/occupation
3. Alcohol/drug usage
4. Postinjury medical complications
5. History of previous brain injury or learning disability
6. Preinjury personality
7. Familial/social support
8. Brain injury education

As previously indicated, emotional and personality changes that occur in individuals who have sustained brain injury depend on, in addition to brain injury itself, a variety of factors such as preinjury adjustment, cognitive loss, and reactions to the cognitive loss. Certainly, negative personality traits that existed before the accident may be accentuated by the injury. In contrast, some rare individuals have experienced a loss of objectionable personality traits secondary to brain trauma. It is often difficult to separate emotional and personality changes that are due to the brain injury from those that are a reaction to the brain injury.

Organic Personality Changes

Significant personality change can result from the brain injury itself, although this is more commonly seen in individuals who have sustained moderate to severe brain injuries than in persons who have suffered mild brain injuries. When an individual sustains a brain injury, particularly if it is a closed head injury, the frontal and temporal lobes are normally affected. The frontal and temporal lobes are involved in emotional behavior, and so one would expect significant changes to occur in personality. Injury to the frontal lobes can produce flat affect, indifference, apathy, and difficulty initiating and completing activities (Damasio & Anderson, 1993). Such individuals, although appearing flat in their affect, will at times show emotionality. Unfortunately, when they do, it is often poorly regulated and poorly directed, and the individual may demonstrate episodic lack of control or "explosive" behavior. Many times, calm individuals with significant frontal lobe injury will show aggressive behavior in an attempt to direct attention to their difficulties or needs. Individuals with frontal lobe injury may also show socially inappropriate behavior. They may be more impulsive in their actions and less aware of the impact of their actions and behaviors on others. This is part of the brain injury, and it is not purposeful. Many times, it is important to allow individuals the freedom to express themselves, understanding that this is a way for them to obtain goals in their environment. The strategy for dealing with objectionable behaviors after frontal lobe injury needs to be first determining the goal of the patient's behavior and then teaching him or her other ways (acceptable behaviors) to achieve that same goal.

Temporal lobe injury may also affect behavior and emotions. Individuals with temporal lobe injury may report heightened emotions ranging from "feeling things more deeply than I did before" to irritability and reduced control of aggressive impulses. The latter, as with frontal lobe injury, partly reflects loss of inhibition. Temporal lobe injury may also produce flattened affect, and may also result in hypersexuality, as seen in the Kluver-Bucy Syndrome (Strub & Black, 1988). A combination of impulsivity and hypersexuality following frontotemporal injury can result in a significant lack of behavioral control.

Reactive Personality Changes

Depression, guilt, anxiety about the future, and feelings of helplessness and hopelessness are often seen in people with brain injury, particularly those with mild to moderate impairment. Many individuals with more severe brain injury do not have an awareness of the severity of their impairments and the impact they will have on day-to-day functioning. Unfortunately, when many therapists see individuals with brain injury who are showing behavior such as depression and anxiety, they think the behaviors are related to adjustment problems independent of the brain injury. The point to be made is that emotional reactions to brain injury, such as depression and anxiety, are perfectly appropriate and expected. Indeed, if they are not present, then the person may not be able to benefit from formal rehabilitation because he or she is unaware of his or her difficulties.

As suggested earlier in this chapter, compromise of adaptive cognitive skills is an important factor in the development of emotional disturbance following brain injury, because of a loss of self-esteem related to reduced ability to perform at preinjury levels. The following scenario is typical of a person who suffers even a mild brain injury. The person may or may not have been hospitalized, but after a week or so, he or she returns to work or school. The individual has been assured by the physician, family, and friends that he or she "looks great." The person feels like "something is missing," but goes ahead with plans to return to work or school. The person "looks good" because there are not obvious fractures, cuts, or scars to remind one of the injury. Because of this, the term "walking wounded" was established and is frequently cited in literature related to survivors of brain injury.

The individual returns to work or school with the assurance that no problems should occur. He or she then goes about interacting with the world as was done in the past. However, the feedback now received from fellow workers, supervisors, teachers, and others is not the same. Whereas challenges were easily met in the past, the feedback now is often negative. The person discovers that he or she has lost or forgotten a message or missed an appointment; performances are not as good on exams; errors are made at work; and if things occur too rapidly, he or she tends to be overloaded and overwhelmed.

Because of these experiences, the individual may feel unsure about his or her capabilities, actions, and judgment. Because the individual has been told that everything is okay, he or she may feel "I am losing my mind." As would be expected, this may produce a great blow to self-confidence and self-esteem. Some of these individuals were perfectionists in the past, and they achieved a great deal of their self-esteem, self-confidence, and self-image from performing at a high level and doing a good job. Now, because of their cognitive difficulties, these individuals may develop anxiety and depression, become socially withdrawn, and become very angry or resentful. Suspiciousness and paranoia may result. Some may cling excessively to family or friends, seeking reassurance that they are still "normal."

Although all of us would have trouble accurately imagining ourselves in this situation, we should try to do it. Your friends say "Nothing is really wrong with you" or "You look great." You have received the impression from your doctors that nothing can be done about the problems, and if you are going to get better, it will just take time. You are a person of average intelligence or above, you have very high expectations of yourself, and you tie your personal accomplishments to your ability to function well in your daily activities. Think of yourself with mild to moderate brain injury. Instead of attending, remembering, and planning quite independently and having things go relatively smoothly in your daily activities at school or at work, you now find that you are thinking more slowly, you are distractible and forgetful, you suffer word-retrieval problems, and you become confused when attempting to meet others' expectations as you confront normal challenges in your daily activities. Your problems may be "mild," but mild can be significant if the demands upon you and your expectations of yourself are high.

Lees-Haley (1987), for example, summed up the impact of memory difficulties on job performance when he observed that "a 10% loss of memory is rated as mild, but employees who forget 10% of what they read in an eight-hour work day may be in 100% trouble" (p. 85). Lees-Haley also made the important observation that for a person of average intellectual ability, a brain injury that lowers IQ by 10 points (this could still be a perfectly normal IQ) could disqualify a person from about 6% of the 24,000 job categories listed by the U.S. Department of Labor. Many of these would be job categories projected to experience high growth in the next decade. Thus, a person with seemingly mild cognitive difficulties might be unable to meet the expectations of past or future employment, and might not be able to acquire the skills needed to obtain jobs with growth potential.

When one considers the effects of the brain injury itself and an individual's reaction to it, it is quite understandable that an individual with even mild cognitive loss may experience significant emotional difficulties secondary to the impact of the cognitive difficulties. With this in mind, we will next discuss the process of psychotherapy with individuals who have sustained mild brain injury.

Psychotherapy for Individuals with Mild TBI

The typical individual who has sustained a mild TBI is of average intellectual ability, has high expectations of himself or herself, and typically ties personal accomplishments to his or her independence and observable achievements. These people are highly motivated to recover from the effects of their injuries, and we rarely see any evidence of malingering types of behavior. Nevertheless, individuals certainly do need to meet certain requirements to benefit from psychotherapy, and these are always considered before beginning that process.

Requirements to Begin Psychotherapy

An obvious criterion is that the individual must, with reasonable probability, demonstrate the capacity to benefit from psychotherapeutic interventions. This is typically not a major problem for people with mild brain injury, because most of them have adequate cognitive awareness to communicate their needs to the therapist and to understand information communicated by the therapist.

A second requirement is that the individual must be aware of his or her cognitive difficulties and behavioral sequelae. He or she must be aware of the impact that these factors are having on his or her ability to interact with and meet the expectations of others. Even in mild brain injury, we will occasionally see people who are not aware of their difficulties (anosognosia), and when this is present, it can thwart the therapists' best intentions. Education and supportive confrontation can be helpful in lessening this syndrome when it is apparent, and typically it will resolve with the passage of time.

Finally, the individual must be highly motivated to participate in the counseling process. Clearly, the individual must be dissatisfied with his or her current status and must desire to make things different in a positive way. Simply realizing that things are not going well is not sufficient. The individual must be so uncomfortable that he or she is willing to work hard to produce positive change. This attitude is measured by regularity in keeping appointments, willingness to discuss difficulties resulting from brain injury, and willingness to do homework if necessary. However, even a desire to produce change is going to be thwarted by cognitive difficulties, and certainly cognitive deficits can place significant limitations on the psychotherapeutic process.

Limits of Cognitive Deficits on Psychotherapy

Most psychologists do not like to do psychotherapy with individuals with brain injuries, even those with mild injuries, because these individuals cannot meet the cognitive demands of psychotherapy. To be successful in psychotherapy, an individual must be able to attend well to the psychotherapist, to maintain a train of thought, and to remember what goes on both within a session and between sessions. Reasoning ability and self-insight must be good, and the patient must be able to generalize issues discussed in therapy to specific instances in his or her everyday life.

This is certainly not the case for many individuals with brain injury. An individual with brain injury typically has trouble sustaining his or her concentration and remembering what happens within and between sessions. Thinking and reasoning ability tend to be quite concrete, and the ability to generalize from a session to "real life" is often impaired. When a patient with a brain injury is required to show insight, deal with feelings, or both, the result may be increased frustration and psychological distress. This is a good example of how treatment can make a person worse. That is, trying to do traditional psychotherapy with individuals with brain injury may make them more distressed than at ease.

A practical way of overcoming obstacles that distractibility produces is for the therapist to take a more active role in counseling sessions and to be certain that what has been said has been accurately interpreted by the individual. This requires the individual to reflect comments back to the therapist. It requires the therapist to write homework to be done, strategies to be used, and actions to be taken after a session is completed. Index cards are often helpful for writing information covered in a session; the patient then takes these home and reviews the information. Tape-recording a session for the individual can also be helpful. In general, the therapist has to be more active and more responsible than is typically the case in psychotherapy with individuals without brain injury.

The Psychotherapeutic Approach: Early Interventions

Psychotherapy with individuals with brain injury needs to address several issues. It also needs to be conducted by a psychotherapist who is well acquainted with brain injury, because an important part of psychotherapy with these individuals is education about the effects of brain injury. Often, the initial intervention includes educating the person about the effects of brain injury through the use of videotapes, handouts, and articles. Community brain injury support groups can also be helpful. Understanding the nature of brain injury is highly beneficial toward removing the "mystique" about it. Education is conducted in either individual or group sessions. Certainly, the group sessions are beneficial in that the individuals support each other and promote feelings of not being alone in the struggle to recover and proceed with the rehabilitation process. Education and information, in addition to their direct benefits, also will decrease the likelihood and severity of secondary psychological reactions related to the individual's lack of information about the effects of brain injury. We generally find that when patients are informed about the normal sequelae of brain injury and the course of recovery, they are less likely to have severe psychological reactions than are individuals seen as long as 1 year or more after the injury, who have received no information about the effects of brain injury. The same is true for family members, and they should be similarly educated. Supportive counseling and education is also provided to family members as needed.

Rather than using a typical psychotherapeutic approach that focuses on self-insight and feelings, psychotherapy with individuals with brain injury focuses on the brain injury and ways to deal with its consequences. The approach is directive and action-oriented, and it attempts to teach coping and compensatory strategies to both patients and family members. The therapeutic approach attempts to help the individual develop effective strategies for coping with emotional problems, and to help the individual understand that cognitive difficulties are going to improve as therapy progresses. However, therapy does not end with simply discussing coping and compensatory strategies. Other issues often arise, including altered peer and family relationships, issues of learned dependency, and long-term adjustment in the face of persisting mild cognitive difficulties.

Family dynamics are often significantly affected by even mild brain injury. This is because the injured person may be different in a variety of cognitive processes and personality attributes. Friends, relatives, and immediate family may abandon the individual, finding that his or her difficulties are too much of a burden. Marital discord and divorce may occur, and it is not uncommon for one therapist to deal with the individual while another therapist is working with the family. Even for individuals with mild brain injury, an important component of recovery is helping the family understand and adapt to the effects of the injury (Rosenthal & Geckler, 1997).

Instead of being abandoned, the individual may have an opposite reaction from family members. The family may take over everything for the injured individual. Because of that, he or she may begin to defer all decisions to family members, and may eventually develop a learned dependency. Even well-meaning rehabilitation counselors or therapists may contribute to learned dependency as they overorganize the life of the individual, make appointments for her or him, and even take the individual to those appointments. Certainly, some patients initially may need this amount of help. The problem is one of excessive involvement. One needs to push the individual as much as possible toward independence, at the same time providing support in case he or she fails. With every step toward greater independence, however, more independence is fostered, and more self-esteem is regained.

The Psychotherapeutic Approach: Later Interventions

Earlier in this chapter, we argued against traditional insight-oriented psychotherapy with individuals with mild brain injury, because many of these individuals cannot engage in such therapy. We would like to qualify that statement by indicating that this should not be an initial focus of psychotherapy. However, as the psychotherapeutic approach progresses, one certainly does need to deal with feelings and insight. As Prigatano (1991) stressed, psychotherapy must at some level confront realities of life. Once an individual has become aware of the difficulties produced by the brain injury, then he or she will need help adjusting to the tragedy of residual problems, even if he or she has sustained only a mild brain injury.

Some of these problems, as indicated earlier, may be abandonment by friends, relatives, and even immediate family. Other losses may include an inability to pursue academic goals, an inability to meet the requirements of one's job, and significant loss of self-esteem and self-worth.

It is important that psychotherapy with such individuals address these losses within a realistic framework. The psychotherapist must be careful to be neither overly optimistic nor pessimistic with the individual. The individual needs to realistically come to grips with his or her altered capabilities, accept them (this does not mean to like them), and move ahead in life within the limits set by the residual deficits. In contrast, it is also important that the individual not overreact to the losses. The person must realize his or her strengths and capabilities and not simply focus on residual problems.

Even after a mild brain injury, a less demanding career may have to be pursued. It may be that plans for higher education are no longer realistic. A person may have to establish a new set of friends and new goals. However, for many individuals, this is not the end of the world. They are capable of productive and self-satisfying lives despite some significant obstacles produced by the brain injury.

When individuals reach this point in their psychological recovery, we generally conclude that they have accommodated to their situation. These individuals are now able to gain a new sense of self rather than mourning for and futilely grasping for the former self. When this occurs, the individual with brain injury has established a new life around the new sense of self, a sense that realistically incorporates new abilities and limitations. Reaching this level of understanding and accommodation is the ultimate goal of psychotherapy with individuals with brain injury, even those with mild injury. Unfortunately, this is often an elusive goal for patients, and it may not occur for years after the brain injury.

Conclusions

In this chapter, we have summarized the emotional consequences of mild TBI, and have discussed psychotherapeutic interventions to be used with individuals with mild brain injury. Certainly, even mild brain injury can cause significant cognitive and emotional symptoms, and unfortunately, some individuals will have persisting symptoms. Emotional and personality changes may result from mild brain injury, and these changes, in conjunction with altered cognitive status, may result in significant career, social, and personal consequences.

The psycotherapeutic approach used with individuals who have sustained mild brain injury needs to focus on education and the development of coping strategies. Insight and feelings orientations should be avoided, at least initially. However, as therapy progresses and if it is clear that the person will have permanent residual difficulties, the focus of therapy must shift to a redefinition of the self. Once an individual recognizes, accepts, and adjusts to the limitations resulting from the brain injury, then a more favorable level of adjustment can occur. This altered sense of self helps the individual to build a new life around a realistic view of his or her strengths and limitations.

References

Bennett, T. L. (1987). Neuropsychological counseling of the adult with minor head injury. *Cognitive Rehabilitation, 5*(1), 10–16.

Bennett, T. L. (1989). Individual psychotherapy and minor head injury. *Cognitive Rehabilitation, 7*(5), 20–25.

Bornstein, R. A., Miller, H. B., & vanSchoor, J. T. (1989). Neuropsychological deficits and emotional disturbance in head injured patients. *Journal of Neurosurgery, 70,* 509–513.

Damasio, A. R., & Anderson, S. W. (1993). The frontal lobes. In K. M. Heilman & E. Valenstein (Eds.), *Clinical Neuropsychology* (3rd ed., pp. 409–460). New York: Oxford University Press.

Dicker, B. G. (1992). Profile of those at risk for minor head injury. *Journal of Head Trauma Rehabilitation, 7,* 83–91.

Goldstein, K. (1942). The effect of brain damage on the personality. *Psychiatry, 15,* 245–260.

Lees-Haley, P. (1987). Mild brain injury. *Trial, 23,* 83–86.

Luria, A. R. (1963). *Restoration of function after brain trauma.* (B. Haigh, Trans.). London: Pergamon Press. (Original work published 1948)

Miller, L. (1993). *Psychotherapy of the brain-injured patient: Reclaiming the shattered self.* New York: Norton.

Prigatano, G. P. (1991, November). *Science and symbolism in neuropsychological rehabilitation after brain injury.* Paper presented at the 10th annual James C. Hemphill Lecture, Rehabilitation Institute of Chicago.

Raymond, M. J. (1989). Major consequences of minor head injury. *JMA Bulletin, 2,*4–7.

Rosenthal, M., & Geckler, C. L. (1997). Family intervention in neuropsychology. In A. M. Horton, Jr., D. Wedding, & J. Webster (Eds.), *The neuropsychology handbook* (2nd ed., pp. 47–72). New York: Springer.

Strub, R. L., & Black, F. W. (1988). *Neurobehavioral disorders: A clinical approach.* Philadelphia: F. A. Davis Company.

Efficacy of Cognitive Rehabilitation in the Treatment of Mild Traumatic Brain Injury

13

Keith D. Cicerone

Despite increasing recognition of the problems that may persist after mild TBI, there have been few descriptions of cognitive rehabilitation developed specifically for these patients. Cognitive impairments are relatively common in the acute days or weeks postinjury, but are expected to improve or resolve in a majority of patients. In clinical practice, providing the individual with mild TBI with information about the nature of the injury, cognitive deficits, and expected course of recovery may be just as effective as initiating specific cognitive interventions. Clinicians should typically encourage patients that their cognitive difficulties will probably improve, without dismissing or minimizing their complaints. Clinicians may provide considerable assistance by monitoring the course of recovery over the initial weeks or months postinjury, fostering realistic attributions and expectations, helping the patient to adapt to initial difficulties and avoid complications, and facilitating the gradual resumption of daily activities without exacerbating symptoms. More active intervention may be necessary when symptoms persist for 2 or 3 months. Although additional cognitive recovery can still be expected at that time, there may be residual changes in functioning. Even when the prognosis for effective resumption of functioning remains good, patients might continue to sense change in the efficiency of their functioning despite continued recovery of their abilities. In the absence of empirical treatment guidelines, clinicians need to be sensitive to patients' needs and use good clinical judgment to determine the most effective timing and form of intervention throughout the course of recovery from mild TBI.

Education, support, and reassurance are commonly believed to be beneficial in the treatment of postconcussive syndrome (PCS), but these interventions have received limited empirical support. Several early reports emphasized the value of support and reassurance (Minderhoud, Boelens, Huizenga, & Saan, 1980) along with mobilization (Relander, Troupp & Bjorkstein, 1972) of the patient during the acute period of hospitalization. Gronwall

(1986) described a program of rehabilitation for nonhospitalized patients with mild TBI who were first assessed within 2 weeks of the injury. Treatment was delivered in three phases: assessment and reassurance, cognitive rehabilitation and stress management, and assisted return to work. Treatment appeared to reduce subjective postconcussive symptoms within the first 3 months postinjury, compared with a control group, although no specific benefits of support, reassurance, and education could be established. Alves, Macciocchi, and Barth (1993) compared the effects of three interventions randomly assigned to patients upon discharge from a 1- to 2-day hospitalization for mild injuries. Patients in the first group (routine treatment) were warned of possible problems indicative of intracranial pathology and were encouraged to return to their usual activities as soon as they felt able, but were not given information about mild TBI. In the second group (information only), patients were given information about the nature, typical sequelae, and prognosis of mild TBI. In the third group (information and reassurance), patients were provided the same information about mild TBI, but were also reassured that recovery would be uncomplicated and complete. These patients were contacted weekly by a clinician until their symptoms had abated or they had fully resumed their usual activities. A significant percentage of patients remained symptomatic at 3-, 6-, and 12-month follow-up. However, there were no differences among the three treatment groups in the relative risk of being symptomatic on follow-up.

Alves et al. (1993) also reported that patients who were symptomatic at hospital discharge were not more likely to remain symptomatic at 3 months; however, patients who were still symptomatic at 3 months after injury were more likely to be symptomatic at 6 or 12 months after injury. This finding is of particular significance for the treatment of persistent cognitive deficits after mild TBI. Whereas the majority of patients sustaining a mild TBI appear to show substantial recovery within the first 3 months postinjury, a significant number of patients may continue to have problems that interfere with or preclude their ability to resume functioning. For those patients, there is a significant risk of persistent postconcussive symptoms and prolonged disability that may extend for 1 year or more. Thus, there is need to provide effective interventions for those patients with persistent cognitive disability.

Mateer, Sohlberg, and Youngman (1990) described five patients with mild concussive or whiplash injuries who received treatment 1 to 5 years after their injuries. The rehabilitation program consisted of individual and group cognitive remediation for attention and memory deficits, along with counseling and vocational rehabilitation, over a period of 8 months. Following treatment, these five subjects made clinically significant gains on 60% of the neuropsychological measures of attention, memory, and general intellectual functioning administered. Mateer (1992) also reported vocational outcomes for 17 mild TBI patients following a similar rehabilitation program.

Of these 17 patients, 5 (30%) were employed at the time of treatment; 3 months after discharge from treatment, 15 patients (88%) were working.

Cicerone et al. (1996) conducted a retrospective, case comparison study of patients referred for neuropsychological treatment due to postconcussive symptoms and functional disability persisting for at least 3 months after their injuries. Two groups of patients were identified based upon their ability to resume productive functioning following treatment. Patients were considered to have a good outcome if they were able to resume work and home responsibilities equivalent to their preinjury status, or if unable to resume their primary preinjury responsibilities, they were engaged in other productive activity that may have been less demanding. Patients who were unable to either resume their primary preinjury responsibilities or attempt other productive activity were considered to demonstrate a poor outcome. All patients received a multidisciplinary neurorehabilitation program including individual cognitive remediation. This treatment included both "paper-and-pencil" and "real-life" activities aimed at improving their ability to focus and sustain attention, maintain task performance in the presence of background noise and distractions, and shift the priority of attention among competing stimuli or tasks. A central aspect of the approach was to address the patients' ability to monitor, recognize, and recover from errors, and to reduce patients' secondary emotional reactions or frustration responses when they experienced difficulty. Most patients learned compensatory strategies for memory difficulties and cognitive–linguistic therapies to improve self-monitoring of language and reading comprehension, and functional communication skills. For the patients who were able to resume productive functioning, neuropsychological rehabilitation was associated with improvements in cognitive functioning and reduction of subjective postconcussive symptoms. Improvements in neuropsychological performance were most apparent in the areas of complex attention and information processing speed. In contrast, the patients who were unable to resume productive activities did not exhibit improvements in neuropsychological functioning or postconcussive symptoms. Patients in the poor outcome group actually demonstrated a decline in functioning on a number of measures at the time of their post-treatment evaluation.

These results suggest that the heterogeneity of symptom presentation after mild TBI influences patients' ability to benefit from treatment and resume productive functioning. The remediation of cognitive deficits after mild TBI requires an understanding of the nature of the dysfunction resulting from the neurologic injury. It is also necessary to consider factors aside from the direct neurologic injury that may influence patients' cognitive functioning after mild TBI. These factors include somatic or emotional factors that may directly affect cognitive functioning, or may contribute to patients' subjective magnification of symptoms.

The Nature of Cognitive Impairments After Mild TBI

Attention deficits are prominent after mild TBI. Patients frequently complain of slowed thinking and difficulty concentrating, being more easily distracted or being unable to return to task after distraction, and difficulty in attending to more than one thing at a time. They may also complain that cognitive functioning is less automatic and requires more effort, or that efforts to concentrate result in additional symptoms such as headache, fatigue, or irritability. Several neuropsychological studies have reported specific impairments of attention after mild TBI. For example, Gentilini et al. (1985) did not find a general neuropsychological impairment in patients 1 month after mild TBI, but they did provide evidence of a specific attention deficit (Gentilini, Nichelli, & Schoenhuber, 1989). Gronwall and Wrightson (1974) related patients' subtle cognitive deficits and postconcussive symptoms to impaired performance on the *Paced Auditory Serial Addition Test* (PASAT; Gronwall, 1977). The PASAT requires both rapid information processing and adequate processing capacity, both of which may be impaired after mild TBI. Slowness of information processing appears to account for many of the attention deficits observed after TBI (Batchelor, Harvey, & Bryant, 1995; Ponsford & Kinsella, 1992). There appears to be an interaction between information processing speed and processing capacity, because slowing is more pronounced as the demand to monitor multiple sources of information is increased (Parasuraman, Mutter, & Molloy, 1991; Ponsford & Kinsella, 1992). Patients with mild TBI are able to adequately perform tests of simple reaction time, but they demonstrate impaired processing speed on more complex reaction-time tasks; their performance may not recover to normal even 3 months after injury (Hugenholtz, Stuss, Stethem, & Richard, 1988). Cicerone (1997) compared the performance of 50 mild TBI subjects who had persistent symptoms with that of normal control subjects, on four measures of attention. Measures of basic attention were relatively insensitive, whereas many subjects with mild TBI had abnormal performances on externally paced tasks that demanded rapid information processing and simultaneously paying attention to multiple sources of information.

An additional aspect of attention is the degree of automatic versus controlled processing required to perform the task. According to Schneider and Shiffrin (1977), automatic processing occurs when long-term memory is activated by the appropriate inputs and proceeds without stressing the capacity of the system, and without necessarily demanding the person's control of attention. Controlled processing refers to search and detection of elements, which requires greater effort and control by the person and is capacity-limited. A number of studies have suggested that tests requiring increased complexity and effortful processing may be necessary to demonstrate the subtle cognitive disturbances of patients with mild TBI. Parasuraman et al.

(1991) demonstrated that patients with mild TBI were able to adequately perform a vigilance task that did not require a lot of effort, but when sustained effortful processing was demanded, the patients showed a marked decline. Bohnen, Jolles, and Twijnstra (1992) found that patients tested within 2 weeks of sustaining a mild TBI showed increased slowing and differed from neurologically normal control subjects on a modified interference task of the *Stroop Color–Word Test* (Stroop, 1935), which required shifting between color naming and word reading. However, there was no difference between groups on the standard interference task. Impaired performance on the modified interference task was also related to the persistence of postconcussive symptoms (Bohnen, Twijnstra, & Jolles, 1992). Newcombe, Rabbit, and Briggs (1994) found no differences at 1 month postinjury between a group of patients with mild head injuries and matched control subjects on standard measures of intelligence and story recall, and a slower version of the PASAT. However, the group with head injuries was significantly worse than the control group on an experimental working memory task that assessed ability to keep track of several variables simultaneously (a paradigm that also reflects a common, subjective, cognitive complaint among mild TBI patients). Cicerone (1996) evaluated specific attentional deficits in 17 patients with persisting postconcussive symptoms at least 6 months after mild TBI, compared with matched control subjects. All of the patients demonstrated generally intact test performance on a standard neuropsychological battery. The study used an extended version of the *Ruff 2 & 7 Test* (Ruff, Evans, & Light, 1986), a measure of automatic and controlled attention, which required subjects to focus attention in the presence of irrelevant background noise and during simultaneous, dual-task demands. No differences were observed between the mild TBI patients and control subjects on the standard or non-relevant distraction conditions. However, the mild TBI patients had significantly reduced processing speed on the primary task when also required to perform a relevant, secondary task. The decline in processing speed was particularly apparent when the primary task required controlled processing. Reductions in processing speed under the extended conditions were related to a number of postconcussive symptoms, including slowed thinking, poor concentration, sensitivity to noise, fatigue, and decreased frustration tolerance. In general, it appeared that the patients with mild TBI needed increased mental effort even on tasks that required relatively automatic processing, while showing disproportionately greater declines in functioning on tasks that required effortful processing.

Schmitter-Edgecombe (1996) suggested that a number of cognitive deficits exhibited by persons with TBI may be due to the reduction of attentional resources available for task performance. The effects of reduced attentional resources would include (a) greater impairment when performing cognitive operations that require effortful versus automatic processes, (b) impairment when two tasks are simultaneous and must share effortful processing resources, and (c) prolonged time to automatize new cognitive processes. The need to rely primarily on effortful cognitive processes may underlie a number of the difficulties experienced by individuals with mild TBI in their daily functioning, such as sometimes being able to perform activities with relative efficiency whereas at other times, the activities are difficult or impossible to perform. Stuss et al. (1989) have suggested that the reliance on effortful processing could be responsible for patients' inability to maintain a consistent level of performance with repeated demands. They demonstrated that patients with mild concussion exhibited both an impaired level of performance and increased variability over time on reaction-time tasks. Bleiberg, Garmoe, Halpern, Reeves, & Nadler (1997) examined the within- and across-day performance variability of six patients with mild or moderate TBI and matched control subjects. The patients and control subjects performed at generally equivalent levels on a single administration of a neuropsychological test battery. However, the mild TBI patients exhibited increased variability of performance across days, including instances of worsened performance, on specific measures of information processing speed and efficiency. These findings were for mild TBI patients who were 12 to 30 months postinjury, demonstrated intact neuropsychological test performance, and had achieved excellent social and vocational recovery, which suggests that reduced stability of performance is an enduring aspect of patients' cognitive functioning. Bleiberg et al. (1997) suggested that "the very absence of predictable patterns of performance across days may be a primary symptom for some patients with [mild] TBI" (p. 252).

Complaints of poor memory are also common after mild TBI. Mutter, Howard, Howard, and Wiggs (1990) demonstrated that individuals with mild TBI, tested within 3 weeks of injury, had memory deficits similar to those in amnesic patients. That is, memory was impaired on tasks that required deliberate, conscious recall of information, but not on measures of implicit memory. Guilmette and Rasile (1995) evaluated performance on a number of verbal memory measures between 16 patients with mild TBI and a group of matched control subjects. Subjects were seen from 1 month to over 6 years postinjury, and all of the patients were symptomatic at the time of testing. The patients showed significant impairments on measures of acquisition, immediate and delayed list recall, and immediate and delayed paragraph recall. Measures of information acquisition without a conceptual context appeared particularly sensitive, suggesting that patients had difficulty in efficiently processing and encoding new information. Zappala and Trexler (1992) also measured impaired acquisition and recall of verbal information for 11 mild TBI patients admitted to post-acute rehabilitation. Qualitative analysis of performance demonstrated that the patients were impaired in their use of a semantic encoding strategy during delayed recall. These results suggest that reduced organization of material, or deficiency in the use of active learning strategies, contributes to the memory difficulties of individuals with mild TBI.

Impairments of attention and information processing speed are likely to contribute to reduced acquisition and recall, and may underlie many of the memory problems experienced after mild TBI. In similar fashion, reduced processing speed and rate of acquisition may underlie complaints of decreased reading and verbal comprehension. Comprehension deficits may be further complicated by reduced processing of multiple stimuli or task demands, as evidenced by reports of difficulty reading in noisy environments or attempting to write and listen simultaneously.

Executive deficits may also be prominent after mild TBI. Two aspects of executive functioning, verbal fluency and abstract conceptual reasoning, were impaired in persons with mild TBI who exhibited persisting symptomatology (Leininger, Gramling, Farrel, Kreutzer, & Peck, 1990). Raskin and Rearick (1996) also evaluated the nature of verbal fluency deficits after mild TBI. At least 1 year after their acceleration/deceleration injuries, 25 patients were compared with 22 normal control subjects, on measures of phonemic and semantic fluency. The total number of responses, organization (clustering) of responses, and perseverative or intrusive errors were measured. The mild TBI subjects produced fewer responses, were less likely to organize responses according to semantically related clusters, and produced a greater number of errors, compared to the control subjects. Semantic fluency was also related to a measure of verbal learning, as were measures of semantic clustering on both the fluency and memory tasks. Impairments of verbal and behavioral fluency may also be related to slowed information processing and slowed access to information after mild TBI, particularly with demands to initiate and sustain effortful processing.

Two additional studies (Stablum, Leonardi, Mazzoldi, Umilta, & Morra, 1994; Stablum, Mogentale, & Umilta, 1996) suggest disturbance of executive functioning after mild TBI. Although patients in the initial study (1994) had sustained severe acceleration/deceleration brain injuries, all demonstrated good recovery with no neurological abnormalities or neuropsychological impairments on standard testing. Despite their apparent good recovery, the patients continued to exhibit postconcussive complaints, including difficulty with concentration or memory, fatigue, irritability, and difficulty performing daily tasks. Subjects were assessed on tasks designed to reflect the framework of executive control proposed by Norman and Shallice (1986). According to this model, there are two modes of control over attention and action. The first, "contention scheduling," operates under most routine conditions, in response to habitual situations. The second, the "supervisory attentional system," is required when habitual responses are inappropriate or ineffective, and it is necessary to produce a novel response; for example, when planning, correcting errors, or solving problems. The performance of the TBI subjects was adequate on routine tasks, but was impaired on tasks that required the strategic monitoring and control of processing, such as coordinating two responses or shifting responses to anticipate a change. In a subsequent study, Stablum et al. (1996) evaluated the performance of mild TBI subjects on similar tasks. The results were similar to those of the 1994 study, demonstrating executive deficits in persons with mild TBI. The deficits were especially apparent in subjects who were over age 30 at the time of injury, and they were seen in subjects who were more than 2 years postinjury. These findings suggest that remediating executive functioning deficits may be an important aspect of rehabilitation for patients who do not completely recover after mild TBI.

The findings of Stablum et al. (1994, 1996) and Raskin and Rearick (1996) are consistent with the suggestion that a deficiency in the active application of strategies contributes to the poor memory performance of patients with mild TBI. The impairment of executive functioning observed by Stablum et al. (1994) was also related to slowed processing speed. Cicerone (1996) also found a relationship between reduced processing speed during simultaneous, dual task demands and behavioral perseveration on neuropsychological testing. This may reflect a unitary impairment of working memory on tasks that require attending to multiple aspects of the environment or shifting between aspects of the external situation and internal mental representations.

In summary, there is evidence for the existence of specific impairments of attention, memory, and executive functioning in individuals who have sustained mild TBI. These deficits may be apparent even for several years after the injury, and may not be readily apparent on traditional measures of neuropsychological functioning. Efforts to remediate the cognitive deficits after mild TBI need to be directed at the specific nature of the dysfunction. Impairments of processing speed appear to be prevalent, although this aspect of functioning may be difficult to directly rehabilitate. Attempts to remediate attentional deficits after mild TBI may therefore have to be directed at (a) helping patients to anticipate situations that are likely to require rapid processing, (b) adapting their performance on self-paced tasks and increasing their control over externally presented information, (c) self-monitoring the mental effort associated with various task demands, (d) reducing reactivity to distraction, (e) minimizing multiple or simultaneous task demands, and (f) increasing their active application of organizational strategies. It is also likely that individuals with mild TBI will have to exert more effortful, conscious, and deliberate processing, even on tasks that they were previously able to perform automatically, to compensate for their residual cognitive impairments.

Postconcussive Symptoms and Cognitive Deficits

A significant number of individuals with mild TBI exhibit persistent physical and emotional symptoms, which may interact with cognitive deficits and interfere with daily functioning. It is common in clinics, particularly among patients referred for rehabilitation, for patients to report postconcussive symptoms months or even years postinjury, although these subjective complaints may be greater than expected based on objective neurological findings or neuropsychological testing. Levin et al. (1987) examined the symptoms of 155 patients who were within 1 week of sustaining a mild TBI that required hospitalization. There were several groups of symptoms, including cognitive symptoms plus depression, somatic symptoms, sleep disturbance, disturbances of smell and taste, and irritability and anxiety. Based on these five symptom groups, three types of patients were identified. The largest group of patients reported minimal or no postconcussive symptoms, despite their somewhat poorer performance on neuropsychological tests. A second group of patients had primary symptoms of cognitive impairment and depression. The third group exhibited prominent somatic symptoms. Alves et al. (1993) examined the subjective postconcussive symptoms among 587 patients with uncomplicated mild TBI. Postconcussive symptoms were present in about two thirds of the patients in the first 3 months postinjury and in nearly half of the patients seen between 6 and 12 months postinjury. Headache, dizziness, and memory complaints were the most frequently reported symptoms, although these were present in only about 6% of the patients at 12 months. Cicerone and Kalmar (1995) examined the structure of persistent subjective complaints in 50 patients who were clinically symptomatic at least 3 months after sustaining a mild TBI. They found several distinct sets of complaints representing cognitive symptoms (primarily concentration and memory), headaches, sleep disturbance, other somatic symptoms (primarily dizziness and imbalance), hypersensitivity to noise and light, and affective symptoms (primarily irritability and frustration). Four groups of patients were identified, based on the nature of their subjective complaints. The first group reported generally mild cognitive symptoms, and minimal symptoms in other areas. The second, largest group reported primarily moderate to severe cognitive and affective symptoms. A third group also reported moderate to severe cognitive and affective symptoms; however, this group also had moderate somatic and sensory complaints. A final, small group reported relatively global and severe subjective complaints and a high incidence of posttraumatic psychiatric symptoms including depression, anxiety, and somatization.

Fatigue and headache may be the most common and persistent symptoms reported after mild TBI. Symptomatic fatigue appears to be closely related to cognitive symptoms (Cicerone & Kalmar, 1995) and disability (Wrightson & Gronwall, 1983). In clinical practice, it is common for patients to report fatigue as a disabling symptom after mild TBI, and these complaints often appear related to mental efforts or attempts to sustain concentration and thinking. Posttraumatic headache has been associated with increased cognitive complaints (Packard, Weaver, & Ham, 1993) and neuropsychological impairments (Gfeller, Chibnall, & Duckro, 1994). Complaints of poor memory and concentration are common among patients with chronic pain symptoms (Iverson & McCracken, 1997; Schnurr & MacDonald, 1995). However, even among patients with chronic pain, a history of head and neck injury is related to neuropsychological impairments, especially on measures of complex attention (Schwartz et al., 1987).

Cognitive symptoms may occur with injury other than damage to the brain, for example, craniocervical injury. Patients with soft tissue injury to the cervical spine, secondary to acceleration/deceleration (whiplash), exhibit neuropsychological deficits, especially in areas of information processing speed and divided attention (Radanov, Dvorak, & Valach, 1992). Cognitive deficits after cervical injury may be due to damage to the cervical musculoskeletal–proprioceptive system (Gimse, Tjell, Bjorgen, Tyssedal, & Bo, 1997), or secondary to pain (Radanov, Hirlinger, DiStefano, & Valach, 1992). However, patients with upper cervical (cervicoencephalic) injury also exhibit increased loss of consciousness (Radanov, Dvorak, & Valach, 1992), suggesting that the cognitive deficits in these cases may be due to frontobasal cerebral and brain stem structures (Ettlin et al., 1992). Posttraumatic vestibular dysfunction may also be associated with cognitive impairments, particularly complaints of difficulty with concentration while reading, or during functional scanning activities in perceptually complex environments (Grimm, Hemenway, Lebray, & Black, 1986). This may again be related to the co-occurrence of vestibular and cerebral concussion (Griffiths, 1979).

Emotional symptoms are thought to influence cognitive functioning, and many patients with moderate to severe cognitive complaints also have significant emotional complaints, as previously noted. TBI patients with depression or anxiety may complain of more cognitive deficits, even in the absence of impairments on neurocognitive evaluation (Fann, Katon, Uomoto, & Esselman, 1995). Subjective complaints and objective cognitive deficits are most apparent in patients with major depressive disorder (Fann et al.), and an emotional basis for cognitive impairments should be suspected in those mild TBI patients with global subjective complaints, gross neuropsychological impairment, and functional disability that is disproportionate to the severity of neurologic injury. The impact of milder forms of depression on cognitive functioning is less well defined, but still needs to be considered. Situational (state) anxiety may also contribute to impairments of information processing speed and complex attention (Batchelor et al., 1995; Deary et al., 1994). Symptoms of irritability, frustration, and feeling easily overwhelmed may directly result from cerebral injury or cognitive problems, although they are often more closely related to other emotional reactions than to specific cognitive deficits. It is not unusual for clinicians to observe patients for whom increased efforts to concentrate result in increased somatic symptoms, leading to increased emotional distress.

It is evident that cognitive and noncognitive postconcussive symptoms may be interrelated and have multiple causes. The severity of postconcussive symptoms may not mirror the severity of objective neuropsychological deficits, but is related to rehabilitation outcome (Cicerone & Kalmar, 1995; Cicerone et al., 1996). The clinician therefore needs to consider these symptoms to provide effective treatment of cognitive disability after mild TBI.

Remediation of Cognitive Disability After Mild TBI

Interventions for cognitive deficits after mild TBI will be described in relation to differing clinical presentations, through two case examples. Despite the differences in specific interventions, these cases follow a similar course and rationale. The initial course of treatment is devoted to developing a shared concept of the nature of cognitive deficits and their potential impact, through individually prescribed tasks. Treatment tasks are then modified to elicit the patient's deficits and illuminate the conditions that influence the patient's level of competence. This process resembles the concept of the "scaffold" (Wood, Bruner, & Ross, 1976) in allowing the therapist to control elements of the task that are initially beyond the patient's capacity, allowing the patient to discover those elements that are within his or her capacity, and allowing the patient to develop compensatory strategies. The scaffold initially provides maximal support, but it does not ensure errorless performance. Errors will occur as the therapist transfers responsibility for the task to the patient, and these errors provide the principal basis for determining the patient's competence and adjusting the level of intervention. Because some errors are inevitable, the patient is able to practice the anticipation, recognition, and correction of errors as a means of increasing cognitive responsibility and control. Throughout this period, it may be necessary to address somatic or psychological factors that affect the patient's functioning, and these factors may be incorporated into treatment tasks. As the nature of difficulties and related conditions become apparent, the patient is asked to monitor similar problems in his or her daily functioning and bring examples to the sessions. This allows a gradual transition from an emphasis on the patient's performance within sessions to an emphasis on functional application of compensatory strategies.

In the case examples, the design and implementation of individual treatments for cognitive deficits will be emphasized. Although this is a common method of cognitive remediation for individuals with mild TBI, additional treatments within a comprehensive rehabilitation program are often essential to effective treatment. The establishment of a therapeutic setting, including group cognitive and interpersonal therapies, can help patients increase their awareness of deficits and develop functional adaptations. Psychological issues that directly affect the cognitive remediation process will be noted; however, no attempt will be made to provide and in-depth discussion of psychotherapeutic interventions, which may be a central aspect of rehabilitation after mild TBI (see Cicerone, 1991).

Case Example 1: Remediation of Attention and Self-Regulation Deficits

Paul, a 22-year-old man, was in a motor vehicle accident in which he apparently sustained acceleration/deceleration and impact injury to the head, with a brief period of posttraumatic amnesia (PTA) suggestive of a grade 2 cerebral concussion. He sustained soft tissue injury to the cervical spine with slight disc bulging but no herniation, orthopedic injury to his right shoulder, and a fractured right wrist. During the initial weeks of his convalescence, he was constantly fatigued, sleeping 12 or more hours daily; and he exhibited slowed thinking and behavior, rarely initiated activities, and exhibited occasional word finding errors and word substitutions. These behaviors were initially attributed to his physical injuries and pain medications, although when they persisted for 6 weeks, his family became concerned, and he became depressed over the interruption in his life. He was initially referred to a psychologist due to his depression. The psychologist recognized the possibility of a mild TBI and referred him for neuropsychological evaluation and treatment approximately 3 months after the injury.

Paul had graduated third in his class, with an "A" average. He attended college for 2 years, majoring in business, and did well, but left college to get started in his own business. For approximately 9 months before the accident he had been working at a retail store, where he was receiving management training and expected to get promoted shortly. He had also been working at several small business ventures including vending machines, investing, and marketing through the Internet. He had not returned to work due to his physical injuries, and he expressed concerns about the impact of his concentration and memory problems on his ability to work.

At the time of initial neuropsychological evalution, his primary complaints were of short attention span, distractibility, and forgetfulness. He noted that he had more difficulty carrying out procedures on his computer and made frequent errors when he had to keep track of several pieces of information. He reported that at times he would "feel overwhelmed" or "forget what to do," and might simply sit in front of the computer for several hours. He had difficulty remembering appointments or familiar phone numbers, and he forgot to carry out everyday activities such as grocery shopping. He was concerned because he could not remember large parts of movies he had recently seen, although this improved with reminders. He had begun using a planner and writing down daily events and appointments, which he felt had helped. He felt that he was not at all like this prior to the accident, and he was concerned that he would never be like he was before the accident.

In addition to his cognitive symptoms, he reported loss of smell and neck pain, although he believed that his cognitive symptoms were independent of his pain.

On neuropsychological evaluation, he showed significant mild impairments of visual and auditory processing speed, with notable decline in his performance on tasks requiring controlled, effortful mental processing and divided attention. There was evidence of verbal and visual memory disturbance characterized by inefficient acquisition of new information, which affected his later recall of the material and produced numerous distortions of the content. He had difficulty initiating, planning, and organizing tasks that required self-direction in the absence of external structure and feedback. All of these deficits could be considered in terms of a breakdown of processes involved in the dynamic regulation and direction of his attention. His intellectual functioning was in the above-average to superior range. Although the neuropsychological test results were indicative of generally mild impairments, these may have reflected significant decline from his expected level of functioning. He appeared occasionally surprised and expressed consternation when he experienced difficulty with task demands, although he exhibited adequate frustration tolerance.

The course of neuropsychological remediation was directed at improving his attention and processing speed, self-monitoring of responses, and efficiency of encoding information, and was expected to result in functional improvements of his memory. During the initial session, we reviewed his deficits in relation to the nature of his injury, their expected impact, and more general issues of recovery and need to compensate for possible residual deficits. We also reviewed his use of a planner and notebook to compensate for memory difficulties. The initial phase of treatment was intended to explore the circumstances that might correlate with his everyday attention difficulties, with the working hypothesis that these difficulties were most likely to occur when he had to shift his responses between information that was immediately present and information that he had to keep in his mind. This was related to the difficulties he experienced while working on his computer, specifically his tendency to keep several files open simultaneously and then lose track of what information had been entered in each file. In treatment we used a number of working memory tasks, with identical versions that either allowed him to control the rate of presentation (self-paced) or required him to respond to externally paced stimuli. In one treatment activity he was presented with ordinary playing cards in random order, and asked to continuously report the number of the card that had been presented either immediately before the card shown, two cards back, or three cards back. A similar set of auditory tasks used tape-recorded stimuli. We addressed his ability to monitor and respond to multiple sources of information, through a computerized version of a multiple attention, multiple response task that required him to simultaneously monitor up to five gauges and control each gauge with a different response. We used different combinations of tasks across treatment sessions, adapting the principle of contextual interference (Battig, 1972; Hanlon, 1996). This procedure simulates the variability in task demands that is inherent in everyday functioning. Whereas the initial acquisition of competence may be prolonged, the long-term application of skills is facilitated by the patient's generating the appropriate strategy every time a task is presented. The transfer of training to new situations may be facilitated through the need to distinguish the requirements of different tasks and apply different strategies to varied task demands.

Within the first few weeks of treatment, Paul was able to identify situations that were likely to cause lapses of attention, and to identify more precisely the nature of his errors. For example, during self-paced tasks his errors were usually related to his responding too quickly, whereas with externally paced tasks his errors were usually related to internal distractions. Paul's attention and memory lapses were discussed in terms of his tendency to take for granted his cognitive functioning, and the difference between automatic and deliberate mental processes. He began to use self-verbalization, self-pacing, and rehearsal strategies to control his attention and to make more deliberate efforts to remember information, explaining the relevance and use of these strategies in his daily activities. He demonstrated spontaneous transfer of these strategies to the different tasks he was given in sessions. His failure to use an overt strategy resulted in increased errors, whereas with overt verbalization he was able to maintain his performance.

Gradually, we increased the complexity of treatment tasks by adding components that required simultaneous or conceptual processing. For example, he would have to name both the number of the card shown two cards back and the color of the current card, sort each card according to different principles, or generate verbal responses according to a given concept (e.g, nonsense trigrams or semantic fluency tasks). During performance of the multiple attention, multiple response task, he was required to monitor or respond to a conversation. The intent of all of these interventions was the continued application of strategies that would allow him to maintain control over internal and external information. He was able to apply verbalization and rehearsal strategies to the tasks and generalize the strategies to compensate for his everyday lapses of attention, consciously directing and allocating attention in response to environmental demands.

After approximately 2 months of treatment, Paul reported fewer cognitive difficulties in his daily functioning. Formal, biweekly monitoring of everyday attentional difficulties revealed nearly a 50% reduction, although he continued to note occasional memory lapses that appeared secondary to external distractions. Selected neuropsychological evaluation demonstrated mild improvement of processing speed and significant improvements of complex attention. His immediate and delayed recall of complex material were both improved to within normal limits, although possibly still reduced relative to his expected level of performance.

When we modified treatment to introduce several tasks that required complex planning and problem solving, Paul still exhibited a pattern of "thoughtless" responding. This was characterized by lack of relation between his initial response latencies and problem complexity, attempts at a direct solution on problems requiring an intermediate response, and a tendency to repeat the same error on repeated trials. Over the next 6 weeks, we continued to direct treatment at the organization and self-regulation of his behavior, using both verbal mediation and a prediction paradigm (Cicerone & Giacino, 1992) that required him to anticipate the possible responses and errors on a number of verbal and nonverbal planning and problem-solving tasks. We alternated practice on these tasks with discussion of everyday situations where he needed to apply these compensations. We continued to emphasize his identification of variations among task demands, both in treatment sessions and in his daily functioning, and the conscious use of strategies that allowed him to direct and control his attention.

After 3½ months of treatment, Paul demonstrated consistent improvement in his performance and ability to initiate and use compensatory strategies. He simultaneously reported improvement in his functioning and indicated that he felt sharper mentally, as if "no longer on a cloud . . . I feel more like myself now." He reported that he had been using his computer at home more regularly and had learned new applications, which he related to his increased ability to sustain attention and keep track of several trains of thought. He also started a training course in business computer use, which he felt would help him to acquire new skills required to return to work. We reviewed his expected course of recovery, including the possibility of continued neurologic recovery and the potential for persistence of mild "errors" in his daily activities when busy, fatigued, or otherwise under increased demands. On follow-up approximately 1 year after his injury, Paul was working successfully for a small business, running several projects from his home computer, and attending business classes part time. He reported that it was more effortful for him to "juggle" these multiple demands, and he could "not take for granted" his ability to function effectively in every situation. He still noticed occasional lapses in his attention and memory, but did not feel that these significantly impaired his functioning.

Case Example 2: Interaction of Cognitive and Emotional Interventions

Sharon, a 38-year-old woman, was driving her car home from work when she was struck from behind while yielding to enter a highway. She sustained an acceleration/deceleration injury to her cervical spine and struck her head on the steering wheel. There was reportedly a loss of consciousness of about 5 minutes, with posttraumatic and retrograde amnesia of approximately 30 minutes; her first recall was of being questioned by the emergency department nurses who "kept asking my home phone number over and over but I couldn't answer them." She was released from the emergency room after an X-ray of the neck and CT scan of the head were normal. Over the next 2 weeks she experienced continuous headaches, neck pain, dizziness, and nausea. She did attempt to return to her job as a legal secretary in a large law firm but was "dizzy, nauseous, and exhausted" by the commute and unable to do anything when she arrived at work. When this happened again the following day, she was sent home from work and went to see a neurologist, who diagnosed a cerebral concussion and gave her physical therapy for her neck. Six months after her injury she had not resumed work, and continued to experience daily headaches, occasional dizziness (lightheadedness), and forgetfulness. She was referred for cognitive evaluation and treatment. She reported that she was unable to concentrate for more than several minutes and could not remember anything that she had read. This was particularly disconcerting, as she had previously been an avid reader, had been required to manage large amounts of professional documentation on her job, and had been used to "doing 12 things at a time." She also reported a marked decline in her ability to manage her daily affairs, such as taking care of her personal finances. Sharon reported that her work had been a major source of life satisfaction for her, providing her with a sense of accomplishment and recognition for her intellectual achievements, even though she "only had a high school diploma." She had always viewed herself as exceptionally responsible and competent, so that her present difficulties seemed intolerable.

During the initial assessment and treatment, she exhibited markedly slowed processing and attention deficits, with no obvious relationship between her level of performance and task difficulty. For example, she made as many errors when required to attend to a single target as when required to attend to five targets on an auditory attention task. Memory was well below her expected level of functioning, primarily due to her severely impaired immediate recall of both visual and verbal information. She became frustrated in response to the experience of her deficits, and was then unable to recover from her errors, which further interfered with her attempts to function effectively. We initiated treatment with a variety of attention training tasks, which required her to listen to auditory tapes or read a page while detecting one or more letters or words, both with and without distractors (similar to the attention training tasks described by Mateer et al., 1990). There was no attempt to present these tasks within a structured hierarchy, but rather the tasks were continuously varied between simpler and more difficult tasks, and she was provided with feedback regarding her performance. The primary focus of the clinical intervention was to increase Sharon's self-monitoring of her secondary emotional reactions (e.g., anxiety, frustration, and feeling overwhelmed) and their impact on her performance, with no attempt to remediate her attention per se. We discussed a verbal mediation strategy to reduce her emotional "flooding" and return her attention to the task even after she made errors. Over the course of 8 weeks, her emotional reactivity decreased, and her attention and processing speed (as monitored by the PASAT) showed significant improvement (from 3 standard deviations below the mean to slightly above average). Her response to this intervention was taken as evidence for a clear relationship between the cognitive and emotional determinants of her performance, which continued to be a theme throughout treatment. We did not try to dismiss her cognitive deficits as an emotional disorder, but simply to continue and provide feedback about the impact of these factors on both her objective performance and subjective feelings of competence and control. At this time, we discussed her difficulties with reading comprehension and balancing her checkbook in relation to the difficulties observed during treatment tasks, and she was instructed to monitor her performance and emotional reactions while performing these activities. She was then able to recognize that she tended to continually "regress" during these activities (reread the same material or repeatedly perform the same calculation) because she was uncertain if she had understood the material or made a mistake. With further self-monitoring, she was able to see that her regressions when doing the checkbook were unrelated to whether her calculations were actually correct. Her regressions were typically accompanied by heightened anxiety. She also tended to push to complete these activities long after she began to feel confused and ineffective, which contributed to her feeling of being overwhelmed, exacerbation of headaches and dizziness, and abandonment of the whole activity after 15 or 20 minutes. She was assisted in developing a compensation for doing her checkbook, where she would check every calculation, once and only once, and then continue with the task. She also practiced the verbal mediation strategy (previously developed during attention training) to control her subjective sense of uncertainty and anxiety while performing functional tasks. To address her feelings of being overwhelmed, she was prescribed activities and instructed to work for no more than 10 minutes and then take a 5-minute break ("whether she needed it or not"), so that her breaks from task were no longer contingent on her becoming symptomatic. Following this intervention, she was eventually able to increase her time performing a task to over 60 minutes, with a reduction in her emotional and physical symptoms.

In sessions we emphasized improving her reading proficiency, after discussing the role of her concentration deficits and emotional reactivity in this area. We discussed a comprehension monitoring strategy that required her to mark the reading material when she felt she did not understand it, and then to paraphrase that section before proceeding. She was instructed to make a summary statement, even if she was unsure of what she had read. She was initially unable to implement this strategy, and would either regress over the same sentence or continue reading long after she failed to understand the material. At that time, we instituted a response-cost procedure, which required her to immediately contribute $1 to a "reading fund" whenever she failed to implement the comprehension monitoring strategy or claimed that she "had no idea" what she had read. She was then able to implement the strategy fairly quickly, and her factual comprehension was probed at the completion of each paragraph and indicated at least 90% accuracy. Several additional psychological issues emerged at this time. For one, her self-assessment of her comprehension accuracy was consistently below her objective performance. We actively addressed the meaning of this discrepancy. It also became apparent that she experienced discomfort with this strategy (which also may have contributed to her initial resistance to its use) because it required her to make a conscious effort to perform activities that had previously been automatic, and as a result these previously enjoyable activities had become quite onerous. Although her discomfort was acknowledged, this process was discussed in the context of the distinction between automatic and controlled processing. The analogy was that much of her cognitive processing had previously been conducted "behind the scenes," whereas now almost all of her thinking was done "at center stage." Sharon was reassured that it was possible (although not guaranteed) that with continued practice her reading comprehension might become "re-automatized." At that point, we reviewed a number of less restrictive advance organizers that could increase her reading comprehension, including the "predict, read, and prove" (Cook & Mayer, 1983) and PQRST (Glasgow, Zeiss, Barbera, & Lewinsohn, 1977) strategies. For example, in the "predict, read, and prove" approach, she would read the initial sentence of a paragraph, predict what she thought the paragraph was about, and then use the information in the paragraph to prove or disprove her prediction, then apply the same strategy to each ensuing paragraph. Eventually, we transferred these strategies to her comprehension of auditory material using a number of commercial books-on-tape. She was to stop the tape and summarize the material as soon as she felt that she did not comprehend the material. This was a more difficult task, and she initially had to stop the tape every sentence or less. Eventually, she progressed to making a summary statement while the tape continued to play, initially aloud and then covertly, and finally to applying a "predict, listen, and prove" strategy to the auditory information. She at times required each of these strategies, depending on the interest level and complexity of the material. Once again, she was required to formally self-monitor her application of these strategies to various situations during her daily activities, including conversations and phone calls, reading the newspaper, and reading material she had previously needed for her work.

In the final phase of treatment, she was required to integrate all of the previously practiced strategies during tasks that demanded recall of material or problem solving. Initially, she again experienced increased frustration and tended to underestimate her actual performance during these tasks. We again addressed this through verbal mediation of her secondary emotional reactions and objective feedback. In addition, I would simultaneously perform the identical task and ask Sharon to evaluate my performance. She was then able to see that her evaluations of her own performance were typically below her evaluations of my performance, even when they were objectively the same. This allowed her to appreciate the personal significance of her residual difficulties (both actual and perceived) and their impact on her daily functioning.

Sharon received cognitive remediation for over 6 months. She continued to experience a reduction in her functioning and a sense of loss from her previous level of competence, but was also able to recognize her ability to successfully complete many activities. Her cognitive difficulties were still apparent, particularly when she needed to perform activities that required extensive planning or had increased time pressure. The reduced consistency of her functioning remained one of her major concerns. For example, although she believed that she was "still intelligent," she complained that her "brain couldn't be relied on" to perform "on demand." As a result, her everyday functioning remained more restricted and routine. However, she gradually shifted over the course of treatment from a vigilance and emotional reactivity toward her residual symptoms to an appreciation of her residual abilities. She did not return to her previous employment, but performed clerical activities as a volunteer and continued to participate in psychotherapy, to adapt to the changes in her functioning. Over 2 years after her injury, she began working part time as a secretary in the offices of a local community college. Her return to work was critical to her establishing a feeling of productivity in her life, although she did not have the same sense of intellectual accomplishment and satisfaction as she did prior to the injury.

Conclusions

The treatment of cognitive disability after mild TBI continues to represent a clinical challenge. This may be due to the subtle nature of the cognitive deficits and functional limitations that appear to be disproportionate to the patients' obvious deficits and injuries. The interaction of subtle cognitive dysfunction, heightened vigilance and emotional sensitivity to symptoms, concurrent somatic symptoms, and poor performance may contribute to the maintenance of functional disability following a mild TBI. On the other hand, patients with relatively mild cognitive deficits often retain the capacity for insight into the nature of their difficulties and the ability to independently apply compensatory strategies, which may increase their potential to benefit from cognitive remediation. In addition to these patient characteristics, the clinical effectiveness of cognitive remediation after mild TBI will depend upon the therapist's understanding of the specific nature of the individual's cognitive deficits, the meaning and significance of the deficits to the individual, and the relevance of cognitive limitations to the individual's everyday functioning.

References

Alves, W., Macciocchi, S. N., & Barth, J. T. (1993). Postconcussive symptoms after uncomplicated mild head injury. *Journal of Head Trauma Rehabilitation, 8*(3), 48–59.

Batchelor, J., Harvey, A. G., & Bryant, R. A. (1995). Stroop Colour Word Test as a measure of attentional deficit following mild head injury. *The Clinical Neuropsychologist, 9,* 180–186.

Battig, W. F. (1972). Intratask interference as a source of facilitation in transfer and retention. In R. F. Thompson & J. F. Voss (Eds.), *Topics in learning and performance* (pp. 211–228). New York: Academic Press.

Bleiberg, J., Garmoe, W. S., Halpern, E. L., Reeves, D. L., & Nadler, J. D. (1997). Consistency of within-day and across-day performance after mild brain injury. *Neuropsychiatry, Neuropsychology, and Behavioral Neurology, 10,* 247–253.

Bohnen, N., Jolles, J., & Twijnstra, A. (1992). Modification of the Stroop Color Word Test improves differentiation between patients with mild head injury and matched controls. *The Clinical Neuropsychologist, 6,* 178–184.

Bohnen, N., Twijnstra, A., & Jolles, J. (1992). Performance in the Stroop Colour Word Test in relation to the persistence of symptoms following mild head injury. *Acta Neurologica Scandinavica, 85,* 116–121.

Cicerone, K. D. (1991). Psychotherapy after mild traumatic brain injury: Relation to the nature and severity of subjective complaints. *Journal of Head Trauma Rehabilitation, 6*(4), 30–43.

Cicerone, K. D. (1996). Attention deficits and dual task demands after mild traumatic brain injury. *Brain Injury, 10,* 79–89.

Cicerone, K. D. (1997). Clinical sensitivity of four measures of attention to mild traumatic brain injury. *The Clinical Neuropsychologist, 11,* 266–272.

Cicerone, K. D., & Giacino, J. T. (1992). Remediation of executive function deficits after traumatic brain injury. *Neurorehabilitation, 2*(3), 12–22.

Cicerone, K. D., & Kalmar, K. (1995). Persistent post-concussive syndrome: Structure of subjective complaints after mild traumatic brain injury. *Journal of Head Trauma Rehabilitation, 10*(3), 1–17.

Cicerone, K. D., Smith, L. C., Ellmo, W., Mangel, H. E., Nelson, P., Chase, R. F., & Kalmar, K. (1996). Neuropsychological rehabilitation of mild traumatic brain injury. *Brain Injury, 10,* 277–286.

Cook, L. K., & Mayer, R. E. (1983). Reading strategies training for meaningful learning from prose. In M. Pressley & J. R. Levin (Eds.), *Cognitive strategy research: Educational applications* (pp. 87–131). New York: Springer-Verlag.

Deary, I. J., Ebmeier, K. P., MacLeod, K. M., Dougall, N., Hepburn, D. A., Frier, B. M., & Goodwin, G. M. (1994). PASAT performance and the pattern of $^{99\,m}$Tc-exametazinme in brain estimated with single photon emission tomography. *Biological Psychology, 38,* 1–18.

Ettlin, T. M., Kischka, U., Reichmann, S., Radii, E. W., Heim, S., Wengen, D., & Benson, D. F. (1992). Cerebral symptoms after whiplash injury of the neck: A prospective clinical and neuropsychological study of whiplash injury. *Journal of Neurology, Neurosurgery, and Psychiatry, 55,* 943–948.

Fann, J. R., Katon, W. J., Uomoto, J. M., & Esselman, P. C. (1995). Psychiatric disorders and functional disability in outpatients with traumatic brain injuries. *American Journal of Psychiatry, 152,* 1493–1499.

Gentilini, M., Nichelli, P., Schoenhuber, R., Bortolotti, P., Tonelli, L., Falasca, A., & Merli, G. A. (1985). Neuropsychological evaluation of mild head injury. *Journal of Neurology, Neurosurgery and Psychiatry, 48,* 137–140.

Gentilini, M., Nichelli, P., & Schoenhuber, R. (1989). Assessment of attention in mild head injury. In H. S. Levin, H. M. Eisenberg, & A. L. Benton (Eds.), *Mild head injury* (pp. 163–175). New York: Oxford University Press.

Gfeller, J. D., Chibnall, J. T., & Duckro, P. N. (1994). Postconcussion symptoms and cognitive functioning in posttraumatic headache patients. *Headache, 34,* 503–507.

Gimse, R., Tjell, C., Bjorgen, I. A., Tyssedal, J. S., & Bo, K. (1997). Reduced cognitive functions in a group of whiplash patients with demonstrated disturbances in the posture control system. *Journal of Clinical and Experimental Neuropsychology, 19,* 838–849.

Glasgow, R. E., Zeiss, R. A., Barbera, M., & Lewinsohn, P. M. (1977). Case studies on remediating memory deficits in brain-damaged individuals. *Journal of Clinical Psychology, 33,* 1049–1054.

Griffiths, M. V. (1979). The incidence of auditory and vestibular concussion following minor head injury. *Journal of Laryngology and Otology, 93,* 253–265.

Grimm, R. J., Hemenway, W. G., Lebray, P. R., & Black, F. O. (1986). The perilymph fistula syndrome defined in mild head trauma. *Acta Otolaryngalogica, 464,* 1–40.

Gronwall, D. (1977). Paced auditory serial addition task: A measure of recovery from concussion. *Perceptual and Motor Skills, 44,* 367–373.

Gronwall, D. (1986). Rehabilitation programs for patients with mild head injury: Components, problems and evaluation. *Journal of Head Trauma Rehabilitation, 1*(2), 53–62.

Gronwall, D., & Wrightson, P. (1974). Delayed recovery of intellectual function after minor head injury. *Lancet, 2,* 995–997.

Guilmette, T. J., & Rasile, D. (1995). Sensitivity, specificity, and diagnostic accuracy of three verbal memory measures in the assessment of mild brain injury. *Neuropsychology, 9,* 338–344.

Hanlon, R. E. (1996). Motor learning following unilateral stroke. *Archives of Physical Medicine and Rehabilitation, 77,* 811–815.

Hugenholtz, H., Stuss, D. T., Stethem, L. L., & Richard, M. T. (1988). How long does it take to recover from a mild concussion? *Neurosurgery, 22,* 853–858.

Iverson, G. L., & McCracken, L. M. (1997). 'Postconcussive' symptoms in persons with chronic pain. *Brain Injury, 11,* 783–790.

Leininger, B. E., Gramling, S. E., Farrel, A. D., Kreutzer, J. S., & Peck, E. A. (1990). Neuropsychological deficits in symptomatic minor head injury patients after concussion and mild concussion. *Journal of Neurology, Neurosurgery and Psychiatry, 53,* 293–296.

Levin, H. S., Gary, H. E., High, W. J., Mattis, S., Ruff, R. M., Eisenberg, H. M., Marshall, L. F., & Tabaddor, K. (1987). Minor head injury and the postconcussional syndrome: Methodological issues in outcome studies. In H. S. Levin, J. Grafman, & H. M. Eisenberg (Eds.), *Neurobehavioral recovery from head injury* (pp. 263–275). New York: Oxford University Press.

Mateer, C. (1992). Systems of care for post-concussive syndrome. In L. Horn & N. Zasler (Eds.), *Post-concussive disorders: State of the art reviews in physical medicine and rehabilitation* (pp. 143–155). Philadelphia: Hanley Belfus Medical.

Mateer, C., Sohlberg, M. M., & Youngman, P. K. (1990). The management of acquired attention and memory deficits. In R. L. Wood & I. Fussey (Eds.), *Cognitive rehabilitation in perspective* (pp. 143–160). New York: Taylor & Francis.

Minderhoud, J. M., Boelens, M. E., Huizenga, J., & Saan, R. J. (1980). Treatment of minor head injuries. *Clinical Neurology and Neurosurgery, 82,* 127–140.

Mutter, S. A., Howard, D. V., Howard, J. H., & Wiggs, C. L. (1990). Performance on direct and indirect tests of memory after mild closed head injury. *Cognitive Neuropsychology, 4,* 329–346.

Newcombe, F., Rabbit, P., & Briggs, M. (1994). Minor head injury: Pathophysiological or iatrogenic sequelae? *Journal of Neurology, Neurosurgery, and Psychiatry, 57,* 709–716.

Norman, D. A., & Shallice, T. (1986). Attention to action: Willed and automatic control of behavior. In R. J. Davidson, G. Schwartz, & D. Shapiro (Eds.), *Consciousness and self-regulation* (pp. 1–18). New York: Plenum Press.

Packard, R. C., Weaver, R., & Ham, L. P. (1993). Cognitive symptoms in patients with post-traumatic headache. *Headache, 33,* 365–368.

Parasuraman, R., Mutter, S. A., & Molloy, R. (1991). Sustained attention following mild closed-head injury. *Journal of Clinical and Experimental Neuropsychology, 13,* 789–811.

Ponsford, J., & Kinsella, G. (1992). Attentional deficits following closed-head injury. *Journal of Clinical and Experimental Neuropsychology, 14,* 822–838.

Radanov, B. P., Dvorak, J., & Valach, L. (1992). Cognitive deficits in patients after soft tissue injury of the cervical spine. *Spine, 17,* 127–131.

Radanov, B. P., Hirlinger, I., DiStefano, G., & Valach, L. (1992). Attentional processing in cervical spine syndromes. *Acta Neurologica Scandinavica, 85,* 358–362.

Raskin, A. A., & Rearick, E. (1996). Verbal fluency in individuals with mild traumatic brain injury. *Neuropsychology, 10,* 416–422.

Relander, M., Troupp, H., & Bjorkstein, G. (1972). Controlled trial of treatment for cerebral concussion. *British Medical Journal, 4,* 777–779.

Ruff, R. M., Evans, R. W., & Light, R. H. (1986). Automatic detection vs. controlled search: A paper-and-pencil approach. *Perceptual and Motor Skills, 62,* 407–416.

Schmitter-Edgecombe, M. (1996). Effects of traumatic brain injury on cognitive performance: An attentional resource hypothesis in search of data. *Journal of Head Trauma Rehabilitation, 11*(2), 17–30.

Schneider, W., & Shiffrin, R. M. (1977). Controlled and automatic human information processing: I. Detection, search and attention. *Psychological Review, 84,* 1–126.

Schnurr, R. F., & MacDonald, M. R. (1995). Memory complaints in chronic pain. *The Clinical Journal of Pain, 11,* 103–111.

Schwartz, D. R., Barth, J. T., Dane, J. R., Drenan, S. E., DeGood, D. E., & Rowlingson, J. C. (1987). Cognitive deficits in chronic pain patients with and without history of head/neck injury: Development of a brief screening battery. *The Clinical Journal of Pain, 3,* 94–101.

Stablum, F., Leonardi, G., Mazzoldi, M., Umilta, C., & Morra, S. (1994). Attention and control deficits following closed head injury. *Cortex, 30,* 603–618.

Stablum, F., Mogentale, C., & Umilta, C. (1996). Executive functioning following mild closed head injury. *Cortex, 32,* 261–278.

Stroop, J. R. (1935). Studies of interference in serial verbal reaction. *Journal of Experimental Psychology, 18,* 643–662.

Stuss, D. T., Stethem, L. L., Hugenholtz, H., Picton, T., Pivik, J., & Richard, M. T. (1989). Reaction time after head injury: Fatigue, divided and focused attention, and consistency of performance. *Journal of Neurology, Neurosurgery, and Psychiatry, 52,* 742–748.

Wood, D., Bruner, J. S., & Ross, G. (1976). The role of tutoring in problem solving. *Journal of Child Psychology and Psychiatry, 17,* 89–100.

Wrightson, P., & Gronwall, G. (1983). Time off work and symptoms after minor head injury. *Injury, 12,* 445–454.

Zappala, G., & Trexler, L. (1992). Quantitative and qualitative aspects of memory performance after minor head injury. *Archives of Clinical Neuropsychology, 7,* 145–154.

14 The Medical Management of Noncognitive Sequelae of Mild Traumatic Brain Injury

Gerald C. McIntosh

There has been a continuing controversy about whether the symptom complex that typifies the typical residual difficulties of many individuals with mild TBI, often called postconcussive syndrome (PCS), exists as an organic, psychogenic, or mixed disorder (Miller, 1961; Rutherford, Merrett, & McDonald, 1977; Symonds, 1962). The currently more accepted view of this symptom complex is that even in mild concussion, there is some structural damage to the deep white matter of the brain, usually consisting of diffuse axonal injury somewhat concentrated in the upper brain stem regions (Alexander, 1995; Selzer, 1995). The PCS reported to follow mild TBI includes headache, dizziness and impaired balance, tinnitus and other auditory symptoms, neck pain and back pain, loss of smell (anosmia), tremor, a variety of visual symptoms, and seizures or other dissociative episodes. Other reported sequelae include less definable symptoms, including cognitive difficulties such as impaired concentration, memory disturbance, attention disorder, and mood disturbances (e.g., fatigue, irritability, anxiety, and depression). This chapter focuses on the medical management of some of these posttraumatic symptoms, especially headaches, seizures, and dizziness and imbalance. The treatment of these symptoms is usually thought to fall within the neurologist's domain, but patients with PCS often are seen initially by the primary care physician.

Reprinted, with changes, from "Medical Management of Noncognitive Sequelae of Minor Traumatic Brain Injury," by Gerald C. McIntosh, 1997, *Applied Neuropsychology, 4*(1), pp. 62–68. Copyright 1997 by Lawrence Erlbaum Associates, Inc.

Posttraumatic Headache

Medical management of headache associated with mild TBI can be very trying, as so-called posttraumatic headache frequently fails to respond to traditional therapeutic measures. For the purposes of this discussion, the International Classification of Headache Disorders will be used (Headache Classification Committee of the International Headache Society, 1988). The International Classification of Headache Disorders has a special category for chronic posttraumatic headache, and divides this into headache with (a) significant head trauma and/or confirmatory signs and (b) minor head trauma and no confirmatory signs. Moderate and severe TBI are less commonly associated with headaches than is mild TBI, for reasons that are not entirely clear (Haas, 1993). Unfortunately, the type of headache associated with minor head trauma in the International Headache Society classification system does not have any definable characteristics other than the clinical association with mild TBI. Many of the headaches that occur after mild TBI fit the pattern typical for migraine, either with or without aura. Another large group of posttraumatic headaches are more of the tension type. A third group seems to be associated with disorder of the cervical spine that occurs in conjunction with the head injury. This discussion on posttraumatic headache will be based on the clinical presentation of headache type using migraine, tension, and cervicogenic headache models. Management of posttraumatic headache should follow a treatment plan designed for the type of headache the clinical presentation most closely resembles. This presentation may very well be a mixture of migraine and tension, tension and cervicogenic, migraine and cervicogenic, or all three together.

Epidemiologic studies have shown a fairly consistent frequency of headaches after TBI—in the range of 25%—from the 1930s to the present (Brenner, Freidmann, Merritt, & Denny-Brown, 1944; Russell, 1932). Somewhere around 50% of individuals with mild TBI have headaches in the acute phase, and half of those improve spontaneously. Because headaches are a relatively ubiquitous disorder, it may be more appropriate to compare headache frequencies before and after brain injury. In one such study, headache frequency increased 24% postinjury (Jensen & Neilsen, 1990). Overall, the 25% figure remains reliable for the frequency of headache in mild TBI.

It is my experience that the most typical headache after mild TBI is of the migraine type. Several authors have made similar observations (Jensen & Neilsen, 1990; Weiss, Stern, & Goldberg, 1991). A cervicogenic component due to whiplash headaches has also been reported (Winston, 1987). Individuals with whiplash headaches also may report some visual symptoms associated with their cervical pain, and may experience headache of the migraine type. Neck pain and stiffness is initially noted just after the accident and then persists, often in a chronic pattern, and accompanies the headache, which may be unilateral (migraine type) or bilateral (tension type). Over 50% of posttraumatic headaches are of the mixed type.

The treatment of posttraumatic migraine may include prophylactic medications such as beta adrenergic blockers (Propranolol), antidepressants (Amitriptyline, Nortriptyline), calcium channel blockers (Verapamil), and anticonvulsants (Valproic Acid) (Tfelt-Hansen & Welch, 1993). Reversal therapy may be accomplished by using Sumatriptan, various Ergotamines (DHE, Ergotamine Tartrate), and a variety of nonsteroidal anti-inflammatory drugs (Ibuprofen, Naproxen). Prophylactic treatment is indicated if headaches occur more than once a week, and the attacks are severe enough to impair normal activities at home or at work. At times with posttraumatic migraine, the headaches may be less frequent or less severe than described above, but psychologically difficult for the individual, and therefore may require prophylactic treatment. Prophylactic treatments also may be indicated if reversal therapies are ineffective. Relatively intensive, multifaceted treatment programs for posttraumatic migraine are frequently quite effective and necessary, because programs based solely on reversal or prophylactic medications may be ineffective (Medina, 1992). Such multidimensional headache treatment programs frequently include, in addition to medications, stress management and biofeedback therapy, and a good headache educational program (Medina). Generally, it is best to introduce therapies one at a time rather than to begin multiple therapies simultaneously.

Treatment of posttraumatic tension headache often uses antidepressant medication (Amitriptyline, Nortriptyline, Trazodone) for prophylaxis, and nonsteroidal anti-inflammatory drugs (Ibuprofen, Naproxen) for symptomatic treatment. Muscle relaxants are not usually beneficial and often cause lethargy or drowsiness, which may worsen other PCS symptoms. A broad-based headache management program, such as the one just discussed for migraine, is also useful in the management of posttraumatic tension headaches.

Posttraumatic cervicogenic headache is often amenable to physical measures such as physical therapy or biofeedback therapy. The addition of nonsteroidal anti-inflammatory medications is frequently beneficial. Not infrequently, migraine or tension headaches and cervicogenic headaches overlap, and treatment is a blend of physical measures and measures specific to migraine and/or tension headache.

Analgesics can be prescribed for symptomatic relief, but in general, narcotic analgesics should be avoided (Warner & Fenichel, 1966). Even if non-narcotic analgesics are used, they should be used with caution to avoid the development of analgesic abuse or "rebound" headache. Initially in the treatment of posttraumatic headaches, it is often beneficial to use some analgesics for relief of pain, because if pain is not relieved early in the therapeutic relationship, the overall therapeutic effectiveness of the treatment program may be undermined. However, continued regular use of analgesics, especially daily, frequently will perpetuate headaches. This pepetuation of headache is called rebound. The typical pattern is relief of headache with analgesics or reversal therapies for several hours, followed by recurrence of headache and relief again with analgesics (Couch, 1995). A rebound pattern can develop over as short a time as several days. Although antidepressant medications are often helpful in the treatment of posttraumatic headache, anxiolytic medications should be avoided (Haas, 1993). A typical treatment program for posttraumatic headache will consist of a prophylactic medication, usually beginning with a trial of antidepressants; appropriate physical measures if there is a cervicogenic component; reversal measures if migraine symptoms are present; and prudent use of analgesics. Flexibility in the application of treatment measures frequently aids the development of a successful treatment program.

Posttraumatic Seizures

The incidence of posttraumatic epilepsy is approximately 10% in all TBI, but in mild TBI it is considerably less (Caveness, 1976). One of the major clinical problems in the management of mild TBI can be discerning whether episodes of dissociation or interruption of the conscious state are actually caused by electrocerebral discharges, and are therefore seizures. Family, friends, or health care workers may report episodes of inattention, various types of staring spells, or strange automatisms, but the injured individual is usually not aware of any interruption in the conscious state. EEG may be normal in epileptic conditions no matter what the cause. A high percentage of the time, in individuals having posttraumatic seizures, a single EEG will not be abnormal in a typical epileptic pattern, although a minor background abnormality may be present. In these situations EEG will fail to answer the clinical question of seizure presence. It is best to know the stereotypical symptoms suggestive of temporal lobe or frontal lobe localization, because these brain regions are more frequently traumatized in TBI. In the case of frontal lobe localization in posttraumatic epilepsy, typical associated symptoms are postural changes, speech arrest, or vocalizations prior to the actual seizure. Occasionally abnormalities of olfaction or other physical automatisms may occur. With temporal lobe localization, the variety of associated symptoms is broader and may include epigastric discomfort, nausea, flushing, fear, panic, and olfactory, gustatory, or vertiginous symptomatology. If the history is atypical for seizures, a repeat EEG, EEG monitoring, or ambulatory EEG may clear up the clinical dilemma. If the EEG is abnormal, brain imaging studies, CT, or MRI are necessary to address the possibility of chronic subdural hematoma or cerebral contusion.

Because seizures associated with TBI are usually either simple partial or complex partial seizures, with or without secondary generalization, the therapy of choice is either Carbamazepine, Phenytoin (MacDonald & McLean, 1986), or the recently introduced anticonvulsants Gabapentin (U.S. Gabapentin Study Group No. 5, 1993) or Lamotrigine (Messenheimer, Ramsay, & Willmore, 1994). If there are accompanying cognitive impairments, then Carbamazepine or Gabapentin are favored therapies, as they are associated with less cognitive disruption. When anticonvulsants are used to treat posttraumatic seizures, the patient needs to be followed closely for side effects to the medication or potential drug interaction or reaction. Monitoring of anticonvulsant levels in the serum is frequently useful in seizure management. Usually one drug works as well or better than several together, and the patient experiences fewer side effects (Wilder, 1987).

Nonepileptic dissociative episodes are not generally amenable to treatment with medication. Various treatment plans can facilitate these individuals' increased awareness of their inattention, and can often be helpful if the attention deficits interfere with activities of daily living.

Posttraumatic Dizziness

After headache, dizziness is the second most common symptom associated with mild TBI (Rutherford et al., 1977). Frequently associated symptoms such as frank vertigo (spinning sensation), diplopia, and nausea accompany the complaint of dizziness. These symptoms tend to support the association that some localized injury in the brain stem occurs with relatively high frequency in mild TBI. In an analysis of postconcussive dizziness with brain stem auditory evoked potentials, inter-peak latencies have been prolonged, indicating disruption at the brain stem level for this particular symptom complex (Rowe & Carlson, 1980).

Unfortunately, medical management of dizziness is problematic. Medications such as Meclizine, which is typically used for motion sickness, tend to be sedating and often don't help the symptomatology. Anxiolytic drugs such as Benzodiazepines have also been used with some efficacy, but somnolence and relatively low efficacy are big problems with these medications. Of the Benzodiazepines that can be used in this clinical situation, Clonazepam has perhaps been most useful. To avoid the sedative side effects, a good starting dosage plan is a low starting dose of 0.5 mg at bedtime, carefully increasing to 0.5 mg twice a day. The medication is initiated at bedtime to help the patient build tolerance to the sedative side effects.

Occasionally, vestibular exercises, which involve periodic changes in body posture or head turning to stimulate the vestibular system, can be effective. When repeatedly stimulated peripherally, the vestibular system shows central suppression. Vestibular exercises are much more effective for peripheral disorders, and posttraumatic dizziness is mainly brain stem (central) in etiology. Thankfully, posttraumatic dizziness tends to gradually and spontaneously improve. Those patients with posttraumatic dizziness may gain confidence by working on gait and balance, initially with a physical therapist and later with a home exercise program.

Posttraumatic Tinnitus and Hearing Impairment

Tinnitus and/or hearing impairment are two symptoms reported after mild TBI that may be noted just after the injury, or not until several weeks after the injury. Hearing impairment after TBI usually remains persistent and is not amenable to hearing augmentation. One of the dilemmas in managing these cases occurs when the patient reports a hearing impairment, but audiometric testing fails to identify a disorder. This may represent problems with central auditory processing, and in this context, it is interesting to note the relatively high incidence of abnormality in brain stem auditory evoked responses in individuals with mild TBI (Rowe & Carlson, 1980). Generally speaking, hearing augmentation with hearing aid devices is not useful after TBI. However, masking of an ear that is sensitive to auditory stimulation can be beneficial in individuals with posttraumatic auditory impairments involving hypersensitivity. Individuals who have central auditory processing disorders and normal routine audiograms frequently show difficulties following directions, sensitivity to loud noises, or increasing confusion in noisy places; treatment remains problematic for these individuals. A more detailed study of this phenomenon is being considered, as attention problems, especially auditory distractibility, may be associated with auditory sensitivity.

Tinnitus is a frequent symptom associated with TBI. Masking with low intensity, pure auditory tone will assist individuals with tinnitus. Medications are generally ineffective in the treatment of either tinnitus or other auditory disorders that occur after mild TBI. In some situations, however, anxiolytic medications such as Benzodiazepines are effective in reducing associated anxiety and thereby reducing awareness of tinnitus. Sedation and/or dependence need to be considered before these medications are used for a protracted period.

Posttraumatic Anosmia

Although posttraumatic anosmia was probably recognized in the 19th century, the first case reports of major disorders after head injury occurred when war injuries were analyzed (Leigh, 1943). The incidence of anosmia, hyposmia, and dysosmia in TBI is generally 5% to 10% (Summer, 1964). Generally, the degree of dysfunction is associated with the severity of trauma. Cases of total anosmia have been reported in minor TBI, but usually relative hyposmia is typical. Disorders of taste usually accompany relative anosmia or dysosmia.

Posttraumatic anosmia may result from shearing of the fine fila olfactoria as they pass through the cribriform plate. This is thought to occur when the brain accelerates or decelerates in the calvarian at the time of the injury. A recent study showed that in five cases of posttraumatic anosmia, attempts for the olfactory epithelium to regenerate were curtailed by fibrotic healing of the cribriform plate, which prevented re-establishment of contact with olfactory bulb neurons (Jafek, Eller, Esses, & Moran, 1989).

In the future, microsurgical intervention might be possible in the region of the cribriform plate. Restoration of the sense of smell with such a technique would be theoretically possible. At this time, however, none of the proposed medication interventions, such as the use of zinc or vitamins, especially B vitamins, has proven to be effective in reestablishing or even improving the sense of smell once it has been absent for longer than 6 months. Frequently in mild TBI there is an improvement from an hyposmic state to a less hyposmic state, for which the affected individual is quite thankful.

Posttraumatic Tremor

TBI has been associated with the development of intention tremor. The amplitude of tremor associated with head injury is usually low, and the tremor often does not interfere with activities. A relatively recent report describes seven cases of tremor associated with mild TBI (Biary, Cleeves, Findley, & Koller, 1989). The interval between the head trauma and the onset of symptoms varied from 1 to 4 weeks. Usually the tremor involves the upper extremities and sometimes the head, without signs of other neurologic impairment. Some myoclonic jerking can also be present.

In the treatment of posttraumatic tremor, Clonazapem in doses of 0.5 mg twice a day may be helpful. Some individuals may respond to treatment with Propranolol. Posttraumatic tremor is often a permanent residual symptom. Interestingly enough, Ethanol, which frequently decreases essential tremor, has little or no effect on posttraumatic tremor.

Posttraumatic Neck Pain and Back Pain

Individuals with mild TBI frequently experience cervical pain, sometimes radiating into the shoulders and upper extremities, and lumbar localized back pain, sometimes radiating into the buttocks and proximal lower extremities. The pain is unassociated with any structural pathology of the cervical or lumbar regions. Such pain is especially likely after motor vehicle accidents where there have been significant flexion/extension injuries to the neck or lumbar region (Yarnell & Rossie, 1988). In these cases, neck and back pain are frequently accompanied by migratory paresthesias in the upper extremities and the lower extremities. Abnormalities of sensory, motor, or reflex examination suggest nerve root irritation, and are indications for imaging studies. An MRI of the spine is especially useful to address possible disc herniation, or less frequently, spinal fractures, not seen on screening radiographs. Unless signs of nerve root injury are present on exam, further evaluation or costly imaging studies of the neck and back are not indicated.

In general, physical measures and nonsteroidal anti-inflammatory medications are the best approaches to neck and back pain when they are associated with mild TBI. Unnecessary surgical intervention should be avoided; surgery should be considered only when there is evidence of nerve root impingement. As in the management of posttraumatic headache, avoidance of analgesics, especially narcotic analgesics, is essential for optimal long-term management.

After an initial gentle introduction to physical therapy, a neck and/or back conditioning program will facilitate long-term symptom improvement. A delay in treatment or exposure to forceful manipulative therapies, such as chiropractic, often prolong the symptoms and can, in some cases, aggravate the disability. Both narcotic analgesics and manipulative therapies should be avoided in the management of neck and/or back pain associated with mild TBI. Neck pain and posttraumatic headache are frequently associated and require complementary treatment programs.

Posttraumatic Visual Symptoms

Diplopia and visual blurring are reported in approximately 10% of individuals with mild TBI. The therapeutic approach to these symptoms is often problematic. It is not uncommon to see patients who have had several changes in their visual correction in attempts to improve visual acuity. These changes in correction seldom show lasting benefit.

Therapies that teach coping strategies for visual deficits have shown some efficacy. These are especially beneficial if the patients report disorders of reading and concentration along with their visual symptoms. However, there is danger of costly overcommitment to a vision therapy program, and there have been cases where vision therapy was recommended for up to a year, with several visits a week. Because the efficacy of this type of therapy is questionable at best, lengthy treatment plans should be avoided.

Posttraumatic Depression and Emotional Lability

Depression and emotional lability are not uncommon after mild TBI (Dikmen & Reitan, 1977; Kwentus, Hart, Peck, & Kornstein, 1985). Usually these symptoms are not seen initially, but develop gradually when associated symptoms disrupt functional capacity. Although there may be no change in physical skills, performance in daily functioning may be significantly affected. Attempts to cope with home and work activities tend to be associated with a wide range of emotions, but most typically irritability, emotional lability, fatigue, and feelings of detachment. There may also be associated sleep disorder, and sleep deprivation may further impair the overall functional performance.

Usually a treatment program for these symptoms consists of reassurance, education, and support. However, if the vegetative symptoms typical of depression are prominent, or if the emotional lability is so uncontrollable that it is interfering with work or home activities, then treatment with antidepressive medications needs to be considered. Medications that may be helpful in this setting are not without problems for these patients.

Tricyclic antidepressants are often associated with an increase in anticholinergic symptoms such as drowsiness, dry mouth, weight gain, or constipation. Therefore, these medications are not usually well tolerated in every individual who suffers emotional lability or depression after TBI. On the other hand, if emotional lability is a prominent symptom, then some of the newer serotinergic antidepressants such as Fluoxetine HCL, Sertraline, or Paroxetine may induce a hyperexcitability syndrome. In general, the tricyclic antidepressants such as Amitriptyline, Nortriptyline, or Doxepin are most effective for individuals who have sleep disorder with prominent insomnia, or poor appetite with weight loss. When depression is associated with headache or spinal pain, then tricyclics are also preferred. The serotinergic antidepressants are more effective for individuals who have prominent inanition or withdrawal symptomatology. When individuals with posttraumatic depression are treated with medications, patients must be closely monitored for potential side effects and responses to treatment. When posttraumatic depression is associated with posttraumatic headache, the therapy programs can be complementary. For example, if headaches improve, depression may improve, or vice versa.

Management of Sports-Related Injuries

Somewhat unfortunately, the approach to sports-related mild TBI is generally based on isolated and anecdotal experiences. Concussion is especially common in football and boxing, but does occur in other sports where collisions or falls may occur. Protective equipment and rule changes seem to have had a limited impact on the problem. It was estimated that 250,000 concussions occur annually (Cantu, 1988), and that approximately 20% of high-school players suffer a concussion in a single season (Gerberich, Priest, Boen, Straub, & Maxwell, 1983).

Acute management and management of noncognitive sequelae are essentially no different for sports-related mild TBI, except that repeat injury is possible. Because catastrophic outcome with permanent disability or even death has been reported, this can be an important matter for consideration (Kelly et al., 1991). Therefore, it has been recommended that even when the athlete has a minor concussion without loss of consciousness, he or she be removed from play and only returned if amnesia or other symptoms do not occur for at least 20 minutes. A thorough neurologic evaluation with imaging studies is indicated for concussion with loss of consciousness. Return to contact sports and its timing remain controversial. Usually if any noncognitive or cognitive sequelae persist, athletes should be withheld from contact sports.

Conclusions

There are a wide variety of noncognitive sequelae of mild TBI that are amenable to treatment. An enlightened medical practitioner can be an important part of the treatment team. Medical treatment alone, however, does not usually facilitate the best overall recovery. Cognitive and adjustment issues often dominate and are best managed outside the medical setting.

References

Alexander, M. P. (1995). Mild traumatic brain injury: Pathophysiology, natural history, and clinical management. *Neurology, 45,* 1253–1260.

Biary, N., Cleeves, L., Findley, L., & Koller, W. (1989). Posttraumatic tremor. *Neurology, 39,* 103–106.

Brenner, C., Freidmann, A. P., Merritt, H. H., & Denny-Brown, D. E. (1944). Posttraumatic Headache. *Journal of Neurosurgery, 1,* 379–391.

Cantu, R. C. (1988). When to return to contact sports after a cerebral concussion. *Sports Medicine Digest, 10,* 1–2.

Caveness, W. E. (1976). Epilepsy, a product of trauma in our time. *Epilepsia, 17,* 207–215.

Couch, J. R. (1995). Post-concussion (post-trauma) syndrome. *Journal of Neurologic Rehabilitation, 9,* 83–89.

Dikmen, S., & Reitan, R. M. (1977). Emotional sequelae of head injury. *Annals of Neurology, 2,* 492–494.

Gerberich, S. G., Priest, J. D., Boen, J. R., Straub, C. P., & Maxwell, R. E. (1983). Concussion incidences and severity in secondary school varsity football players. *American Journal of Public Health, 73,* 1370–1375.

Haas, D. C. (1993). Chronic posttraumatic headache. In J. Olesen, P. Tfelt-Hansen, & K. M. A. Welch (Eds.), *The headaches* (pp. 629–638). New York: Raven Press.

Headache Classification Committee of the International Headache Society. (1988). Classification and diagnostic criteria for headache disorders, cranial neuralgias and facial pain. *Cephalgia, 8,* 1–96.

Jafek, B. W., Eller, P. M., Esses, B. A., & Moran, D. T. (1989). Posttraumatic anosmia: Ultrastructural correlate. *Archives of Neurology, 46,* 300–304.

Jensen, O. K., & Neilsen, F. F. (1990). The influence of sex and pre-traumatic headache on the incidence and severity of headache after head injury. *Cephalgia, 26,* 515–516.

Kelly, J. P., Nichols, J. S., Filley, C. M., Lillehei, K. O., Rubinstein, D., & Kleinschmidt-DeMasters, B. K. (1991). Concussion in sports: Guidelines for the prevention of catastrophic outcome. *Journal of the American Medical Association, 266,* 2867–2869.

Kwentus, J. A., Hart, R. P., Peck, E. T., & Kornstein, S. (1985). Psychiatric complications of closed head injury. *Psychosomatics, 26,* 8–15.

Leigh, A. D. (1943). Defect of smell after head injury. *Lancet, 11,* 38–40.

MacDonald, R. L., & McLean, M. J. (1986). Anticonvulsant drugs: Mechanism of action. *Advances in Neurology, 44,* 713–736.

Medina, J. L. (1992). Efficacy of an individualized outpatient program in the treatment of chronic posttraumatic headache. *Headache, 32,* 180–182.

Messenheimer, J., Ramsay, R. E., & Willmore, L. J. (1994). Lamotrigine therapy for partial seizures: A multicenter, placebo-controlled, double-blind, cross-over trial. *Epilepsia, 35,* 113–121.

Miller, H. (1961). Accident neurosis. *British Medical Journal, 1,* 919–925.

Rowe, M. J., & Carlson, L. (1980). Brainstem auditory evoked potentials in posttraumatic dizziness. *Archives of Neurology, 37,* 679–683.

Russell, W. R. (1932). Cerebral involvement in head injury. A study based on the examination of 200 cases. *Brain, 55,* 549–603.

Rutherford, W. H., Merrett, J. D., & McDonald, J. R. (1977). Sequelae of concussion caused by minor head injuries. *Lancet, 1,* 1–4.

Selzer, M. E. (1995). Introduction: Epidemiology and pathophysiology of traumatic brain injury. *Journal of Neurologic Rehabilitation, 9,* 55–60.

Summer, D. (1964). Posttraumatic anosmia. *Brain, 87,* 107–120.

Symonds, C. (1962). Concussion and its sequelae. *Lancet, 1,* 1–5.

Tfelt-Hansen, P., & Welch, K. M. A. (1993). General principles of pharmacological treatment. In J. Olesen, P. Tfelt-Hansen, & K. M. A. Welch (Eds.), *The headaches* (pp. 299–304). New York: Raven Press.

U.S. Gabapentin Study Group No. 5. (1993). Gabapentin as add-on therapy in refractory partial epilepsy: A double-blind, placebo-controlled, parallel-group study. *Neurology, 43,* 2292–2298.

Warner, J. S., & Fenichel, G. M. (1966). Chronic posttraumatic headache often a myth. *Neurology, 46,* 915–916.

Weiss, H. D., Stern, B. J., & Goldberg, J. (1991). Posttraumatic migraine: chronic migraine precipitated by minor head or neck trauma. *Headache, 31,* 451–456.

Wilder, B. J. (1987). Treatment considerations in anticonvulsant monotherapy. *Epilepsia, 28,* S1–S7.

Winston, K. R. (1987). Whiplash and its relation to migraine. *Headache, 27,* 452–457.

Yarnell, P. R., & Rossie, G. V. (1988). Minor whiplash head injury with major debilitation. *Brain Injury, 2,* 255–258.

Outpatient Rehabilitation Program for Individuals with Persisting Mild to Moderate Symptoms Following Mild Traumatic Brain Injury

15

Christy Dittmar

The diagnosis of mild TBI has received considerable attention in recent years, and continues to need clarification among health professionals, the rehabilitation community, and third-party payers. Rehabilitation professionals who subscribe to the definition of mild TBI as drafted by the Mild Traumatic Brain Injury Committee of the Head Injury Interdisciplinary Special Interest Group of the American Congress of Rehabilitation Medicine (1993) agree with the general consensus that mild TBI can result in either little or no sequelae for some individuals, but in significant and long-lasting disability for others. For those who are left with significant deficits, the success of their rehabilitation depends largely on the validation of such factors as changes in cognition, personality, and behavior.

Mild TBI comprises between 70% and 85% of all head injuries reported by hospitals (Kraus & Nourjah, 1988). Rehabilitation professionals are increasingly faced with the treatment of this population and challenged by the unique set of problems. Rimel, Giordani, and Barth (1981) documented three primary problem areas following mild TBI: (a) physical (e.g., headache, vertigo, excessive fatigue, disturbed sleep patterns), (b) cognitive (e.g., concentration, memory, reduced information processing ability, slowed reaction time, and (c) emotional (e.g., irritability, depressed or labile affect). These issues must be considered holistically and as they relate to the client's individual lifestyle.

In this chapter, I present a model of an outpatient interdisciplinary program that focuses on each client's individual needs following TBI. The Brain Injury Recovery Program (BIRP) in Fort Collins, Colorado has evolved over

---

Reprinted, with changes, from "Outpatient Rehabilitation Program for Clients with Persisting Mild to Moderate Symptoms Following Traumatic Brain Injury," by Christy Dittmar, 1997, *Applied Neuropsychology, 4*(1), pp. 50–54. Copyright 1997 by Lawrence Erlbaum Associates, Inc.

the last decade and embraces a neuropsychological foundation for medically based rehabilitation. Treatment goals originate from the problems encountered following a TBI, rather than from the nature of the acute event. We have found that long-term TBI outcomes are best clarified by assessing the post-acute consequences of the injury. During the last 10 years, we have had contact with approximately 2,000 individuals and their families who have experienced the effects of what was initially diagnosed as mild brain injury. Many times individuals with mild TBI are discharged from a hospital emergency room without any perceived need for formal rehabilitation. Although these individuals do not appear impaired to medical personnel and family, many of them experience great difficulty when they attempt to resume their responsibilities at home, work, or school.

Consistent with other research (e.g., Leininger & Kreutzer, 1992), our findings indicate complex, yet subtle, symptomatology. As noted in this literature review, we also observe that deficits appear mostly in the form of altered attention, concentration, information processing speed, memory, and reasoning. Language, sensory, motor, and visual abilities may be affected as well. Relationships with family, peers, and coworkers often suffer, and psychological stability may be at risk. Fatigue and irritability are common problems that contribute to lack of success at work, home, or school.

As discussed by Bennett, Dittmar, and Ho (1997), there are a constellation of cognitive, emotional, personality, and noncognitive symptoms that interact to produce the postconcussive syndrome (PCS). Factors to consider include the effect of diffuse injury in producing decreased speed and efficiency of thinking, difficulty ignoring nonrelevant environmental information, and increased difficulty in retrieval processes. These deficits, in turn, disrupt dependent cognitive processes such as attention, learning and memory, perception, communication, problem solving, and general intelligence.

Authors such as Rimel et al. (1981) and Leininger, Gramling, and Farrell (1990) discuss subtle, but measurable, neuropsychological deficits and persisting postconcussive symptoms that represent central nervous system (CNS) dysfunction. However, it is critical to screen for the disproportionate cognitive deficits that accompany chronic pain and psychological distress (e.g., psychological factors, anxiety, depression, posttraumatic headaches, epilepsy, sensory deficits). Psychological support and neurological management are key factors in completing the rehabilitation picture of these individuals.

Critical Features of Rehabilitation

A comprehensive team approach is essential in maximizing functional ability and preventing the magnification of postconcussive symptoms. The client and family are initially provided education and support, in conjunction with a systematic evaluation of skills for daily living, schooling, and work. The team, in which the client and family are integral members, shares one goal: the client's rehabilitation and reentry into the community.

The course of rehabilitation with TBI has been conceptualized by many authors (e.g., Goldstein & Ruthven, 1983; Kreutzer & Wehman, 1990; Ylvisaker & Gobble, 1987) as a process of integrating the frames of reference from neuropsychology, physical therapy, occupational therapy, speech and language pathology, and clinical psychology. In addition, Gronwall (1986) identified four elements of rehabilitation that are important after mild head injury: reassurance, education, support, and regular monitoring of progress. These elements of treatment should be included in all regular rehabilitation sessions, and addressed separately in individual or group counseling meetings.

- **Reassurance.** Validation of symptoms is needed. Deficits in functioning may exist even when physical appearance is normal. Coping with normal home and work activities may be overly stressful. A faster recovery is promoted by reassurance from professionals and others with injuries that symptoms will improve.

- **Education.** Explanation of findings, reason for therapy schedule, and expectations empowers the client. Practical changes, such as possible changes in sleep patterns, fatigue, and memory gaps, are discussed, as is avoiding further injuries by not drinking or engaging in contact sports.

- **Support.** Clients may need assistance in decision making and problem solving, or support from outside agencies, such as Consumer Credit Counseling. According to Miller and Jones (1990), if individuals with mild TBI have access to sympathetic and informed advice and supervision, they might avoid much anxiety and have fewer other problems.

- **Regular monitoring.** The client's participation is encouraged by regular progress reviews that involve the client and family in goal setting, and active involvement at each session. New problems are quickly identified and resolved. This creates an open, trusting rapport between the client and rehabilitation team. Feedback from the therapist and peers ensures that generalization is occurring.

- **Compensation and remediation.** In addition to the preceding four elements, we would add that rehabilitation should emphasize the processes of compensation and remediation. Cognitive rehabilitation is thought to be restorative (developing a reorganization of partially damaged neurocognitive systems) or compensatory (developing behaviors to accomplish goals without depending on damaged neurocognitive systems). Successful adaptation to the changes produced by a mild head injury involves an integration of both processes. Therapy is geared toward improving functional outcome.

Following the learning of a new strategy, the client has an opportunity to try it in simulated or real-life environments (home, work, or community). For example, a person with memory problems may receive training to improve attention and therefore memory capacity (remedial training). He or she is also taught strategies to counteract the memory deficit, such as a personal memory book, mnemonics, note-taking, verbal rehearsing, and using timers and alarms (compensatory).

The program described in this chapter is a comprehensive integrated approach, as described by Prigatano, Fordyce, and Zeiner (1986), Ben-Yishay and Prigatano (1990), and Malec, Schafer, and Jacket (1992). With this approach, the problems of individuals with TBI are addressed in a coordinated, organized, and integrated manner. An actual working system of multidisciplinary treatment is needed for success.

Program Design

The program at BIRP, diagrammed in Figure 15.1, is a product of many years of experience and information gathering with survivors, families, and other providers. The model includes an interdisciplinary program consisting of cognitive rehabilitation, occupational therapy, speech and language pathology, physical therapy, neuropsychological counseling, biofeedback, vocational rehabilitation, and neurology, which are provided through individualized treatment plans. It is a distributed-practice approach that emphasizes the rehabilitation of functional skills.

The program and physical facilities allow individuals with mild or moderate TBI to choose a comfortable level of integration with others who are recovering from more severe TBI. We accomplish this by using multiple sites for treatment and flexible programming. We plan schedules to encourage adequate rest, peer support, and social opportunities, as appropriate for all. Community-based treatment facilitates combined sharing, mutual learning, support, and companionship.

Neuropsychology is the primary focus when the client enters the program and provides an assessment of all symptoms. Using this neuropsychological information, we can comprehensively assess all appropriate disciplines. Following the assessment, we develop treatment goals and a plan at a meeting with the client and family. Each plan is individualized and based on the unique strengths and weaknesses of each client. Neuropsychological counseling (psychotherapy) may also be indicated on entrance to the program, to provide emotional support and to assist the client in distinguishing TBI symptoms from psychological issues. The family is included in this education and support through individual or group settings. This approach is very specialized and has been developed in consideration of the needs of previous clients.

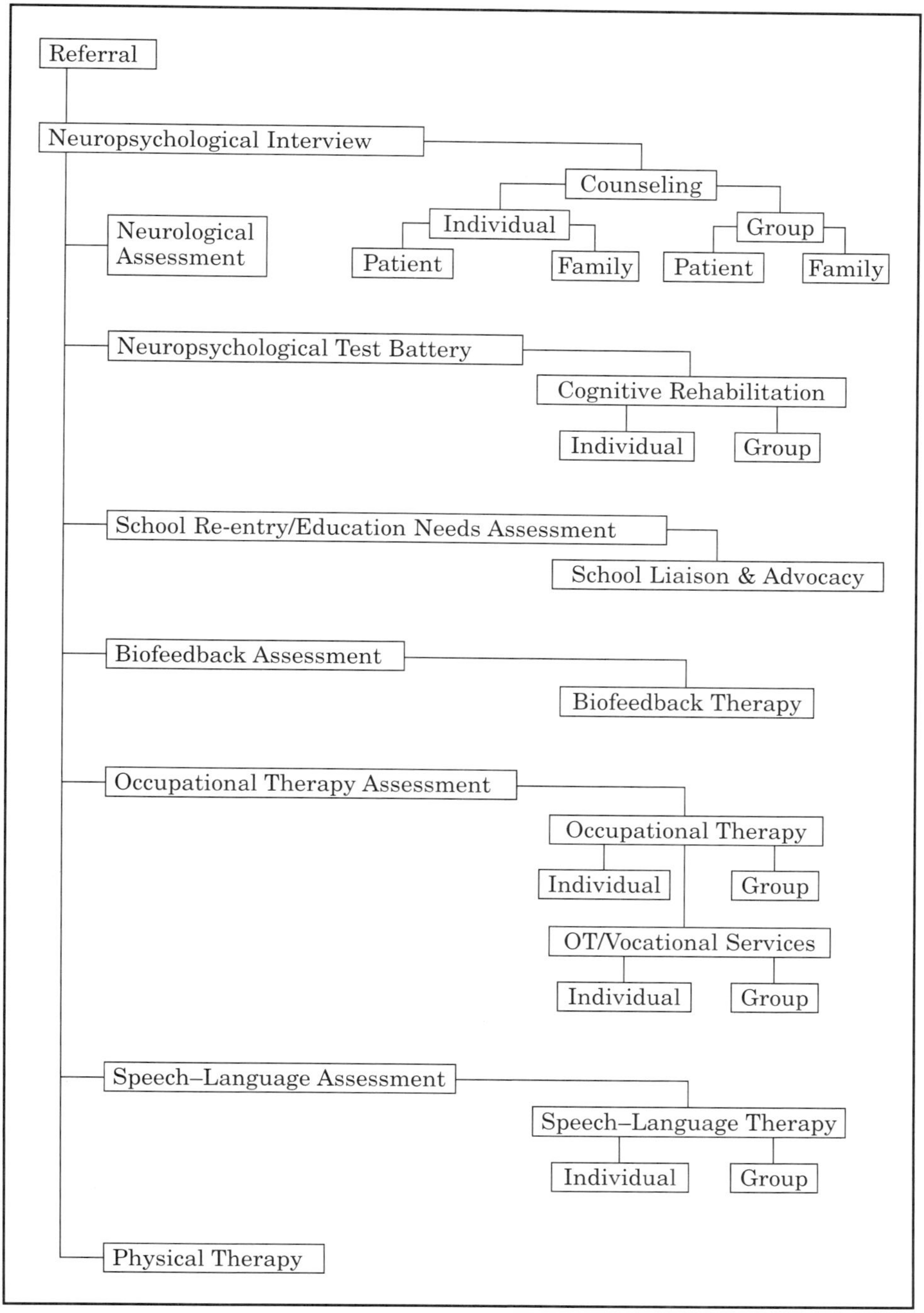

Figure 15.1. Services flow chart for the Brain Injury Recovery (BIRP) program.

Biofeedback is particularly effective when musculoskeletal problems are producing pain and when the client is experiencing posttraumatic stress. We incorporate autogenic training, visualization, and relaxation training in pain and stress management. Biofeedback therapy will interact with physical therapy.

We develop cognitive rehabilitation goals from the neuropsychological assessments. Deficit areas may include attention, concentration, memory, learning, flexibility of thinking, speed of processing, and executive skills. The cognitive therapist may be a specialist in cognitive rehabilitation, a speech–language pathologist, or an occupational therapist. Cognitive goals are often included in the related goal areas of speech or occupational therapy. We always emphasize practical application of remediation to real-life situations.

The occupational therapist addresses higher level functional skills referred to as *activities of daily living.* Typically, the person with mild TBI will independently perform basic daily activities, such as dressing, bathing, grooming, and cooking, but will have difficulty sequencing these activities at a real-life pace. The client may be able to complete each task individually but unable to integrate and prioritize tasks into a full day of activities. Generally, some form of memory and organization problem is the interfering factor. Normal environmental distractions and demands exaggerate memory and organization problems, and may interfere with previously used strategies. Time management and organization strategies may need to be modified to ensure safety and success. Other strategies for compensation of memory, organization, and executive skills are woven into the remedial training with cognitive rehabilitation.

Occupational therapists also provide vision screenings to assess convergence, acuity, and binocular functioning. Vestibular programs are often needed when there is damage to this system. This usually follows an evaluation by an otology specialist. Driving assessments are initiated by an occupational therapist who is familiar with diagnostic sequelae, driving skill testing, and with motor vehicle department or driver control regulations. A careful evaluation and cooperation from the treating physician are essential in this process.

When physical therapy (PT) is needed, a referral is made and included in the full plan. The physical therapist works as a member of the rehabilitation team to address problems of mobility, musculoskeletal dysfunction, pain, and motor control skills. PT treatment relies heavily on appropriate exercise, along with manual techniques and other more traditional modalities, to remediate deficits. It may be necessary to hold back on other therapies until these somatic or pain problems are successfully managed. For best results, the physical therapist should have experience with the sequelae of mild TBI, such as fatigue and overload.

The speech–language pathologist addresses those deficits that are language based. Practical language problems may be observed or determined from family information. Treatment may be individual or in groups, and it targets problems found in formal assessment of oral motor skills, swallowing, memory, attention, reading, communication, comprehension, and writing skills.

Vocational issues are often the most critical and of highest priority for clients and their families. This service begins as soon as the client has resolved the majority of pain problems and has manageable fatigue with appropriate emotional stability. We use information from the comprehensive team evaluation to develop a return-to-work plan or to maintain existing employment. Careful timing and education of employers will result in job retention. Job analysis may be needed to make changes to the work environment or work tasks.

The return-to-work phase is the most demanding part of recovery and requires an experienced vocational specialist. It is critical to provide ongoing vocational services as clients resume employment.

Other specialists who often participate in the treatment include behavioral optometrists, otolaryngologists for vestibular or balance problems, central auditory processing specialists, driver education trainers, endocrinologists, dieticians, and massage therapists.

The person with mild TBI has unique confidentiality concerns, and the staff must be particularly mindful of this during community-based treatment. For example, name tags are removed in sensitive situations, and clients may need to anonymously observe from a distance in some cases. Public acknowledgement of an injury is handled in a sensitive and confidential manner. Return-to-work issues are individualized by the client and employer. The employment plan includes education of coworkers at a level that does not jeopardize long-term working relationships.

Pediatric rehabilitation needs are unique and require additional specialists. The school reentry program, directed by a school psychologist, provides services to meet the special needs of children and adolescents with brain injuries. Services include remediation and improvement of cognitive, sensory/perceptual, physical/motor, and communication deficits. We will also coordinate therapy and school district services, such as homebound teaching. We provide the student with skills (cognitive and social interactive) to meet the demands of school. Education of school personnel and special education services regarding the student's needs is critical for successful reentry.

Our observations match those of another study (Gerber & Schraa, 1995) in which participants with mild TBI showed a decline in somatic symptoms but an increase in the average number of cognitive symptoms at 6-month follow-up. This finding is consistent with research that shows awareness of subjective cognitive symptoms may increase over time as individuals with mild TBI are challenged by their environments.

Rehabilitation occurs in an outpatient setting that uses community and home-based activities as much as possible. The program atmosphere is relaxed and nonmedical, and promotes maximum functioning through individual and group activities. The treatment environment is perceived as a safe place to practice skills with others who understand the person's needs. Purposeful rehabilitation extends beyond the clinic into community sites (e.g., gyms, pools, health clubs, malls, restaurants, grocery stores, work, or home). Schedules for individual therapy vary from one to three sessions per week to less contact, as needed, after a transition back to work or school, or on completion of the program. Terminology of *client* versus *patient* reflects the expectation that the client will be an active partner in the program.

Efficacy of Treatment

The BIRP asserts that the ultimate measure of the success of a rehabilitation program for mild TBI is an increase in independent daily living skills. Through holistic rehabilitation, clients participate in a program that includes a blend of remedial and compensatory training.

Using clients from the BIRP, Ho and Bennett (1997) investigated the efficacy of cognitive rehabilitation in clients with mild to moderate TBI. They studied 36 clients who participated in cognitive rehabilitation from 1988 to 1992. All participants met stringent selection criteria on age, injury, cognitive impairment severity, etiology of injury, postinjury to initial assessment interval, neuropsychological measures obtained, rehabilitation program components received, and rehabilitative status.

Selected tests from the fully administered *Halstead-Reitan Neuropsychological Battery* (HRNB) were used in the data analysis. Modified rating scales were used to assess cognitive and behavioral processes related to activities of daily living. The scales were modified to address the levels of cognitive functioning model proposed by Bennett (1992), as well as other measures deemed important to daily living skills. Four cognitive scales assessed speed of processing, attention, memory, and executive functions in the client's daily activities. Five scales addressed behavioral processes related to cognitive ability, and included vocational and educational status, social and interpersonal interactions, leisure activities, emotional adjustment, and cognitive stamina.

Comparison of neuropsychological test scores before and after rehabilitation indicated significant improvement ($p \leq .05$) on most of the measures considered. The posttest was administered 6 to 12 months after the pretest so there would be no practice effect. There was also a significant improvement in functional performance as indicated by ratings on the behavioral scales. That is, individuals who participated in rehabilitation treatment showed a significant improvement in their activities of daily living and in their cognitive functioning on the selected neuropsychological tests.

As emphasized in this study, the assessment tools that we have available for clients with mild injuries do not accurately measure the significant impact that these injuries have on cognitive functioning and daily living skills. There is an ongoing need for an assessment that is more sensitive to the impact on functioning and that will contribute to the research base.

Other informal outcome data from BIRP indicate that individuals with TBI make greater gains when the therapy is spread over time and intensity is gradually reduced so that transfer to real-life situations can occur. The extension of rehabilitation over months rather than weeks is difficult to accomplish with managed care restraints. This challenge will require creativity, communication at a different level with insurance resources, and rehabilitation that is efficient and consumer-oriented.

Conclusions

The rehabilitation of the person with mild TBI has made great strides during the last decade. As we move toward improved diagnostic tools and better descriptions, we must also improve the design of service delivery for these individuals. The needs of this population dictate a unique model of an interdisciplinary, distributed-practice approach in an outpatient environment. Recovery should be aimed at improving functional problems and driven by the perceived purposefulness to the client. Program effectiveness should be measured by the client and his or her support system. In this chapter, I described a model interdisciplinary outpatient program that promotes the community reintegration of the individual who has experienced major difficulty from a mild TBI. This program uses a neuropsychological foundation for community-based rehabilitation. Results of an efficacy study indicate significant improvement in most measures considered.

References

Bennett, T. L. (1992). Conceptualizing traumatic brain injuries. *The Journal of Head Injury, 3,* 21–28.

Bennett, T. L., Dittmar, C., & Ho, M. (1997). The neuropsychology of traumatic brain injury. In A. M. Horton, D. Wedding, & J. Webster (Eds.), *The neuropsychology handbook: Treatment issues and special populations* (2nd ed., pp. 123–172). New York: Springer.

Ben-Yishay, Y., & Prigatano, G. P. (1990). Cognitive remediation. In M. Rosenthal, E. R. Griffith, M. R. Bond, & J. D. Miller (Eds.), *Rehabilitation of the adult and child with traumatic brain injury* (pp. 236–247). Philadelphia: Davis.

Gerber, D. J., & Schraa, J. C. (1995). Mild traumatic brain injury: Searching for the syndrome. *Journal of Head Trauma Rehabilitation, 10,* 28–40.

Goldstein, G., & Ruthven, L. (1983). *Rehabilitation of the brain damaged adult.* New York: Plenum.

Gronwall, D. (1986). Rehabilitation programs for patients with mild head injury: Components, problems, and evaluation. *Journal of Head Trauma Rehabilitation, 1,* 53–62.

Ho, M. R., & Bennett, T. L. (1997). Efficacy of neuropsychological rehabilitation following mild-moderate traumatic brain injury. *Archives of Clinical Neuropsychology, 12,* 1–11.

Kraus, J. F., & Nourjah, P. (1988). The epidemiology of mild, uncomplicated brain injury. *Journal of Trauma, 28,* 1637–1643.

Kreutzer, J. S., & Wehman, P. (1990). *Community integration following traumatic brain injury.* Baltimore: Brookes.

Leininger, B. E., Gramling, S. E., & Farrell, A. D. (1990). Neuropsychological deficits in symptomatic minor head injury patients after concussion and mild concussion. *Journal of Neurological Neurosurgery Psychiatry, 53,* 293–296.

Leininger, B. E., & Kreutzer, J. S. (1992). Neuropsychological outcomes of adults with mild traumatic brain injury: Implications for clinical practice and research. In L. J. Horn & N. D. Zasler (Eds.), *Physical medicine and rehabilitation: State of the art reviews* (pp. 169–182). Philadelphia: Hanley & Belfus.

Malec, J., Schafer, D., & Jacket, M. (1992). Comprehensive-integrated postacute outpatient brain injury rehabilitation. *NeuroRehabilitation, 2*(3), 1–11.

Mild Traumatic Brain Injury Committee of the Head Injury Interdisciplinary Special Interest Group of the American Congress of Rehabilitation Medicine (1993). Definition of mild traumatic brain injury. *Journal of Head Trauma Rehabilitation, 8,* 86–87.

Miller, J. D., & Jones, P. A. (1990). Minor head injury. In M. Rosenthal, E. R. Griffith, M. R. Bond, & J. D. Miller (Eds.), *Rehabilitation of the adult and child with traumatic brain injury* (2nd ed., pp. 236–247). Philadelphia: Davis.

Prigatano, G., Fordyce, D. J., & Zeiner, H. K. (1986). *Neuropsychological rehabilitation after brain injury.* Baltimore: Johns Hopkins University Press.

Rimel, R., Giordani, B., & Barth, J. (1981). Disability caused by minor head injury. *Neurosurgery, 9,* 221–228.

Ylvisaker, M., & Gobble, E. M. (1987). *Community reentry for head injured adults.* Boston: Little, Brown.

About the Editors

Michael J. Raymond, PhD, ABPN, received his PhD from Florida State University in 1981. For the past 12 years he has been director of neuropsychological/cognitive services at Allied Services, John Heinz Institute of Rehabilitation Medicine, Wilkes-Barre, Pennsylvania. He is also a consultant neuropsychologist for Monmouth Neuropsychological Associates, Red Bank, New Jersey. Dr. Raymond teaches graduate neuropsychology courses and serves as a clinical surveyor (brain injury programs) for the Commission on Accreditation of Rehabilitation Facilities (CARF). He is an examiner for the American Board of Professional Neuropsychology and New Jersey State Board of Psychologists. He is a fellow of the National Academy of Neuropsychology and the American College of Professional Neuropsychology. He is a diplomate of the American Board of Professional Neuropsychology. He has authored and co-authored numerous peer reviewed articles and book chapters, presented at national and international conferences, and serves on editorial boards.

Thomas L. (Tim) Bennett, PhD, ABPN, ABPP is a Professor Emeritus of psychology at Colorado State University where, in 1996, he was named the University Honored Scientist by Sigma Xi. He was named the distinguished graduate educator by the College of Natural Sciences in 1998. He is clinical director of the multidisciplinary Brain Injury Recovery Program in Fort Collins, Colorado. He is the author or co-author of over 135 publications including *Brain and Behavior* (1977), *The Sensory World: An Introduction to Sensation and Perception* (1978), *The Psychology of Learning and Memory* (1979), *Introduction to Physiological Psychology* (1982), *The Neuropsychology of Epilepsy* (1992), *Brainwave-R: Cognitive Strategies and Techniques for Brain Injury Rehabilitation* (1997), and *Psychology Video Teaching Modules: The Brain, Second Edition* (1997). He is board certified in neuropsychology (American Board of Professional Neuropsychology) and rehabilitation psychology (American Board of Professional Psychology). He is currently president of the American Board of Professional Neuropsychology. In the past he has served as a member of the board of directors and the annual conference coordinator for the National Academy of Neuropsychology. He is a fellow of the National Academy of Neuropsychology, the American Psychological Association, and the American Psychological Society.

Lawrence C. Hartlage, PhD, ABPN, ABPP, has served as president of the National Academy of Neuropsychology, the American Board of Professional Neuropsychology, and American Psychological Association Division of Neuropsychology. He has also authored more than 200 books, invited chapters, and articles. In the forensic arena, he has been court-appointed expert witness in more than 3,000 hearings, and has testified as expert witness in more than 30 jurisdictions in the United States and Canada. His degrees are from Ohio State University and the University of Louisville.

C. Munro Cullum, PhD, ABPP, received his PhD from The University of Texas at Austin and obtained residency training in clinical neuropsychology at the University of California-San Diego and the San Diego VA Hospital. He currently is associate professor of psychiatry and neurology and director of neuropsychology at The University of Texas Southwestern Medical Center at Dallas. He is a diplomate of the American Board of Professional Psychology/American Board of Clinical Neuropsychology and is actively involved in clinical practice, research, and teaching in neuropsychology at the doctoral and post-doctoral level. He is president of the National Academy of Neuropsychology and was the executive director of that organization for 6 years. He served as a delegate to The Houston Conference on Specialty Training and Education in Neuropsychology and is a member-at-large of Division 40 (Clinical Neuropsychology) of the American Psychological Association. He has been the recipient of a number of federally and foundation-funded research grants, with much of his research in the area of neuropsychological functions in aging and dementia. Dr. Cullum has authored and co-authored more than 60 articles and two books. He serves on the editorial boards of several neuropsychology journals and is a reviewer for multiple journals in psychology, psychiatry, and neurology.

Author Index

Abbott, R. D., 82, 83
Abildskov, T. J., 26
Abrams, 213
Ackley, A., 120
Ackley, B., 41
Adams, J. H., 32, 213
Adams, L., 123
Adams, R. L., 53, 166, 174
Adams, W., 96
Albert, J., 99
Alexander, M. P., 12, 37, 41, 138, 255
Allen, C., 78
Alves, W. M., 31, 34, 41, 49, 124, 232, 239
Aman, M., 99
Amato, R. C. d'. *See* D'Amato, R. C.
American Academy of Neurology, 33, 120, 121, 124, 138
American Academy of Pediatrics, 121
American Psychiatric Association, 163, 168, 177, 188
American Psychological Association, 161, 167
Amparo, E., 141, 208
Anastasi, A., 167
Anderson, C. V., 19, 23, 26
Anderson, S. W., 222
Annegers, J. R., 64, 135
Ardila, A., 79
Armsden, G., 34, 209, 210, 212
Arnold, L. E., 99
Asarnow, R. F , 99
Assessment of Brain SPECT, 23
Augustiny, K. F., 32
Ayers, A. J., 83

Bachen, N. I., 125
Bagby, R. M., 178
Bailey, B. J., 26
Ball, J. D., 82
Balla, D. A., 90
Bandeen-Roche, K., 123, 126
Barbera, M., 248
Barkley, R. A., 98
Barona, A., 173
Barth, C. Leon-. *See* Leon-Barth, C.
Barth, J. T., 1, 6, 34, 34–35, 41, 64, 77, 78, 80, 83, 87, 101, 102, 103, 117–118, 120, 124, 138, 139, 141, 159, 162, 163–164, 203, 232, 239, 240, 267, 268
Bass, A. E., 36, 211
Batchelor, E. S., 79, 82, 83, 85, 91
Batchelor, J., 234
Battig, W. F., 244
Bauer, R. M., 83, 86
Bayre, A. D. Hinton-. *See* Hinton-Bayre, A. D.
Beck, L. H., 99
Becker, D. P., 136
Becker, T., 126
Beeson, J. A. O., 172, 174
Bell, I., 139
Bell, K., 23–26
Benedict, R. H. B., 99
Benfante, P., 138
Bennett, A., 121, 140
Bennett, T. L., 4, 6–7, 7, 70, 219, 268, 274
Benson, D. F., 32, 240
Benton, A. C., 139
Benton, A. L., 31, 63, 64, 65, 78, 119
Ben-Yishay, Y., 270
Bergstrand, G., 122
Bernard, B. A., 172
Berninger, V. W., 82, 83
Berry, D. T., 174
Beverly, D., 123
Biary, N., 261
Bigler, E. D., 5, 11, 12, 14, 16, 19, 23, 26, 32, 37, 77, 83, 85, 91, 92, 96, 96–98, 98, 99
Bijur, P. E., 101
Binder, H., 23
Binder, L. M., 34, 172, 177, 178, 189
Bixby-Hammett, D. M., 126
Bjorgen, I. A., 240
Bjorkstein, G., 231
Black, F. O., 240
Black, F. W., 222
Black, M. A., 64
Blair, J., 172
Blatter, D. D., 14, 19, 23, 26
Bleiberg, J., 236
Bo, K., 240
Boelens, M. E., 231
Boen, J. R., 118, 263
Bohnen, N., 31, 32, 35, 235
Boll, T. J., 1, 64, 77, 78, 80, 82, 83, 87, 90, 92, 99, 100, 101, 102, 103, 117–118, 120, 124, 138, 139, 141, 203
Bolter, J. F., 86, 174
Bond, M. R., 2, 204, 205
Bornstein, R. A., 220
Bortolotti, P., 234
Bossuyt, A., 23
Botscheller, M. L., 140
Bouman, D. E. , 173
Bourke, D., 173
Bowen, J. D., 121
Bowers, S., 64
Bowman, K. M., 205, 207, 209
Branch, W. B., 85, 89, 96
Bransome, E. D., 99

Brenner, C., 256
Brenner, R., 136
Breslau, N., 79
Brewer, M. Carson-. *See* Carson-Brewer, M.
Briggs, J. R., 139
Briggs, M., 235
Brink, J. D., 86
Brockett, D.R., 140
Brooks, D. N., 101, 102
Brooks, N., 123
Brown, D., 136, 141
Brown, D. E. Denny-. *See* Denny-Brown, D. E.
Brown, G., 90, 102, 173, 174
Brown, L. M., 36, 164
Brown, R., 127
Bruner, J. S., 241
Brunt, R. T. van. *See* Van Brunt, R. T.
Bryan, J. E., 173
Bryant, R. A., 234
Buchsbaum, M. S., 119
Burnett, B., 19, 23, 26
Burns, H. J., 37
Burr, R. B., 14, 16
Burrows, L., 35
Bushnell, D. L., 23, 70
Butcher, J. N., 179
Butler, R., 123

Callahan, C. D., 173
Callahan, T. S., 96
Campbell, D. A., 174
Cantu, R. C., 120, 124, 263
Carico, G. A., 120
Carlson, L., 259
Carpenter, G. S., 174
Carson-Brewer, M., 123
Carter, A., 99
Casat, C. D.
Casey, R., 102
Casson, I. R., 122
Cavallo, M., 31
Caveness, W. E., 258
Caveness, W. F., 1, 135
Celentano, D., 123, 126
Chadwick, O., 79, 90, 94, 99, 102
Chapman, R. W., 136
Chase, R. F., 233
Chastain, R. L., 173
Chelune, G. J., 100, 175, 176
Cheng, C. L., 136
Chibnall, J. T., 239
Chitooran, M. M., 80
Christensen, B., 99
Christman, C., 136
Chun, M., 23–26
Chung, D. G., 23
Cicchetti, D. V., 88, 90
Cicerone, K. D., 7, 119, 233, 234, 235, 238, 239, 241, 242, 245
Clark, K., 139
Clark, L., 81, 87
Claussen, B., 141
Clavette, K., 121
Cleeves, L., 261
Clikeman, M. Semrud-. *See* Semrud-Clikeman, M.
Cobbs, L. Ewing-. *See* Ewing-Cobbs, L.
Cochrane, R. H. B., 174
Cohen, M. J., 85, 89, 96, 98
Cole, M., 122
Collins, L. F., 166, 176
Collins, M. W., 41
Collinson, D., 126
Committee on Ethical Guidelines for Forensic Psychologists, 165, 167
Conners, C., 99
Conroy, C., 101
Cook, L. K., 248
Coonley-Hoganson, R., 64
Corrigan, S. K., 196
Couch, J. R., 258
Craig, P. L., 174
Crane, M. Uddo-. *See* Uddo-Crane, M.
Crawford, J. R., 172, 174
Crockett, D. D., 139
Crossen, J. R., 173
Crouch, J. A., 119
Crovitz, H. F., 205
Cullum, C. M., 5, 41, 136

Dacey, R. G., 31, 212
Dahlstrom, W. G., 179
Damasio, A. R., 222
D'Amato, R. C., 79, 80, 82, 83, 89, 103
Dane, J. R. , 240
Daniel, M. S., 207, 210
Daniel, W. F., 205
Das, J. P., 83, 91
Daubert v. Merrell Chemical Co., 153, 192
Davidoff, D. A., 210
Davis, M. E., 147
Davison, L. A., 92
Day, D., 99
Dean, R. S., 78, 79, 82, 83, 91, 139, 140
Deary, I. J., 240
Deecke, L., 23
DeFilippis, N. A., 135
DeGood, D. E., 240
DeLacey, G., 172
DeLee, J. C., 123
Delis, D. C., 177
DeMasters, B. K. Kleinschmidt-. *See* Kleinschmidt-DeMasters, B. K.
Denckla, M. B., 100
Denker, P. G., 209
Denny-Brown, D. E., 256
Deno, S. L., 94
DePompei, R., 102
Desai, B. T., 64
Deviaene, C., 212, 214
Dickens, S. E., 178
Dicker, B. G., 204, 208, 221
Dieter, J., 138
DiGiulio, D. V., 36, 211
Dikmen, S., 34, 36, 37, 39, 40, 63, 64, 67, 120, 138, 139, 141, 172, 205, 206, 207, 208, 209, 210, 212, 262–263
Di Stefano, G., 32, 240
Dittmar, C., 7, 268
Dixon, C., 119
Dixon, C. E., 140–141
Dodrill, C. B., 164
Dolezal-Wood, S , 36
Donders, J., 91
Dooneief, G., 23–26
Dotan, M., 91
Dougall, N., 240
Doyle, D., 213
Drenan, S. E., 240
Duckett, S., 119
Duckett, S., 119
Duckro, P. N., 239
Duff, K., 6
Duffy, J., 23

Duncan, G. W., 138, 139
Dvorak, J., 240

Earnest, K., 36
Ebmeier, K. P , 240
Edgecombe, M. Schmitter-. *See* Schmitter-Edgecombe, M.
Edgell, D., 50, 77, 82, 84, 86
Edman, G., 122
Einhaus, S. L., 32
Eisenberg, H. M., 5, 31, 32, 34, 37, 49, 64, 64–65, 65, 67, 70, 96, 119, 120, 139, 141, 208, 212, 239
Eliason, M. J., 99
Eller, P. M., 261
Ellmo, W., 233
Ely, P., 139
Endicott, J., 178
Enz, B. E., 136
Eppinger, M. G., 174
Erdal, K., 35
Eriksson, E., 121, 122, 125
Esselman, P. C., 240
Esses, B. A., 261
Ettlin, T. M., 32, 240
Evans, R. W., 138, 235
Ewing-Cobbs, L., 81, 82, 96
Ezrachi, O., 31

Fahy, J. F., 209
Falasca, A., 234
Fan, X., 92
Fann, J. R., 240
Farney, W. C., 123
Farrell, A. D., 33, 206, 237, 268
Faust, D., 159
Fay, G. E., 82, 83
Feinsod, M., 5
Felix, R., 123
Felten, R., 123
Fenichel, G. M., 257
Fennell, E. B., 83, 86
Ferris, L. M., 98
Fichera, S., 35
Fife, D., 101, 212
Filley, C. M., 33, 264
Filippis, N. A. de. *See* DeFilippis, N. A.
Findley, L., 261
Finlayson, M. A. J., 52
Fisher J., 3
Fisher J. M., 164
Fletcher, J. M., 77, 81, 83, 85, 86, 89, 96, 105, 166
Fletcher–Janzen, E., 86, 103, 104, 105
Ford, I., 213
Fordyce, D. J., 139, 270
Forsythe, W., 123
Foster, J. B., 126
Fox, D. D., 36
Fox, J. H., 172
Francis, J. P., 6
Frankowski, R. F., 1, 37, 120, 135
Franks, W., 23
Franzen, M. D., 96, 177, 189
Fraser, R., 141, 209
Freidmann, A. P., 256
French, L. R., 141
Frier, R. M., 240
Frye, D., 99
Frye v. United States, 153, 192
Fuchs, L. S., 94
Fullerton, L., 126
Funke, W., 123

Gaddes, W. H., 50, 83, 84
Galanty, H. L., 125
Galbraith, S., 123
Gale, S. D., 16, 19, 26
Gandy, S., 121
Garmoe, W. S., 236
Garrett, A. L., 86
Gary, H. E. Jr., 174, 210, 239
Gbadebo, D. M., 141
Gean, A. D., 11
Geary, D. C., 94
Geckler, C. L., 227
Geffen, G., 41, 121
Gennarelli, T. A., 3, 32, 33, 119, 136, 139, 213
Gentilini, M., 64, 67, 138, 234
Gerber, D. J., 273
Gerberich, S. G., 118, 124, 263
Gfeller, J. D., 239
Giacino, J. T., 245
Gibbs, N., 126
Gilger, J. W., 94
Gillberg, C., 96
Gilley, D. W., 172
Gimse, R., 240
Giordani, B., 1, 34, 34–35, 64, 117–118, 120, 124, 138, 139, 141, 203, 267, 268
Giuliano, A. J., 162, 163–164
Glasgow, R. E., 248
Glucksman, C. E., 85
Gobble, E. M., 269
Goethe, K. E., 139, 141
Goldberg, J., 256
Golden, C. J., 92, 94
Goldenberg, G., 23
Golding, J., 101
Goldman, P. S., 86
Goldman-Rakic, P. S., 86
Goldstein, F. C., 174
Goldstein, G., 269
Goldstein, K., 219
Good, D. E. de. *See* DeGood, D. E.
Goodwin, G. M., 240
Gordon, B., 123, 126
Gouvier, W. D., 36, 164, 174
Grabow, J. D., 64, 135
Grady, M. S., 136
Graham, D. I., 213
Graham, D. L., 14, 32
Graham, J. R., 179
Graham, P., 79
Gramling, S. E., 33, 206, 237, 268
Grant, I., 37, 38, 41, 52, 55, 169, 174
Gray, B. G., 23
Gray, J. A., 80
Gray, J. W., 78, 79, 82, 83, 91
Green, G. A., 125
Green, J., 138
Gresham, F. M., 88, 103
Griffiths, M. V., 240
Grigsby, J. P., 139
Grimm, R. J., 240
Grisell, J., 173
Gronwall, D., 34, 36, 64, 67, 120, 204, 207, 210, 211, 214, 231–232, 234, 269
Gronwall, G., 239
Grossier, D. B., 100
Grossman, R. G., 34, 63, 78, 139, 209
Guildburd, J. M., 5

Guilmette J., 175, 176, 236
Guinto, F. C., 32, 34
Guse, C. E., 121
Gustavson, J. L., 94
Guthkelch, A. N., 204
Gutkin, T. B., 173

Haak, R. A., 77, 101, 105
Haas, D.C., 256
Haase, R. F., 41
Haban, G., 207
Hadley, M., 5
Haglund, Y., 121, 122, 125
Hale, W. R., 86
Haley, P.R. Lees-. *See* Lees-Haley, P. R.
Hall, C., 123, 126
Hall, D. E., 102
Hall, D. F., 37
Hallett, M., 11
Halperin, J. M., 79, 99
Halpern, E. L., 236
Ham, L. P., 239
Hamilton, M. G., 126
Hamm, R. J., 141
Hammett, D. M. Bixby-. *See* Bixby-Hammett, D. M.
Hanlon, R. E., 244
Hansen, P. Tfelt-. *See* Tfelt-Hansen, P.
Harbaugh, R. E., 141
Hardman, J. M., 122
Harrington, D. E., 119
Harris, A. E., 99
Harris, P., 86
Hart, K. J., 178
Hart, R. P., 262–263
Hartlage, L. C., 6, 80, 84, 85, 135, 136, 137, 138, 139, 140, 141
Hartshorne, M. F., 11
Harvey, A. G., 234
Haslum, M., 101
Hathaway, R., 168
Haut, J. S., 96
Haut, M. W., 96
Hawk, G. L., 139, 159, 162, 163–164
Hawryluk, G. A., 212, 214
Hayes, R. L., 119, 140, 140–141
Hazard, H., 126
Headache Classification Committee of the International Headache Society, 256
Heaton, R. K., 37, 38, 41, 52, 55, 100, 169, 172, 174, 175
Heilbronner, R. L., 123, 171, 189, 193
Heilbrun, K., 168, 170
Heim, S., 32, 240
Helton, K., 174
Hemenway. W. G., 240
Henry, G. K., 123
Hepburn, D. A., 240
Herman, D. O., 169, 173
Hessol, N., 64
Hickman, J. A., 84
Hiemenz, J. R., 84
High, W. M., Jr., 5, 32, 34, 37, 64–65, 67, 120, 141, 208, 239
Hillerud, L., 140
Hilmer, V. F., 174
Hilton, D. L., 32
Hinton-Bayre, A. D., 41, 121
Hirlinger, I., 240
Hirsch, A. E., 33
Hiscock, C. K., 178
Hiscock, M., 178
Ho, M., 268, 274
Hoganson, R. Coonley-. *See* Coonley-Hoganson, R.
Holbourn, A., 3
Holzgraefe, M., 123
Hooper, S. R., 77, 79, 82, 89
Hopkins, R. O., 26
Horn, L. J., 139
Horn, R. W., 205
Horn, S., 19, 23
Horwich, M., 121
Houston, A., 123
Howard, D. V., 236
Howard, J. H., 236
Howieson, D. B., 92
Huerta, M., 11
Hugenholtz, H., 139, 207, 234, 236
Huizenga, J., 231
Hutchison, J., 123
Hutton, J. T., 141
Hynd, G. W., 79, 82, 85, 86, 89, 96, 100, 101
Ichise, M., 23
Ingels, M., 23
International Neuropsychology Task Force, 161–162
Isaac, G., 23
Isaac, W., 100
Iverson, G. L., 177, 189, 240

Jabour, B. A., 125
Jacket, M., 270
Jacobs, A., 23
Jacobs, B. A., 121
Jacobson, R. R., 31
Jadcobs, A. R., 121
Jafek, B. W., 261
Jagger, J., 64, 212
Jane, J. A., 1, 2, 31, 41, 49, 64, 117–118, 120, 124, 138, 141, 203
Janzen, E. Fletcher-. *See* Fletcher-Janzen, E.
Jarman, R. F., 83, 91
Jastak, S., 173
Jenkins, A., 5
Jenkins, L. W., 140
Jennett, B., 4, 64
Jensen, O. K., 256
John, E. R., 11
Johnson, K. A., 52
Johnson, S. C., 14, 16, 19, 23, 26
Johnstone, B., 173
Jolles, J., 31, 32, 35, 235
Jones, C. L., 205, 208, 209
Jones, P. A., 269
Jordan, B. D., 119, 121, 122, 124, 126, 127
Jordan, S. E., 125

Kade, H. D., 86, 103, 104, 105
Kaemmer, B., 179
Kagan, J., 99
Kah, D., 23
Kalmar, K., 239, 241
Kalven, H., 198
Kamphaus, R. W., 84, 90, 91, 98, 99, 101, 103
Kane, R., 167
Kanik, A., 121
Kant, L., 23
Kapila, C. J., 173
Kaplan, E., 88
Kaplan, R. M., 167

Karavidas, T., 171
Karp, S., 98–99
Karpakka, J., 123
Karzmark, P., 174
Kastner, M. P., 175, 176
Katon, W. J., 240
Katz, H., 119
Kaufman, A. S., 56, 91, 173
Kaufman, N. L., 91
Kay, T., 31, 102
Kelly, J. P., 33, 37, 41, 120, 264
Kemp, P., 123
Kepler, K., 102
Kern, R. A., 99
Kertesz, A , 168
Kessler, H. R., 210
Khayrallah, M.
Kibby, M., 2, 6, 206, 214
Kinsbourne, M., 80, 91
Kinsella, G., 174, 234
Kirby, J. R., 8 , 91
Kirchner, P., 23
Kirsh, J. C., 23
Kischka, U., 32, 240
Kixmiller, J. S., 139, 140
Klein, F. C., 136
Klein, K., 52, 55
Kleinschmidt-DeMasters, B. K., 33, 264
Klesges, R. C., 174
Klonoff, H., 81, 87, 102, 139
Kluge, J., 41, 120
Knowlton, S., 64
Knutson, N., 94
Koller, W., 261
Kontos, H. A., 140
Kornstein, S., 262–263
Krach, L., 86
Kramer, H., 177
Kraus, J. F., 1, 3, 64, 101, 267
Krauss, J., 135
Kreutzer, J. S., 33, 102, 206, 237, 268, 269
Kriel, R., 86
Krug, D. K., 140
Krull, K. R., 174
Kukull, W. A., 121
Kurland, L. T., 64, 135, 138
Kurth, S., 19, 23
Kurtzke, J. F., 138
Kwentus, J. A., 262–263

Lacey, G. de. *See* DeLacey, G.
Laibstain, D. F., 210
Laing, L. C., 164, 166
LaMarche, J. A., 77, 78, 80, 83, 87, 101, 102, 103
Lampert, P. W., 122
La Rochelle, S., 139
Larrabee, G. J., 172
Larson, E. B., 121
Laws, E. R., Jr., 64, 135
Lebray, P. R., 240
Lee, J. C. de. *See* DeLee, J. C.
Lees-Haley, P. R., 36, 127, 209, 224
Lehr, E., 87, 103
Leibrook, L. G., 94
Leiderman, J., 86
Leigh, A. D., 260
Leiguarda, R.., 126
Leininger, B. E., 33, 206, 237, 268
Lemberger, A., 5
Lemme, W., 123
Leon-Barth, C., 138
Leonardi, G., 237
Lesser, R., 123, 126
Leu, P. W., 83
Levi, L., 5
Levin, H. S., 5, 31, 32, 34, 37, 39, 49, 63, 64, 64–65, 65, 67, 70, 78, 81, 96, 119, 120, 122, 138, 139, 174, 205, 206, 208, 209, 210, 214, 239
Levine, J. I., 64
Levine, M. J., 208, 212
Lewine, J. D., 11
Lewinsohn, P. M., 248
Ley, P., 64
Lezak, M. D., 92, 98, 167, 173
Liberman, J., 123, 126
Lidvall, H. F., 204, 207, 211, 212
Light, R. H.
Lighthall, J. W., 32
Lillehei, K. O., 33, 264
Linderoth, B., 204, 207, 211, 212
Lipke-Molby, T., 174
Lishman, W. A., 210, 214
Little, S. G., 103
Livingston, R. B., 77, 105
Loftus, E. F., 37
Long, C. J., 2, 6, 52, 55, 85, 86, 164, 166, 174, 176, 206, 207, 208, 209, 210, 211, 214
Lontos, H. A., 119
Lorentzon, R., 126
Lottenberg, S., 119
Lovell, M. R., 41
Low, M. D., 81, 87
Lowery, R., 91
Ludwig, S., 102
Luria, A. R., 78, 83, 85, 99, 100, 219
Lyeth, B. G., 140
Lynch, J. K., 172, 173, 174

Macanamara, S. E., 26
Macciocchi, S. N ., 34, 41, 117, 120, 124, 127, 139, 141, 232, 239
MacDonald, M. R., 240
MacDonald, R. L., 258
Machamer, J. E., 34, 40, 120, 206
MacLeod, K. M., 240
Macleod, M., 123
MacPhearson, P., 5
Magnes, S. A., 124
Mahone, R. H., 33
Malec, J., 119, 270
Mandelbaum, B. E., 125
Mangel. H. E., 233
Manshadi, F. F., 70
Marcincin, R. P., 32
Marder, K., 23–26
Marion, D. W., 140
Mark, D. H., 121
Mark, V. H., 210
Markow, T., 99
Marlowe, W., 98, 100
Marshall, I. A., 79
Marshall, L. F., 37, 64–65, 67, 119, 120, 209, 210, 214, 239
Martin, R. P., 101
Marwitz, J. H., 102
Matarazzo, J. D., 83, 169, 172, 173
Mateer, C. A., 98, 100, 232, 246
Matheson, L. N., 195
Matier, K., 79
Matser, E., 122

Matthews, C. G., 37, 38, 52, 55, 169, 174
Mattis, S., 37, 64–65, 67, 120, 138, 239
Maxwell, R. E., 118, 263
Maxwell, W. L., 14
Mayer, R. E., 248
Mayeux, R., 23–26
Mayfield, J. W., 82, 88, 103, 104
Mazzoldi, M., 237
McAlister, T. W., 70
McArdle, C. B., 5, 208
McCaffrey, R. J., 6, 41, 164, 166, 170, 172, 173, 174
McCormick, J. A., 99
McCormick, M., 102
McCormick, W. C., 121
McCracken, L. M., 177, 189, 240
McCrea, M., 41, 120
McCunney, R. J., 121, 122
McDonald, J. R., 35, 213, 255, 259
McFarland, K., 41, 121
McGhee, D. E., 99
McGuire, T. L., 102
McIntosh, G. C., 7
McIntosh, T. K., 141
McKay, K. E., 79
McKinlay, W., 101, 102
McKinley, J. C., 168
McLatchie, G., 123
McLaughlin, A. M., 102
McLean, A., 36, 63, 67, 120, 138, 139, 141, 172, 173, 206, 207, 209, 212
McLean, M. J., 258
McLellan, D. R., 213
McMillan, T. M. , 85
MEDICODE, Inc., 188–189
Medina, J. L., 257
Meier, M. J., 161
Melville, I., 123
Melvin, J. W., 32
Mendelson, G., 139
Meric, A. L., 32
Merli, G. A., 234
Merola, J. L , 86
Merrett, H. D., 213
Merrett, J. D., 35, 255, 259
Merritt, H. H., 256
Messenheimer, J., 258–259
Mild Traumatic Brain Injury Committee of the Head Injury Interdisciplinary Special Interest Group of the American Congress of Rehabilitation Medicine, 4, 5, 32, 65–66, 119–120, 162–163, 267
Miller, B., 141, 209
Miller, D. G., 37
Miller, E. S., 189
Miller, H., 213, 255
Miller, H. B., 220
Miller, J. D., 269
Miller, L., 221
Miller, L. P., 140
Miller, L. T., 79
Miller, W. G., 189
Minderhoud, J. M., 231
Mirsky, A. F., 99
Mittenberg, W., 35, 36, 189, 193, 211
Moehle, K. A., 175, 176
Mogentale C., 237, 238
Molby, T. Lipke-. *See* Lipke-Molby, T.
Molfese, D. L., 79
Molloy, R., 234
Montelpare, W. J., 126
Moore, A. D., 212, 214
Moore, J. W., 160
Moran, D. T., 261
Morra, S., 237
Morris, J. M., 91
Mortimer, J. A., 141
Murelius, O., 122
Mutter, S. A., 234, 236

Nadler, J. D., 236
Naplin, A., 37
Nathan, M., 23
Naugle, R. I., 40
Neilsen, F. F., 256
Nelson, H. E., 172
Nelson, P., 233
Nelson, W. E., 41, 124
Nemeth, S. J., 207, 209, 211
Nevin, N., 4
Newcombe, F., 175, 176, 235
Newman, B., 31
Newman, R., 160, 166, 167
Nichelli, P., 64, 67, 139, 234
Nichols, J. S., 33, 264
Nickel, V. C., 86
Nies, K. J., 177, 178, 189–190, 193
Nilsson, P., 140
Nolet, V., 94
Noll, R. B., 88
Norlin, B., 204, 207, 211, 212
Norman, D. A., 237
Nourjab, P., 1, 3, 64, 267
Novack, T. A., 207, 210
Nuechterlein, K. H., 99
Nussbaum, N. L., 80, 83, 92, 96, 98

Ober, B. A., 177
O'Brien, C., 126
Obrzut, J. E., 79, 82
Oder, W., 23
O'Donnell, V. M., 34
Ogloff, J. R. P., 191–192
O'Hara, C., 210
Okiyama, K., 141
Oltman, P., 98–99
O'Meara, E. S., 121
Ommaya, A. K., 32, 33, 119
Oppenheimer, D. R., 4, 71, 140
Orchard, J., 126
Oreland, L., 122
Orrison, W. W., 11
Ortega, A., 41
Osborn, A. G., 11, 23

Packard, R. C., 239
Palav, A., 6
Palmer, A. M., 140
Pankratz, L., 177, 178
Panser, L., 86
Paolo, A. M., 174
Parasuraman, R., 234, 234–235
Park, M. R., 32
Parker, D. M., 172, 174
Parker, N., 19, 23
Parker, R. S., 172
Parsons, O. A., 52, 88, 174
Passler, M., 100
Patton, R. M., 120
Peck, E. A., 33, 206, 237
Peck, E. T., 262–263
Pelletier, R., 126
Pendleton, M. G., 175

Pennington, B. F., 40, 100
Perrin, S., 36, 211
Persson, H. E., 123
Peters, L. C., 212, 214
Pethybridge, R., 123
Petito, C., 121
Pfanschmidt, M., 121
Phillips, W., 99
Pieter, W., 126
Picton, T., 236
Pirier, C., 139
Pivik, J., 236
Podereka, I., 23
Pompei, R. de. *See* DePompei, R.
Ponsford, J., 234
Ponten, U., 140
Popper, J. S., 138
Povlishock, J. T., 14, 119, 136, 140
Price, J. R., 6
Prichard, J. W., 23
Priest, J. D., 118, 263
Prigatano, G. P., 52, 88, 101, 139, 219, 227, 270
Prior, M., 174
Put, E., 23
Put, T., 23

Rabbit, P., 235
Radanov, B. P., 32, 240
Radii, E. W., 32, 240
Rakic, P. S. Goldman-. *See* Goldman-Rakic, P. S.
Ramsay, R. E., 258–259
Ramsey, M. C., 96
Randall, R., 123, 126
Randolph, C., 41, 120
Rapaport, I. R., 6
Rasile, D., 236
Raskin, A. A., 237, 238
Raskin, E., 98–99
Rattan, G., 91, 136, 137
Ravdin, L. D., 121
Rayls, K. R., 35
Raymond, M. J., 6–7, 7, 219
Rearick, E., 237, 238
Reeves, D. L., 236
Reichmann, S., 32, 240
Reitan, R. M., 3, 5–6, 41, 49, 50, 52, 53, 54, 56, 60, 61, 62, 63, 66–67, 67, 68, 70, 83, 84, 92, 139, 168, 178, 205, 208, 212, 262–263
Relander, M., 231
Relkin, N., 121
Reschley, D., 88, 103
Resnick, M., 31
Resnick, P. J., 189, 192, 193
Rey, A., 178
Reynolds, C. R., 6, 80, 82, 83, 84, 85, 86, 87, 90, 91, 92, 94, 96, 96–98, 99, 103, 104, 106, 173
Rezai, K., 23
Reznick, J. S., 99
Rhodes, R. L., 83
Riccio, C. A., 6, 80, 84, 91, 92, 94, 104
Richard, M. T., 139, 207, 234, 236
Richardson, J. T. E., 163
Richardson, R. E. L., 166
Richman, L. C., 99
Rimel, R. W., 1, 2, 31, 34–35, 41, 64, 117–118, 120, 124, 138, 139, 141, 203, 267
Ris, M. D., 88
Risser, A., 77, 82, 86
Roberts, M. A., 70
Roberts, R., 23
Robertson, J. T., 32
Roche, K., Bandeen-. *See* Bandeen-Roche, K.
Rochelle, S. La. *See* La Rochelle, S.
Rogers, R., 178, 189, 193
Rohling, M. L., 172
Rojas, D. C., 70
Rokaw, W., 64
Roselli, M., 79
Rosenbaum, G., 173, 174
Rosenblood, L. K., 52
Rosenblum, A., 172
Rosenthal, B. L., 84
Rosenthal, M., 102, 227
Rosman, B. L., 99
Ross, G., 241
Ross, R. J., 122
Rossie, G. V., 3, 261
Rosvold, H. E., 99
Rothenberg, M. B., 102
Rothlisberg, B. A., 79, 82, 83, 89, 103
Rotholc, A. , 189, 193
Roueche, J. R., 139
Rourke, B. P., 40, 50, 80, 83, 88, 89
Rowan, J., 5
Rowe, M. J., 259
Rowlingson, J. C., 240
Rubinstein, D., 33, 264
Ruchinskas, R. A., 6
Ruesch, J., 205, 207, 209
Ruff, R. M., 35, 37, 64–65, 67, 119, 120, 138, 178, 189, 209, 210, 214, 235, 239
Russel, W. R., 208
Russell, E. W., 172, 189, 193
Russell, N. R., 137
Russell, W. R., 203, 256
Russo, A. A., 26
Russo, P. K., 121, 122
Rutherford, W. H., 35, 213, 255, 259
Ruthven, L., 269
Rutter, M., 79, 86, 90, 102, 139
Ryan, A. J., 121
Ryan, J. J., 173, 174
Ryan, T. V., 41, 77, 78, 80, 83, 87, 101, 102, 103, 139, 159, 162, 163–164
Ryser, D. K., 26

Saal, J., 120
Saan, R. J., 231
Saccuzzo, D. P., 167
Sachs, C., 122
Saks, M. J., 160
Sam, J. Woo-. *See* Woo-Sam, J.
Sampson, H., 67
Sanchez, V. E., 174
Sanders, J. A., 11
Sandoval, J., 88
Sano, M., 23–26
Sarason, I., 99
Sattler, J. M., 173
Satz, P., 40, 85, 86
Saunders, R. L., 141
Schafer, D., 270
Schellenberg, G. D., 121
Schmidt. M., 189
Schmitt, F. A., 174
Schmitter, M. E., 164

Schmitter-Edgecombe, M., 235
Schneider, R. C., 120
Schneider, W., 234
Schnidrig, A., 32
Schnurr, R. F., 240
Schoenhuber, R., 64, 67, 138, 139, 234
Schofield, P. W., 23–26, 121
Schoor, J. T. van. See van-Schoor, J. T.
Schraa, J. C., 273
Schuman, L. M., 141
Schwartz, D. R., 240
Schweitzer, J. B., 32
Sciabassi, R. J., 140
Scott, J. G., 174
Seemiller, L. Smith-. *See* Smith-Seemiller, L.
Segalowitz, S. J., 136, 141
Seger, S., 123, 126
Seidel, U., 79
Selnes, O., 123, 126
Selzer, M. E., 255
Semrud-Clikeman, M., 82, 85, 101, 101–102
Seward, H., 126
Shaffer, D., 90, 102
Shallice, T., 237
Shapiro, E. G., 91
Shapiro, S., 2
Sharma, V., 79
Shaw, S. R., 87, 94
Shechter, A., 123, 126
Shell, D., 120
Sheppard, L., 121
Sherer, M., 53, 174
Sheslow, D , 96
Shiffrin, R. M., 234
Shinn, M. R., 94
Shurtleff, H. A., 82, 83
Siegel, O., 122
Silverstein, A. B., 174
Simon, D., 123, 126
Sisler, G. E., 139
Skilbeck, C., 99
Smith, A., 164, 208
Smith, D. H., 141
Smith, L. C., 233
Smith, R. D., 6
Smith, R. S., 210
Smith-Seemiller, L., 23
Snow, J. H., 77
Snyder, J. L., 19, 32, 37
Sohlberg, M. M., 232, 246
Somers, L. M., 119
Sontag, M., 120
Sorenson, S., 135
Soustiel, J. F., 5
Sparrow, S. S., 90
Spatt, J., 23
Sperry, R. W., 91
Spettell, C., 70
Spiers, M., 94
Spitzer, R. L., 178
Spreen, O., 77, 82, 86, 172
Squire, L. R., 141
Stablum, F., 237, 238
Stambrook, M., 212, 214
Standards for Educational and Psychological Testing, 167, 170
Stanford, L. D., 82, 83, 85, 87, 90, 101
Stanton, A. L., 174
Stanton, H. C., 90
Stark, R. M., 126
Staub, C. P., 118
Stavrou, E., 103
Stebbins, G. T., 172
Stefano, G. di, 32
Stein, S. C., 70
Stern, B. J., 256
Stern, Y., 23–26
Stethem, L. L., 234, 236
Stevens, K. B., 6, 207
Stewart, L. E., 172, 174
Stewart, W., 123, 126
Stone, B., 85
Storli, O. V., 125
Straub, C. P., 263
Strich, S., 3
Strider, J. S., 154, 157
Stroop, J. R., 235
Strub, R. L., 222
Sturzenneggerr, M., 32
Stuss, D. T., 33, 139, 207, 234, 236
Sullivan, C., 64
Summer, D., 260
Sundell, R. R., 94
Swedlow, P. E., 140
Sweeney, D., 121
Sweeney, J. R., 32
Sweet, J. J., 177, 178, 189–190, 193
Symonds, C., 2, 255

Tabaddor, K., 37, 64–65, 67, 120, 239
Taft, W. C., 119, 140–141
Talley, J. L., 96
Tang, M., 23–26
Taylor, H. G., 77, 83, 85, 86, 89, 105
Taylor, S. J., 196, 199
Teasdale, E., 123
Teasdale, G., 4, 5
Teeter, P. A., 82, 85, 101, 101–102
Tegner, Y., 126
Tellegen, A. M., 179
Telzrow, C. F., 80, 85
Temkin, N. R., 34, 36, 63, 67, 120, 138, 139, 141, 172, 206, 207, 208, 209, 210, 212
Temple, C. M., 77, 105
Tennant, W., 35, 178, 189
Teri, L., 121
Texas Rules of Civil Procedures, 197
Tfelt-Hansen, P., 257
Thatcher, R. W., 11
Thibault, L. B., 32
Thomas, M. J., 141
Thompson, C. J., 32
Thompson, J. D., 121
Thompson, L. L., 5, 37, 100, 136
Tilley, P., 126
Timmermans, S. R., 99
Tjell, C., 240
Tonelli, L., 234
Torg, J. S., 124
Torgesen, J. K., 100
Torkelson, R. D., 94
Torres, F., 2
Trammer, R. I., 126
Tramontana, M. G., 79, 82, 89
Traub, M., 90
Tremont, G., 35
Trexler, L., 236
Troster, A. I., 119, 174
Troupp, H., 231
Trueblood, W., 189
Tsushima, W. T., 138
Tucker, D. M., 80

Tuokko, H., 77
Tupper, D. E., 52, 77
Turbott, S. H., 99
Tusa, S., 123, 126
Twijnstra, A., 35, 235
Tyssedal, J. S., 240
Tysvaer, A. T., 125

Uddo-Crane, M., 36, 164
Ueno, K., 32
Umilta, C., 237, 238
Ungerstalt, U., 140
U.S. Gabapentin Study Group No. 5, 258
Uomoto, J. M., 240
Urbina, S., 167

Valach, L., 240
Van Brunt, R. T., 154, 157
vanSchoor, J. T., 220
Varney, N. R., 23, 119, 136
Varney, R. N., 119, 136
Vaughn, G. W., 136
Vaughn, M., 101
Vega, A., 52
Veneklasen, J., 174
Verhey, F. R , 32
Vernon, P. A., 79
Vogt, A. T., 172
Vygotsky, L. S., 86

Waaland, P. K., 102
Walker, D., 138
Walker, W., 23
Warner, J. S., 257
Wasserman, J., 96
Weaver, R., 239
Webbe, F., 125
Wechsler, D., 56, 170
Wedding, D., 138, 159
Wehman, P., 269
Wei, E. P., 140
Weiner, R. L., 5, 208
Weiss, H. D., 256
Welch, K. M. A., 257
Wells, C. E., 138, 139
Wells, G. L., 37
Welsh, M. C., 100
Wengen, D., 32, 240
Westervelt, H. J., 170
Wetter, M. W., 196
Weyandt, L. L., 85, 89
Whinnery, A. M., 33
Whinnery, J. E., 33
White, R. P., 32
Whitman, D., 173
Whitman, S., 64
Whitten, C. J., 80
Wiens, A. N., 173
Wiggs, C. L., 236
Wilder, B. J., 259
Wilen, S., 85
Wilhelm, K. L., 173
Wilkinson, G. S., 173
Williams, A. D., 164, 166
Williams, B. L., 139, 140
Williams, D., 98, 100
Williams, D. H., 5, 32, 34, 49, 67, 70, 139, 141, 208, 212
Williams, J., 168
Williams, J. M., 102
Williams, M. A., 92, 99
Willis, W. G., 79, 85, 86, 89, 101
Willson, V. L., 88, 92
Willmore, L. J., 258–259
Wilshire, D., 174
Wilson, J. T. L., 213
Wilson, L., 123
Wilson, R. S., 172, 173, 174, 176
Winn, H. R., 31, 34, 212
Winn, R., 120
Winston, K. R., 256
Witkin, H. A., 98–99
Witol, A., 125
Wolfson, D., 3, 5–6, 41, 49, 50, 52, 53, 54, 56, 60, 61, 62, 63, 66–67, 68, 70, 92, 139, 168, 178
Wood, D., 241
Wood, S. Dolezal-. *See* Dolezal-Wood, S.
Woodcock, R. W., 94
Woo-Sam, J., 86
Wrightsman, L. S., 198
Wrightson, P., 34, 67, 120, 204, 207, 210, 211, 234, 239
Wyler, A. R., 67, 139, 206
Wylie, T., 35, 178, 189

Yang, F., 140–141
Yarnell, P. R., 3, 261
Yingst, C. A., 87, 94
Yishay, Y. Ben-. *See* Ben-Yishay, Y.
Ylvisaker, M., 77, 269
Young, C. C., 121
Young, T., 102
Youngjohn, J. R., 35, 196
Youngman, P. K., 232, 246
Yule, W., 79

Zappala, G., 236
Zarski, J. J., 102
Zasler, N. D., 135, 136, 138, 139
Zazula, T., 122
Zeffiro, T., 11
Zeiner, H. K., 270
Zeisel, H., 198
Zeiss, R. A., 248
Zelazo, P. D., 99, 100
Zemper, E. D., 123, 126
Zielinski, J. J., 177, 178
Zielinski, R. E., 35
Zillmer, E., 94
Zimmerman, R., 122
Zinner, E. S., 82
Ziskin, J., 159

Subject Index

Ability, present, in preinjury functioning measurement, 172–173
Academic achievement, in child assessment, 94–95
Accuracy, of event recall, in mild TBI, 36–37
Acknowledgment, medical, in TBI recovery, 211
Activities of daily living, in outpatient rehabilitation, 272
Adjustment, emotional, in TBI recovery, 210
Age factors, in TBI recovery, 208. *See also* Education factors.
Aikmen, Troy, 117
Alcohol abuse, in TBI, 208
Alterations, electroencephalographic, from mild TBI, 2–3
Alzheimer's disease, neuroimaging findings in, 26
Amnesia
  posttraumatic, 62–63, 204–205
  whiplash, 2–3
Amyloid plaque levels, in boxing injuries, 121–122
Analgesics, in posttraumatic headache, 257–258
Anosmia, posttraumatic, 260–261
Apolipoprotein E levels, in boxing injuries, 121–122
Atrophy
  cortical, 122
  white matter, 14–19
Attention
  deficits in, 40, 234–235
    cognitive remediation of, 242–245
  functions of, 95–98
Attorney(s), civil litigation role of, 195–197
Axonal injury, diffuse, in TBI, 213

Back pain, posttraumatic, 261–262
BASC ADHD Monitor, 99, 101
Base rates, of neuropsychological impairments, 38–40
Behavior Assessment System for Children (BASC), 90
Behavioral domains, in child neuropsychology, 87–88
Behavioral/emotional status, in child assessment, 100–101
Best performance method, in preinjury functioning measurement, 173
Biofeedback, in outpatient rehabilitation, 272
Biomechanical forces, in brain injury, 32–33
Boxing
  mild concussion in, 122–123
  severe brain injury in, 121–122
Brain injury, mild traumatic. *See* Traumatic brain injury, mild.
Brain Injury Recovery Program (BIRP)
  critical features of, 268–270
  efficacy of treatment in, 274–275
  program design for, 270–274
Brouardel, P. C. H., 192

California Verbal Learning Test (CVLT), 177
Callosum, corpus, atrophy of, 14–19
Category Test, in neuropsychological evaluation, 37
CBM (curriculum-based measurement), 94
Child(ren), neuropsychological evaluation of, 77–106
Children's Category Test (CCT), 100
Children's Embedded Figure Test (CEFT), 98–99
Children's Memory Scale (CMS), 98
Claims process, in litigation, 147–149
Cognitive functioning, in child assessment, 91–92
Cognitive impairments
  in mild TBI, 234–238, 240
  postconcussive symptoms of, 238–241
  rehabilitation in
    attention and self-regulation deficits, 242–245
    emotional interventions and, 245–249
Coma. *See also* Glasgow Coma Scale (GCS).
  in documenting TBI, 137–138
  in loss of consciousness, 33–34
  in mild TBI, 11, 63, 119

Compensation
claims for, in TBI recovery, 213
in outpatient rehabilitation, 269
Complaint and answer process, in litigation, 149–150
Computerized tomography (CT), in neuro-imaging, 11
Concussion
in boxing, 122–123
in football, 123–125
in second-impact syndrome, 120–121
Confidentiality issues, in outpatient rehabilitation, 273
Consciousness, loss of. *See* Loss of consciousness (LOC).
Consultant, neuropsychologist as, 192–197
Contention scheduling, in cognitive rehabilitation, 237
Continuous performance test (CPT), in child assessment, 99
Contusions, in TBI, 213
Corpus callosum, atrophy of, 14–19
Cortical atrophy, in boxing injuries, 122
CT (computerized tomography), in neuro-imaging, 11
Curriculum-based measurement (CBM), 94

Defendant(s), civil litigation role of, 197
Defense attorney(s), civil litigation role of, 196–297
Demographic variables, in preinjury functioning measurement, 173
Deposition(s), in testimony, 154–155
Depression, posttraumatic, 262–263
Diagnostic and Statistical Manual of Mental Disorders (DSM), 163, 188
Diffuse axonal injury, in TBI, 213
Digit Memory Test, 178
Discovery deposition, in testimony, 154
Discovery process, in litigation, 150–151
Dizziness, posttraumatic, 259
Documentation
of mild TBI, 137–139
neuropsychologist's role in, 139–141
Drug abuse, in TBI, 208
Dysarthria, in boxing injuries, 121

Education factors. *See also* Age factors.
IQ scores as, 56–58
literature on, 51–53
neuropsychological performance as, 61–73
neuropsychological status as, 53–55
in outpatient rehabilitation, 269
psychological test scores as, 60–61
research in, 66–73
in TBI recovery, 209
WAIS subtest scores as, 58–60
Electroencephalographic alterations, from mild TBI, 2–3
Emotional adjustment, in TBI recovery, 210
Emotional/behavioral status, in child asessment, 100–101
Emotional changes
following TBI, 220–224, 240
posttraumatic, 262–263
Emotional interventions, in cognitive rehabilitation, 245–249
Environmental variables, in child assessment, 101–103
Epilepsy, posttraumatic, 258–259
Event recall, in mild TBI, 36–37
Executive functions, of children, 99–100
Expectations
as psychological factors, 35–36
in TBI recovery, 211–212
Expert opinions. *See* Opinions, expert.

Family/home setting, in child assessment, 102
Family support, in TBI recovery 213–214
Fatigue, after mild TBI, 239–240
Figure Memory Test, in neuropsychological evaluation, 37
Fixed neuropsychological battery, defined, 167
Flexible neuropsychological battery, defined, 167
Football, mild concussion in, 123–125
Forensic aspects, of TBI. *See* Traumatic brain injury (TBI), forensic aspects of.
Frontal lobe injury, in mild TBI, 222
Full Scale IQ, in neuropsychological evaluation, 56–58
Future outcome, expert opinions in, 175–177

General Neuropsychological Deficit Scale (GNDS), 6, 51, 53–55, 70–72
Glasgow Coma Scale (GCS)
in documenting TBI, 137–138
in loss of consciousness, 33–34
in mild TBI, 11, 63, 119

Halstead–Reitan Battery, 52, 53
Halstead–Reitan Neuropsychological Test Battery , 92, 168, 274
Head injury, mild. *See* Traumatic brain injury, mild.

Headache, after mild TBI, 239–240, 256–258
Hearing impairment, posttraumatic, 260
Hemorrhagic lesions, neuroimaging findings of, 23
Horseback riding, head injuries in, 125–126
Hyperactivity/Attention-Deficit Disorder, 40
Hypersexuality, in temporal lobe injury, 222

ICD (International Classification of Diseases), 188–189
Imaging, of brain. *See* Neuroimaging.
Impairment Index, 52
Impeachment, of witnesses, 155–156
Independent medical exam, in litigation, 151–154
Injury(ies), sport. *See* Sports injury(ies).
Intentional malingering, 193–194
Intentional symptom exaggeration, 195
Interface, brain–skull, in neuroimaging, 12–14
International Classification of Diseases (ICD), 188–189
Interventions, emotional,in cognitive rehabilitation, 245–249
IQ scores, in neuropsychological evaluation, 56–58

Junction, white matter–gray matter, in neuroimaging, 14

Kaufman Assessment Battery for Children, 91
Kluver-Bucy Syndrome, in temporal lobe injury, 222

Lability, posttraumatic emotional, 262–263
Lawyer(s), civil litigation role of, 195–197
Learning functions, of children, 95–98
Lesions, hemorrhagic, neuroimaging findings of, 23
Litigation
  process(es) in
    claims as, 147–149
    complaint and answer as, 149–150
    discovery as, 150–151
    independent medical exam as, 151–154
    testimony as, 154–156
  roles in
    of attorney, 195–197
    of neuropsychologist, 188–193
    of plaintiff, 193–195
Loss of consciousness (LOC)
  neuroimaging findings of, 23–26
  in residual brain injury, 33–34, 62–63
Luria Nebraska Neuropsychological Battery–Children's Revision, 92–94

Magnetic Familiar Figure Task (MPFT), 99
Magnetic resonance imaging (MRI), in neuroimaging, 11
Malingering
  expert opinion on, 177–179
  intentional, 193–194
  legal implications of
    for attorneys, 195–197
    for defendant, 197
    for trier of fact, 197–199
  neuropsychologist role in
    as consultant, 192–197
    as diagnostician, 188–190
    as expert witness, 159–167, 191–192
    as therapist, 190–191
  plaintiff role in, 193–195
Measurement, curriculum-based, 94
Medical acknowledgment, in TBI recovery, 211
Medical exam, independent, 151–154
Memory, 95–98, 236
Memory Assessment Scales, 168
"Mere conduit-educator," neuropsychologist as, 160–161
Mild traumatic brain injury. *See* Traumatic brain injury, mild.
Minnesota Multiphasic Personality Inventory (MMPI), 168, 178, 179
Misconceptions, forensic, in TBI, 159–179
Monitoring, in outpatient rehabilitation, 269
Montana, Joe, 117
Motor functioning, in child assessment, 92–94

National Adult Reading Test (NART), 172
Neck pain, posttraumatic, 261–262
Neurodevelopmental issues, in child neuropsychology, 85–87
Neuroimaging
  fundamentals of, 12
  permanent vs. transient findings in, 23–26
  quantitative, 19
  SPECT, 19–23
  trauma–associated abnormalities in
    brain–skull interface as, 12–14
    white matter atrophy as, 14–19
    white matter–gray matter junction as, 14

Neurological complications, in TBI recovery, 212–214
Neuropsychiatric history, in TBI recovery, 210
Neuropsychological Deficit Scale for Older Children, (NDS), 60–61
Neuropsychological evaluation. *See also* Traumatic brain injury, mild.
age and education factors in, 45–73. *See also* Age factors; Education factors.
certainty of opinions in, 171–178
of children's skills
academic, 94–95
attention, 98–99
cognitive, 91–92
executive, 99–100
learning, 95–98
motor, 92–94
sensory, 92–94
data generated from, 103–105
diagnostic issues in, 41–43
documentation in, 139–141
emotional/behavioral status in, 100–101
environmental variables in, 101–103
findings in, 37–40
impairment base rates in, 38–40
neurodevelopmental issues in, 85–87
in nonimpact brain injury, 32–33
preinjury status in, 89–91
process of, 80–87
symptomatology in, 33–36
test selection for, 87–88, 167–170
Nonimpact brain injury, 2–33

Observation, structured, in child assessment, 101
Occupational factors, in TBI recovery, 209
Occupational therapy, in outpatient rehabilitation, 272
Opinions
expert
on future outcome, 175–177
on possible malingering, 177–179
on preinjury functioning, 89–91, 172–175
neuropsychological certainty of, 171–178
Organic personality changes, in TBI, 222
Outcome factors
age as, 308–209
alcohol and drug abuse as, 208
compensation claims as, 213
confusion regarding, 206–207
education and occupation as, 209
emotional adjustment as, 210
expectations as, 211–212
family support as, 213–214
neurological complications as, 212–214 neuropsychiatric history as, 210
personality as, 209
postconcussive symptoms as, 34–35, 207
postraumatic
medical acknowledgment as, 211
stress as, 210–211
preinjury as, 208
Outpatient rehabilitation
critical features of, 268–270
efficacy of treatment in, 274–275
program design for, 270–274

Paced Auditory Serial Addition Test (PASAT), 234
Parkinson's disease, in boxing injuries, 121
Pathophysiology, of mild TBI, 3–4
PDRT (*Portland Digit Recognition Test*) 178, 190
Pediatric outpatient rehabilitation, 273
Performance IQ, in neuropsychological evaluation, 56–58, 169
Personality
changes of, 222–224
traits of, in TBI recovery, 209
Phenomenon, shear–strain, in mild TBI, 3–4
Physical therapy, in outpatient rehabilitation, 272
Plaintiff attorneys, civil litigation role of, 195–197
Portland Digit Recognition Test (PDRT), 178, 190
Postconcussive symptoms
cognitive deficits in, 238–241
in mild TBI, 34–35, 207
Posttraumatic sequelae
amnesia as, 62–63, 204–205
anosmia as, 260–261
depression and emotional lability as, 262–263
dizziness as, 259
headache as, 256–258
hearing impairment as, 260
neck and back pain as, 261–262
seizures as, 258–259
sports-related, 263–264
tinnitus as, 260
visual, 262
Preinjury factors, in TBI, 208

Preinjury functioning
expert opinions in, 172–175
status of, in child assessment, 89–91
Present ability measures, in preinjury functioning measurement, 172–173
Preservation deposition, in testimony, 154–155
Program design, for outpatient rehabilitation, 270–274
Psychiatric history, in TBI recovery, 210
Psychological test scores, of children, 60–61
Psychometric issues, in child neuropsychology, 88–103
Psychotherapy, in mild TBI, 224–228
PTA (posttraumatic amnesia), 62–63, 204–205
"Punch-drunk" syndrome, in boxing injuries, 121, 122

Quantitative neuroimaging, in cerebral trauma, 19
Quigley's rule, in multiple concussions, 120

Reactive personality changes, in TBI, 223–224
Reassurance, in outpatient rehabilitation, 269
Recall, event, in mild TBI, 36–37
Recognition, of mild TBI, 135–137
Recovery, from mild TBI, 40–41. *See also* Outcome factors.
Regression equations, in preinjury functioning measurement, 173–174
Rehabilitation
cognitive
in attention and self-regulation deficits, 242–245
emotional interventions and, 245–249
outpatient
critical features of, 268–270
efficacy of treatment in, 274–275
program design for, 270–274
Reitan–Indiana Neuropsychological Battery, 92
Remediation, in outpatient rehabilitation, 269
Resonance imaging, magnetic, in neuroimaging, 11
Rey 15–Item Test, 178, 190
Ruff 2 & 7 Test, 235

SAC (*Standardized Assessment of Concussion*), 120–121
Schedule of Affective Disorders and Schizophrenia (SADS), 178
School setting, in child assessment, 102–103
Second-impact syndrome, 33, 120
Second opinion, in litigation, 151–154
Seizures, posttraumatic, 258–259
Self-regulation deficits, cognitive remediation of, 242–245
Sensory functioning, in child assessment, 92–94
Sequelae, posttraumatic. *See* Posttraumatic sequelae.
Severity, of brain injury, 204–210
Shear-strain phenomenon, in mild TBI, 3–4
SIRS (*Structured Interview of Reported Symptoms*), 178
Skull–brain interface, in neuroimaging, 12–14
Soccer, concussion in, 125
Societal impact, of mild TBI, 2
SPECT imaging, 19–23
Speech difficulties, in boxing injuries, 121
Speech–language therapy, in outpatient rehabilitation, 272–273
Sports injury(ies)
in boxing, 121–122
in football, 123–125
in horseback riding, 125–126
in soccer, 125
posttraumatic, 263–264
Standardized Assessment of Concussion (SAC), 120–121
Story Memory Test, in neuropsychological evaluation, 37
Stress, in TBI recovery, 210–211
Stroop Color–Word Test, 235
Structured Interview of Reported Symptoms (SIRS), 178
Structured observation, in child assessment, 101
Subpoena, in litigation, 150–151
Supervisory attentional system, in cognitive rehabilitation, 237–238
Support, in outpatient rehabilitation, 269
Syndrome(s)
Kluver-Bucy, 222
postconcussive, 34–35
"punch drunk", 121, 122
second-impact, 33, 120

Temporal lobe injury, in mild TBI, 222
Test of Memory and Learning (TOMAL), 96–98

Test selection, in neuropsychology, 87–88, 167–170
Testimony, in litigation, 154–156
Therapist, neuropsychologist as, 190–191
Tinnitus, posttraumatic, 260
TOMAL (*Test of Memory and Learning*), 96–98
Tomography, computerized, in neuroimaging, 11
Trail Making Test, in neuropsychological evaluation, 37
Traumatic brain injury, mild. *See also* Neuropsychological evaluation.
  biomechanical forces in, 32–33
  in children, 77–106
  deficit(s) from
    attention, 40, 234–235
    cognitive, 234–238
    executive, 237
    memory, 236
  defined, 6–7, 62–66, 119–121, 162, 203–204
  diagnosis of
    errors in, 41–42
    false–positive and false–negative issues in, 42–43
  emotional changes following, 220–224
  forensic aspects of
    documentation as, 137–139
    litigation as, 147–157. *See also* Litigation.
    misconceptions in, 159–179
    recognition as, 135–137
  lower limits of, 203
  neuroimaging in, 11–27. *See also* Neuro imaging.
  nonimpact, 32–33
  pathophysiology of, 3–4
  posttraumatic sequelae of, 256–264. *See also* Posttraumatic sequelae. psychotherapy in, 224–228
  recovery from, 40–41
  research in, 2–3
  severity of, 204–210
  societal impact of, 2
  in sports, 117–126. *See also* Sports injury(ies); and specific sports.
  symptoms of
    base rates of, 35–36
    event recall problems as, 36–37
    neuropsychological impairments as, 38–40
    unintentional exaggeration of, 195
  upper limits of, 203
Tremor, posttraumatic, 261
Trier of fact, civil litigation role of, 197–199

Verbal IQ, in neuropsychological evaluation, 56–58, 169
Vineland Adaptive Behavior Scale, 90, 101
Visual symptoms, posttraumatic, 262
Vocational issues, in outpatient rehabilitation, 273

Wechsler Adult Intelligence Scale (WAIS), 41, 50, 56, 169,173–174
Wechsler Intelligence Scale for Children (WISC), 50, 58–60
Wechsler Memory Scale–Revised (WMS–R), 170
Western Aphasia Battery, 168
Whiplash amnesia, from mild TBI, 2–3
White matter, 14–19
Wide Range Achievement Test–Revised (WRAT–R), 172–173
Wide Range Assessment of Memory and Learning (WRAML), 96–97
WISC (*Wechsler Intelligence Scale for Children*), 50, 58–60
Wisconsin Card Sorting Test (WCST), 100
Witness(es),
  expert, neuropsychologist as, 159–167, 191–192
  impeachment of, 155–156
Woodcock-Johnson Psychoeducational Battery, 94
WRAML (*Wide Range Assessment of Memory and Learning)* 96–97
WRAT–R (*Wide Range Achievement Test–Revised*), 172–173